Global Governance and Public Health

Global Governance and Public Health

Obstacles and Opportunities

Geoffrey B. Cockerham

ROWMAN &
LITTLEFIELD
INTERNATIONAL
London • New York

Published by Rowman & Littlefield International Ltd
Unit A, Whitacre Mews, 26–34 Stannary Street, London SE11 4AB
www.rowmaninternational.com

Rowman & Littlefield International Ltd.is an affiliate of Rowman & Littlefield
4501 Forbes Boulevard, Suite 200, Lanham, Maryland 20706, USA
With additional offices in Boulder, New York, Toronto (Canada), and Plymouth (UK)
www.rowman.com

British Library Cataloguing in Publication Data

A catalogue record for this book is available from the British Library

ISBN HB 978-1-7866-0848-2
PB 978-1-7866-0849-9

Library of Congress Cataloging-in-Publication Data

Names: Cockerham, Geoffrey B., author.
Title: Global governance and public health : obstacles and opportunities / Geoffrey B. Cockerham.
Description: London ; New York : Rowman & Littlefield International, [2018] | Includes bibliographical references and index.
Identifiers: LCCN 2018025561 (print) | LCCN 2018026253 (ebook) | ISBN 9781786608505 (Electronic) | ISBN 9781786608482 (cloth : alk. paper) | ISBN 9781786608499 (pbk. : alk. paper)
Subjects: LCSH: Globalization—Health aspects. | World health.
Classification: LCC RA441 (ebook) | LCC RA441 .C63 2018 (print) | DDC 362.1—dc23
LC record available at https://lccn.loc.gov/2018025561

∞™ The paper used in this publication meets the minimum requirements of American National Standard for Information Sciences—Permanence of Paper for Printed Library Materials, ANSI/NISO Z39.48–1992.

Printed in the United States of America

Contents

Preface and Acknowledgements

The purpose of this book is to introduce students to the politics of global health and global health governance utilizing prominent theories of international relations. To accomplish this objective, the approach I have taken is to familiarize the reader with these theories in the first chapter, and then apply their logic and insight to help better understand various actors and issues in global health. To supplement the content in the chapters, I have also included discussion questions and suggested readings at the end of each chapter. Hopefully, the questions will help facilitate interesting thoughts and engaging discussions in the classroom about the material covered in each chapter, and the suggested readings will provide useful information for those interested in further research on international relations theory and global health. Two lessons, in particular, that I hope the reader will come away with from this book are: 1) although financing, medicine, science, and technology are endemic features of global health, politics frequently dictates their use and influence, and 2) the complex and disaggregated nature of global governance makes it extremely challenging to solve health problems that cut across national borders.

There are many individuals who I would like to thank in the development of this project. Jay DeSart, David Yells, and especially David Connelly of Utah Valley University were all very supportive of travel and leave time for my research and preparation of this manuscript. In addition, I would also like to thank my colleagues in the Department of History and Political Science at Utah Valley University for their support and collegiality, especially my fellow IR colleagues, Baktybek Abdrisaev and Hong Pang for their interest in this project. I also would like to express appreciation to all of the excellent panels that I participated in organized by the Global Health Studies section of the International Studies Association over the last couple of years. In particular, I would like to thank my panel discussants Owain Williams, Vlad Kravtsov, and Stefan Elbe who gave me great feedback on certain portions of this manuscript presented at the conference. I must also thank Lawrence Gostin and Jeffrey Crowley for selecting me for admission to the O'Neill Institute Summer Program on Infectious Diseases and the Law at Georgetown University Law Center in 2015. This program proved to be inspirational and provided me with several ideas on how to approach some of the material in this book. It is also necessary for me to thank Dhara Snowden and Rebecca Anastasi at Rowan and Littlefield International for their support of this book, and tremendous assistance during the proposal and publication process.

This book also would not have been possible without the support of my family. I would like to express my appreciation to my father, William, who was willing to read and make comments on early versions of this manuscript, and my mother Cynthia, who consistently gave me encouragement and advice along the way. Also, my mother-in-law, Linda Hyer, who was willing to provide "emergency" child care as I was racing to meet deadlines. And, of course, I thank my wife, Erin, and my children, Anthony and Michael, for their love and support. I dedicate this book to them.

List of Abbreviations

ACA	Patient Protection and Affordable Health Care Act
ACT	artemisinin-based combination therapy
AFTA	ASEAN Free Trade Area
AIDS	acquired immune deficiency syndrome
AMC	Advanced Market Commitment
ARV	antiretroviral drugs
BCG	Bacillus Calmette-Guérin
BIT	bilateral investment treaty
BWC	Convention on the Prohibition of the Development, Production, and Stockpiling of Bacteriological (Biological) and Toxin Weapons and on Their Destruction
CCM	country coordinating mechanism
CESCR	Committee on Economic, Social, and Cultural Rights
CFC	chlorofluorocarbon
CIA	Central Intelligence Agency
CMH	Commission on Macroeconomics and Health
COP	Conference of the Parties
CRC	Convention on the Rights of the Child
CWC	Chemical Weapons Convention
DALY	disability-adjusted life year
DDT	dichloro-diphenyl-trichloroethane
DOT	directly observed therapy
DPAH	Global Strategy on Diet, Physical Activity, and Health
DSB	Dispute Settlement Body
EBF	extrabudgetary fund
ECOSOC	Economic and Social Council
EU	European Union

FAO	Food and Agriculture Organization
FBI	Federal Bureau of Investigation
FBO	faith-based organization
FCA	Framework Convention Alliance
FCGH	Framework Convention on Global Health
FCTC	Framework Convention on Tobacco Control
FDA	Food and Drug Administration
FDI	foreign direct investment
FTA	free trade agreement
GATS	General Agreement on Trade in Services
GATT	General Agreement on Tariffs and Trade
GDEP	Global DOTS Expansion Plan
GDP	gross domestic product
GEF	Global Environment Facility
GFATM	Global Fund to Fight AIDS, Tuberculosis, and Malaria
GHPPP	Global health public-private partnership
GHSA	Global Health Security Agenda
GMEP	Global Malaria Eradication Program
GOARN	Global Outbreak Alert and Response Network
GPA	Global Programme on AIDS
GPPN	Global Public Policy Network
GRID	gay-related immune deficiency syndrome
H1N1	swine flu
H5N1	avian influenza
H8	Health Eight
HIV	human immunodeficiency virus
HOLN	Health Organization of the League of Nations
IBRD	International Bank for Reconstruction and Development
ICCPR	International Covenant on Civil and Political Rights
ICESCR	International Covenant on Economic, Social, and Cultural Rights
ICRC	International Committee of the Red Cross
ICSID	International Center for Settlement of Investment Disputes
IFC	International Finance Corporation
IFFIm	International Finance Facility for Immunization
IGO	intergovernmental organization
IHD	International Health Division
IHR	International Health Regulations
IMF	International Monetary Fund
IPCC	Intergovernmental Panel on Climate Change
IRS	indoor residual spraying
ISR	International Sanitary Regulations
ITN	insecticide-treated net

ITO	International Trade Organization
ITPMS	International Tobacco Products Marketing Standards
LRTAP	Convention on Long-Range Transboundary Air Pollution
LSF	Liberté Sans Frontières Foundation
MAP	Multicountry HIV/AIDS program
MDG	Millennium Development Goal
MDR	multidrug resistance
MNC	multinational corporation
MSF	Médecins Sans Frontières
NAFTA	North American Free Trade Agreement
NCD	non-communicable disease
NGO	non-governmental organization
NIEO	New International Economic Order
NTD	neglected tropical diseases
OHCHR	Office of the United Nations High Commissioner for Human Rights
OIHP	Office International d'Hygiène Publique
OPCW	Organization for the Prohibition of Chemical Weapons
PAHO	Pan American Health Organization
PEPFAR	President's Emergency Plan for AIDS Relief
PHEIC	public health emergency of international concern
PhRMA	Pharmaceutical Research and Manufacturers of America
PPP	public-private partnerships
RBM	Roll Back Malaria Initiative
SAP	structural adjustments program
SARS	severe acute respiratory syndrome
SDG	Sustainable Development Goal
SPS	Agreement on the Application of Sanitary and Phytosanitary Measures
TAC	Treatment Access Campaign
TB	tuberculosis
TBT	Technical Barriers to Trade Agreement
TFI	Tobacco Free Initiative
TPRB	Trade Policy Review Body
TRIPS	Agreement on Trade-Related Aspects of Intellectual Property Rights
UDHR	Universal Declaration of Human Rights
UN	United Nations
UNAIDS	Joint United Nations Programme on HIV/AIDS
UNCED	United Nations Conference on Environment and Development
UNCITRAL	United Nations Commission on International Trade Law
UNDP	United Nations Development Programme
UNEP	United Nations Environment Programme

UNESCO	United Nations Educational, Scientific, and Cultural Organization
UNFCCC	United Nations Framework Convention on Climate Change
UNICEF	United Nations Children's Fund
UNPFA	United Nations Population Fund
USTR	Office of the United States Trade Representative
WHA	World Health Assembly
WHO	World Health Organization
WMO	World Meteorological Organization
WTO	World Trade Organization

List of Boxes and Tables

BOXES

TABLES

Chapter 1

International Relations Theory and Global Health

On December 6, 2013, a two-year-old boy, named Emile Ouamouno, who lived in a remote village in southern Guinea became seriously ill and died four days later. Over the next few weeks, his mother, sister, and grandmother also died with similar symptoms. The disease soon began to spread outside of the village, crossing over into the neighboring states of Sierra Leone and Liberia. The cause of these deaths was not identified as the Ebola virus until March 2014 as fifty-nine people had died in Guinea by the end of that month (McNeil 2014). Until this point in time, the Ebola virus had been a rare, contagious disease that had mostly been confined to remote areas of Central and East Africa. After the first Ebola outbreak in 1976, 1,590 people had died from this virus (Sack et al. 2014). Nevertheless, it was not until early August 2014, when the World Health Organization (WHO) designated the epidemic as a "public health emergency of international concern." While the WHO faced a good deal of disparagement from critics due to its slow response, at the same time, it "was never intended to be a 'first responder', but rather the 'directing and coordinating authority' in international health" (Kamradt-Scott 2016: 405). The following month, the United Nations (UN) Security Council declared the outbreak to be a "threat to international peace and security" (United Nations Security Council 2014). This action was supplemented by the United Nations General Assembly's decision to direct the Secretary-General to establish the UN's first emergency health mission (United Nations General Assembly 2014). Then in October, the WHO's Director-General Margaret Chan called the outbreak "unquestionably the most severe acute public health emergency in modern times" (Cumming-Bruce 2014). By the end of 2014, 7,905 people had died from this outbreak (Reuters 2014). While almost all the cases of the disease were located in the impoverished countries of Guinea, Sierra Leone, and Liberia, the disease managed to spread globally, including cases in the United States and Europe.

The 2014 Ebola outbreak in West Africa demonstrated how globalization has facilitated the spread of infectious diseases, including unusual and deadly diseases such as Ebola, from a small village in Guinea to two nurses in Dallas, Texas, in a matter of months. Because such diseases cannot be confined to national borders, some measure of global governance is often necessary to stem the growth of the problem. This need is especially strong when epidemics, such as Ebola, originate in poor countries that lack the capacity to efficiently diagnose, control, and treat these diseases. The puzzle regarding global governance in health, or any other area for that matter, is what is the appropriate arrangement for effective governance at the global level, and is sufficient political will to support such an arrangement available in a world structured around independent, sovereign states?

Although global governance in the area of health has undergone some significant changes since 2000, it is by no means a new area of international cooperation. A series of international conferences and treaties were concluded in the nineteenth century to promote interstate cooperation and standardization of procedures to contain the spread of infectious diseases. These diseases are products of nature that are not constrained by national borders. As European powers began to establish more networks around the world as part of their colonization process, such arrangements contributed to the spread of diseases on a global scale. Europeans brought new diseases, such as smallpox, to the Americas, resulting in the deaths of a significant part of the native population. Diseases such as cholera and the plague spread from Asia to other parts of the world killing millions of people. International cooperation to control the spread of these diseases was based on pragmatic interests rather than idealistic principles. During the nineteenth century alone, leading national governments conducted ten international conferences and negotiated eight agreements toward this end. By 1923, these states had also agreed to create two international organizations and one regional organization devoted to health. The extent of this activity in global health made it one of the most active areas of international cooperation during this time (Fidler 1999). The spread of disease is related to globalization. Because disease is a global phenomenon, states have had to continuously work together to manage this problem as the world has become more globalized.

Globalization is a complex process of integration on a worldwide level that affects people's lives in a multitude of ways, including health. It is characterized by specific temporal, spatial, and organizational attributes that impact relationships globally. While globalization is not a new phenomenon, its post–Cold War form features an extensive reach of global relations and networks exhibiting high levels of intensity, velocity, and impact on many aspects of social life (Held and McGrew 2002). However, despite its increasing strength, it is not a uniform process as its effects vary throughout the world (Keohane 2001). That is, some locales are subject to greater degrees of globalization than others. Health is an important aspect of this development in that health and disease have been greatly affected by the pattern of contemporary globalization. The increased interconnections among states and people in the world have created a growing concern over a variety of threats to health that have transcended national borders and the jurisdiction of national governments (Cockerham and Cockerham 2010). At the same time, this process exhibits an inconsistent impact as certain health concerns and threats affect some parts of the world more than others.

A significant aspect of the globalization of health, as with the globalization of any facet of social life, is a lack of regulation. Globalization is not a normative concept in that it is neither inherently good nor bad, but it can exhibit both positive and negative influences on human life. Due to the lack of capacity of individual states to limit the impact of the negative aspects of globalization, some degree of cooperation, coordination, or regulation above the state level is necessary (Woods 2002). Determining the appropriate mode of governance is problematic, given the number of states and types of actors involved. Some scholars are pessimistic on whether globalization can effectively be governed. Rosenau (1990), for example, argues that a multicentric world has risen to challenge the traditional state-centric system that has previously dominated international relations. In particular, he views global governance as a disaggregated authority structure, where the spheres of authority, which are composed of many actors, are the main units of governance. The disaggregated nature of authority in global governance makes the coordination necessary for effective implementation unlikely (Rosenau 2005).

Despite the theoretical complexity of governance at a global level, the concept has received attention by policy-makers in the area of health. In September 2000, the Secretary-General of the UN, Kofi Annan, convened a summit of UN member states to adopt the Millennium Development Goals (MDGs). Endorsed by 189 states, these goals were translated into eight objectives that the UN member states agreed to achieve by 2015. Among these objectives was the goal of stopping the spread of HIV/AIDS, malaria, tuberculosis, and other major diseases, as well as improving child and maternal mortality. The achievements of the MDGs were mixed. On one hand, the number of people living in extreme hunger was reduced by millions, and the number of HIV/AIDS, malaria, and tuberculosis infections substantially declined since 2000. On the other hand, economic and gender inequality, as well as climate change and environmental degradation, still proved to be significant burdens for progress, especially for developing countries. Politically, however, the MDGs were viewed as a positive development, and the key principles maintained widespread support. During the United Nations Sustainable Development Summit held in September 2015, the 2030 Agenda for Sustainable Development and seventeen Sustainable Development Goals (SDGs) were adopted. The SDGs were designed to build upon the MDGs with a much more ambitious and comprehensive set of objectives.

Although the MDGs had a strong moral basis and universal political support in principle, their achievement by 2015 was questionable. With more ambitious objectives, the SDGs may face even greater obstacles. Different levels of socioeconomic development among populations and states, limitations on resources, distribution problems, conflicts of interests among relevant actors, and other issues pose significant obstacles that still need to be overcome. For global health governance to be effective, cooperation, coordination, and regulation issues need to be adequately resolved.

A limitation regarding the MDGs for global health governance was that they were primarily directed at infectious diseases. Chronic or non-communicable diseases did not receive the same level of attention. This relative neglect was taking place despite the fact that in developing countries, 80 percent more lives are lost to chronic diseases than infectious diseases (Mathers and Loncar 2006). UN-affiliated organizations like the WHO have also traditionally focused on infectious disease control rather than chronic disease control. This emphasis, however, began to change as with the WHO's support of the passage of the Framework Convention on Tobacco Control in 2003. Although the tobacco control movement was successful, other risk factors related to the causes of chronic diseases have yet to be addressed in a similar manner. For example, in the WHO's proposed budget for 2018–2019, its top objectives were related to infectious diseases. A fund of US$805 million was allocated to reduce the burden of these diseases, with US$272 million for vaccine-preventable diseases, US$145 million directly for HIV/AIDS, US$124 million for tuberculosis, and US$116 million for malaria. In comparison, burden reduction for all non-communicable diseases was allocated US$351 million (World Health Organization 2017a).

The SDGs, however, provide much more comprehensive targets for global health than the MDGs do. In addition to calling for the end of the epidemics of AIDS, tuberculosis, and malaria by 2030, the SDGs target a one-third reduction in premature deaths from non-communicable diseases and a substantial reduction in deaths from air, water, and soil pollution during this time frame. Objectives of the SDGs also include strengthening the implementation of the Framework Convention on Tobacco Control and improving prevention and treatment of drug and alcohol abuse. Other significant health-related objectives encompass the achievement of universal health coverage, affordable access to essential medicines and vaccines, and a substantial increase in health financing by 2030. While the SDGs indicate even greater political support for global health in 2015 compared to that in 2000, the number and scope of these goals will be a substantial test for global governance.

Many issues are at the center of efforts to enact global health governance. In addition to the cooperation, management, financing, and regulation issues, health care coverage is at stake. Science and law are integral parts of this system, as they act to frame various issues for negotiations. In order to describe, explain, and understand global governance in health or any other area, theories of international relations can be useful tools in attempting to analyze such complex system. Why are international relations theories necessary to improve our understanding of global health? Global health issues transcend national borders and state sovereignty. As a result, a collective response at the international level is necessary to effectively address these problems. This response, however, is not simply based on medical expertise or technology but is largely dependent on politics. Health has become inextricably linked to policies developed by global governance, whether these policies involve the surveillance and the prevention of the spread of infectious disease across borders; the distribution and consumption of goods that pose a health risk through international commerce; the right to quality health for everyone, regardless of a person's country of residence; or the protection of human health from climate change and environmental degradation. International relations theories therefore provide a key analytical tool for understanding the dynamics of the political process in global governance to addressing health issues in an increasingly globalized world.

In its analysis of global health and global health governance, this book will focus on the dominant theories in the study of international relations, realism, and liberalism, as well as two of the leading perspectives outside of the mainstream in constructivism and Marxism. While this focus certainly does not nearly cover every theory of international relations, it does include an analysis of rational approaches (realism and liberalism), as well as its critiques from non-rational (constructivism) and critical theories (Marxism). In this chapter, I will discuss these influential theories of international relations and describe how they relate to the concept of global health governance as background reference material for the other chapters discussing key actors and topics in global health. A brief synopsis of each theory can be found in table 1.1.

REALISM

Realism is the oldest school of thought in international relations studies. It is a paradigm that is associated with several different theories, but the fundamental commonality is a state-centric view of international politics that

Table 1.1. International Relations Theories in Brief

Realism/Neorealism—States, particularly the most powerful, are the dominant actors in international politics. The national interest of the state is the pursuit of power or security. Relationships between states are competitive and often conflictual. Cooperation is a challenge, and international law and organizations have a limited impact on international politics.

Liberalism/Neoliberalism—States may be the primary actors in international politics, but intergovernmental organization (IGO) and non-state actors are influential as well. States have multiple and changing national interests. They are also likely to cooperate with each other due to the prospect of achieving mutual benefits. International law and organizations are important features of the international system, because they can facilitate cooperation and the provision of collective goods.

Constructivism—The behavior of states is based on the social identities of individuals. Their interests are based upon prevailing social norms. Power is not just material but social as well. International institutions play a major role in international politics, because they are both products and purveyors of international norms.

Marxism/Neo-Marxism—Social classes, in particular, the transnational capitalist class, are the dominant actors in the international system. The relationship among states is based on generating wealth and profit-maximizing interests. Globalization creates a significant degree of inequality both between and within states. International law and organizations primarily serve as agents of capitalist interests. Multinational corporations are key actors in promoting these interests and facilitating inequality.

assumes that the power and security interests of states drive the system. The roots of realist thought can be traced back to Thucydides, an ancient Greek historian, who wrote about the conflict between Athens and Sparta in his *History of the Peloponnesian War* during the 400s B.C. (Thucydides 1972). His account revealed a series of interactions among Greek city-states based on power politics and security concerns as motivating factors. Morality was defined by the powerful, and their will was imposed upon weaker entities, by force if necessary. This view of political realism reappears in the work of Niccolo Machiavelli and Thomas Hobbes in the sixteenth and seventeenth centuries.

Realism became integrated with the study of international relations with the work of E. H. Carr and Reinhold Niebuhr who challenged idealistic principles in international affairs. The most significant contribution in the early development of realism in international relations was Hans Morgenthau's seminal text, *Politics among Nations*, originally published in 1948. This book was the first effort to specifically advance realism as a theory of international politics (Wohlforth 2008). Morgenthau's approach, also associated with classical realism, established some influential assumptions about the nature of international politics. His theory assumed that politicians were rational decision-makers, whose actions are guided by the pursuit of power. States were the dominant actors in international relations, and international politics was a struggle for power among these actors. Decision-making and behavior were driven by rationality rather than by universal moral principles (Morgenthau 1967).

Neorealism emerged as a new interpretation of these ideas in the later part of the Cold War. Waltz's (1979) *Theory of International Politics* sought to refine realism's theoretical framework. He focused on the structure of the international system as a primary factor in understanding international politics. This structure consisted of two characteristics. The first is that the international system is based upon anarchy, which means that no central authority exists above the state. The second characteristic of the structure is the distribution of the material power capabilities among the states in the system. Due to a lack of a world government, the condition of anarchy has been a constant feature of international politics. The distribution of power, however, has varied over time as the system exhibited multipolar, bipolar, and unipolar characteristics at different periods in history. According to neorealism, the structure of the system constrains the actions of states and influences their interactions with other states. Another difference between neorealism and classical realism is that neorealists argue that security interests primarily motivate states, not the pursuit of power. That is, power is not an end goal; rather, it is a means for the state to establish and maintain its security.

Although realism has different variations, at its roots it views politics as a product of competition and conflict. This interpretation, of course, leads to an interesting question as to how cooperation can be achieved in such an environment. Neorealism is skeptical about its prospects. Waltz (1979) addresses this point by suggesting that states are concerned about cooperation, because they will be wary about which party is benefiting more from the bargain. Such insecurity inhibits cooperation among states. This situation, known as a *relative gains problem*, results from the greater willingness states have to cooperate with others if they achieve a greater advantage than their partners in the transaction. Cooperation between states, nevertheless, happens. Grieco (1988) suggests that while states are subject to relative gains in international bargaining, this interaction is also influenced by each party's sensitivity to the payoff that the other party will receive. This sensitivity varies depending on the relationship between the parties, as well as the issue area for cooperation. States will be much more sensitive about potential payoffs in interactions with adversaries and in the security than they will have with allies and in areas of low politics. He maintains, however, that regardless of the nature of the interaction, relative gains concerns will have an impact, and some sensitivity about security exists even between close allies.

A key mechanism for cooperation in international relations is institutions. While institutions are regarded as a core concept in international relations theory, studies have not been uniformly clear as to what exactly constitutes an institution. According to Keohane (1989: 32), "Institutions are often discussed without being defined at all, or after having been defined only casually." Mearsheimer (1994/1995: 8) has offered a definition of institutions as a "set of rules that stipulate the ways in which states should cooperate and compete with each other." In assessing the utility of institutions through a neorealist perspective, Mearsheimer finds that institutions have only a limited effect on state behavior. They tend to reflect the interests of the powerful, and they do not usually affect international interactions independent of great power support. As with cooperation, neorealists are pessimistic about institutions. They are constrained by both the uneven power distribution and the relative gains problem that are inherent in international relations.

Although realists are skeptics when it comes to international cooperation and institutions, some realist theorists have sought to account for how international rules, norms, and institutions can develop and be maintained. This explanation is based upon hegemonic stability theory, which posits that the power and leadership of a dominant state, or hegemon, can establish an international order that promotes cooperative mechanisms. Much of the research on hegemonic stability has been used to explain the global economy. Realists have suggested that an open global economic system results from a hegemonic state that is willing to support it as a public good. The hegemon is willing to provide this service because it perceives that its interests will benefit. This state must use its resources and power to manage the system, as well as encourage other states to adhere to the rules and norms of the system. The provision of this international order is dependent on the power and willingness of a hegemonic state (Krasner 1976; Gilpin 1987). The United States' support of the Bretton Woods institutions after World War II to stabilize international trade and monetary relations has often been used as an example of hegemonic stability theory.

LIBERALISM AND ITS VARIANTS

Unlike realist theory, liberalism is much more optimistic about the prospects and utility of international cooperation and institutions. Because of this perspective, research based upon liberal theories tends to place much more attention on these concepts. Contemporary liberal theory in international relations is heavily influenced by the work and ideas of Hugo Grotius, Immanuel Kant, and Woodrow Wilson (Karns and Mingst 2015). Grotius (1583–1645) was considered to be the founder of modern international law in the seventeenth century. Although he was a proponent of natural law, Grotius also based his view of the law of nations on the importance of consent. His contribution to the theory, study, and practice of international relations was that states were bound to follow rules, whether natural or contractual, in their interactions with one another. From this perspective, these rules and the practice of following them would contribute to an international society, which would not only constrain the sovereignty of states but also provide more stability in international relations.

Grotius also believed that war was not an inherent right of states. It was subject to the limitations of law. Kant (1724–1804), however, focused on the achievement of a foundation of peace based on three components: representative democracy as a norm for government, the establishment of a federation of free states, and world citizenship. Kant argued that representative democracies would be more prone to peace than other forms of government. These states would be more peaceful, because the decision to go to war would be based on the consent of citizens and the rule of law, rather than the will of authoritarian leaders. Democracy by itself, nevertheless, would not guarantee peace. Democratic states also needed to agree to a contract for peace and commit themselves to resolving their disputes peacefully through the creation of a federation devoted to this purpose. World citizenship among the people of the world would also be an important factor in establishing a lasting peace. Increases in interactions across borders in areas such as trade, commerce, transportation, communication, and tourism could facilitate the development of a cosmopolitan identity that would make citizens of democratic states much less likely to support going to war with one another.

Wilson's contribution to liberalism was his attempt to institute these liberal ideas into practice following the devastating consequences of World War I. The principles of the rule of law, peaceful dispute resolution, and a federation of states devoted to peace were incorporated into the Treaty of Versailles ending the war and the Covenant of the League of Nations. Wilson spearheaded this move toward liberalism in international relations. The lack of commitment by the member states of the League of Nations to respond effectively to acts of aggression leading to World War II caused liberalism to be met with a great deal of skepticism in the mid-twentieth century. The ideas, however, continued to live on through the establishment of the UN to promote international peace and security and the Bretton Woods institutions (i.e., International Monetary Fund [IMF] and World Bank) to support international economic cooperation.

Although realism emerged as the dominant paradigm in international relations after the war, liberalism continued to have relevancy with the global movement toward establishing international organizations. Functionalism was a variant of liberalism developed to account for this trend, especially with the early stages of European integration, as well as the founding of technical organizations in the UN system, such as the WHO and the Food and Agriculture Organization. In his essay "A Working Peace System" Mitrany (1966) posits that peace among states can be achieved by bringing them together through cooperation in areas of low politics and technical matters, such as health and labor standards, which would not pose much of an infringement on sovereignty and may provide for mutual benefits. In theory, functional cooperation would become more habitual over time and eventually spillover into higher areas of politics such as security. Functionalism's contribution to liberalism was in providing a logical explanation for international politics that went beyond the dominance of the state and the constraints posed by nationalism emphasized by realists.

The weaknesses of functionalist theory are based on its lack of precision. It does not specify the conditions necessary for cooperative spillover into high politics to be achieved. It also does not take into account potential costs or constraints that could be presented with higher forms of political cooperation. Other than assuming that habits of cooperation will deepen over time, the connection and the form of a lasting peace are not well specified. Neofunctionalism and its main proponent Ernst Haas refined the theory by focusing more on the calculus of cooperation, particularly regionally rather than globally, instead of a pathway to peace. Haas (1958) views the major actors in the process of integration to be supranational institutions and domestic interest groups rather than the state. The supranational institutions desire to promote deeper cooperation among member states in order to expand their influence. Interest groups within the state also wish to promote integration to further their interests, especially when they are not sufficiently met by the national government's existing policies. Rational self-interest by these actors, rather than the achievement of mutual gains and harmony espoused by functionalists, distinguishes this approach.

Instead of driving integration, the state plays a reactionary role to the other actors. The process of integration is based on functional and political spillovers. Functional spillover is based on the integration of particular economic sectors. Because some industrial economic sectors are interdependent, integrating these sectors will require their dependent sectors to also become more integrated in response. This form of spillover takes place without the pressures by interest groups. Political spillover involves the political changes brought about by the interactions of the supranational institutions, the national governments, and the interest groups. As the institutions and groups promote their agendas, the states become socialized and begin to adopt more integrative policies as such policies become perceived as in the state's best interest. For spillover to take place, neofunctionalists retained the assumption that it begins in areas of low politics. While neofunctionalism goes further than functionalism in explaining the process of integration and the role of international organizations, it also does not specify the conditions when political spillover will take place and when group interests to integrate will be incorporated into the interests of the national governments.

While functional theories had some success explaining the creation of technical IGOs and the early stages of European integration, neoliberal institutionalism emerged as the primary liberal challenge to realism in international relations, particularly in regard to economic matters. Despite some important differences, neoliberal institutionalists share certain assumptions with realists, such as the important role of the state, the view of the state as a rational actor, and the exogenous interests of the state. They primarily differ with realists on the relative dominance of state in international affairs and the emphasis that realists place on relative gains in cooperation. Neoliberals emphasize the importance of international institutions and international law in enhancing cooperative relationships based on mutual gain. Neoliberal institutionalists view international relations as less conflictual and more ordered than realists do.

Neoliberal institutionalism developed as a revision of neofunctionalism by maintaining the assumption of a natural tendency to cooperate in international relations to achieve mutual benefits but including a much more active and important role for the state in the process. Keohane and Nye's (1977) *Power and Interdependence* described the relationships among states as based on connections of multiple channels, where security is not always the dominant issue, and where military force is not a viable option between states that are highly interdependent. International institutions are key actors in managing interdependence because they serve to define issues of mutual concern, assist states in linking them and coordinating transnational policies. Institutions can also mitigate the power differences between states in affecting outcomes.

Neoliberal institutionalism assumes that states are much more prone to cooperate than realist theories due to their preference of absolute gains over relative gains. This assumption means that states are much more concerned with their individual gains in a mutual transaction than any potential gains that are received by other states. In comparing the propensity of states to favor absolute gains over relative gains, Powell (1991) found that unless the interaction between states is influenced by security interests where use of force between the actors is a possibility, states will be motivated by absolute gains in their relationships with others. Due to their emphasis on absolute gains, neoliberal institutionalists do not view motivation to cooperate as a significant problem. The issue, rather, is how to address the cooperation problems evidenced in the Prisoner's Dilemma, described in box 1.1, such as establishing trust and discouraging cheating.

Although many interactions in international relations involve bargains among actors where each actor receives some form of a benefit, some

BOX 1.1 THE PROBLEM OF INTERNATIONAL COOPERATION AS SEEN THROUGH THE PRISONER'S DILEMMA

Keohane's (1984) *After Hegemony* focused more on the role of international institutions and particularly how they could be effective in addressing the problem of states pursuing self-interested behavior that would impede the achievement of cooperative outcomes that are mutually beneficial. This logical problem of collective action is found in the Prisoner's Dilemma. In this game, two prisoners have mixed motives regarding whether or not to confess to a crime. If one prisoner confesses and the other does not, then the confessing prisoner will go free, while the other prisoner will receive a long prison sentence. If both confess, then they both would receive a medium prison term. If they both remain silent, then the outcome would be a short prison term for both prisoners. The mutually beneficial, or optimal, outcome of this game is for both to remain silent so that each prisoner would serve a short sentence. The dilemma, however, is that both prisoners have an incentive to confess, and therefore cheat their partner, so they can be set free.

Assuming that the prisoners are rational actors, the expectation is that they will confess and not cooperate with one another due to their fear of the possibility of being cheated and serving a long sentence. In the context of such a mixed motive game in international relations, institutions can act as a means to reduce the potential of cheating and promote a more cooperative outcome. By helping to clarify the cooperative solution to a given problem, as well as reducing transaction costs, and increasing transparency of the interaction, institutions may promote the establishment of a cooperative relationship that realists would expect to be unlikely.

cooperative relationships are based on collective goods, or benefits that are received by all regardless of whether each individual contributed to providing the good. This situation, known as *collective action*, can also create a challenge for cooperation. In this instance, the problem is based on "free-riding." Because all members of the group benefit from the good, it is in their self-interest not to contribute to providing the good so they can receive the benefit of it without incurring any costs. The dilemma, however, is that if a significant number of members of the group decide to "free-ride," then the collective good will not be provided. Liberal theories have contributed to potential resolutions to this collective action problem. Olson (1968) argues that the size of the group is related to the feasibility of providing common goods. In smaller groups, it is easier to detect free-riding and compel compliance than in larger groups. Institutions may also play a role as well. In their analysis of why states act through international organizations, Abbott and Snidal (1998) note that organizational structure can make collective actions more efficient by offering mediation and adjudication services to help resolve disputes. Organizations can promote norms and practices of member states so that they will be more unlikely to defect from cooperating in collective action situations.

While international institutions can provide some management over collective goods as a supranational authority, they may not necessarily be the best means to address the collective action problem. Ostrom (1990) finds that private actors can effectively manage common resources. In order to be successful, however, these actors must establish particular rules among themselves such as clearly defined boundaries and a means of monitoring, sanctioning, and dispute resolution. The private actors participate in all the aspects of managing the rules. Rather than following regulations by a superseding authority, development of communication, trust, and inclusiveness among the group may be more effective in alleviating the collective action problem.

CONSTRUCTIVISM

Both realism and neoliberalism share some similarities in that both assume that relevant actors are behaving based on a rational decision-making process and their emphasis on materialism in shaping outcomes of international interactions. Social constructivism provides a different ontological perspective on international relations. Alexander Wendt (1992: 396–397) describes that "a fundamental principle of constructivist social theory is that people act toward objects, including other actors, on the basis of the meanings that the objects have for them." According to this view, international interactions are shaped by ideas and the identities of the actors. In terms of decision-making and behavior of relevant actors, constructivists consider the process to be influenced by identities and norms rather than rational decision-making. Material interests also do not tend to a primary factor in the outcome of international interactions. The emphasis by constructivists on ideas and norms does not suggest that material factors are irrelevant; however, their meaning and influence are interpreted both subjectively by individuals and intersubjectively as shared understandings by groups or communities of individuals. Interpretation, of course, is subject to the changing conditions of time and place.

Because of this feature, the interests of actors, influence of material factors, and the structure of the international system are in a constant state of flux.

Although constructivism provides some useful insights about international relations by incorporating more intangible aspects of the process into its analysis, it has some limitations as well. Checkel (1998), for instance, refers to constructivism more as a method than as a unified theory. Constructivism incorporates the concepts of ideas and identities into the analysis of international politics, but it does not specify the relative significance of international actors and specific causal mechanisms. This limitation constrains constructivism's predictive utility. In assessing a constructivist view on global governance, Hoffmann (2005a) suggests that while constructivism can account for the process of governance, it does not provide a clear set of assumptions as to its design.

Nevertheless, constructivists have identified particular factors such as norms and identities that influence political outcomes in empirical research. Studies by Klotz (1995) and Tannenwald (1999) demonstrated how international norms affect state behavior. Klotz (1995: 14) defines norms as "shared (thus social) understandings of standards for behavior." Norms act as constraints on behavior as a form of social pressure for states to comply with them. She also suggests that norms motivate state behavior by defining a state's national interest. In the case of the apartheid regime in South Africa, she finds that a global norm of racial equality, and not material interests, explain why a large number of states adopted sanctions against the white minority government. In the area of security, Tannenwald found that a norm of a "nuclear taboo" had emerged at the global level, which increasingly restrained the United States from considering the use of nuclear weapons as the norm grew stronger.

Norms have a dynamic life cycle that changes over time. Finnemore and Sikkink (1998) explain this life cycle in three stages: norm emergence, norm cascade, and norm internationalization. In the emergence stage, entrepreneurs try to promote a particular norm, often through international organizations. If the norm is sufficiently accepted, it reaches a "tipping point," then it begins to cascade, which means that more and more states adopt the norm due to international pressure and socialization. At the last stage of the life cycle, the norm becomes internalized and gains an "oughtness" quality where the norm becomes a part of the state's identity and interests. Not all norms successfully complete this life cycle. In fact, many norms fail to reach the "tipping point" where they begin to cascade. For a norm to reach the tipping point, Finnemore and Sikkink suggest that the norm must be accepted by at least one-third of world's national governments. This number, however, may be affected by how many of the more powerful states endorse the evolving norm.

Identity is a critical factor in understanding the behavior of states according to constructivists. In their examination of security communities, Adler and Barnett (1998) suggest that these communities are created through the development of a collective identity. Social interactions and institutions promote social learning among the actors involved that leads to mutual trust. A strong sense of trust then contributes to a common identity or sense of "we-ness" among these previously disparate actors. A fundamental difference between the constructivist interpretation and rationalist approaches, notably realism and neoliberal institutionalism, is that it assumes that interests change due to socialization rather than remaining fixed.

Although constructivism is ontologically and epistemologically different from realism and neoliberal institutionalism, constructivists do find key variables associated with these approaches to be significant, albeit in different ways. Power, as assumed by realists, has been conceptualized as based on material resources and the capacity of a state to use these resources to influence another actor to do something that it would otherwise not do. Barnett and Duvall (2005), however, argue that while power is a major factor in international relations, the realist conceptualization is limited because it omits the social aspect of power. They suggest that power comes from four different forms: compulsory, institutional, structural, and productive. Compulsory refers to a type of power where one actor directly controls another. This type of power fits closest with the realist view. Institutional power is indirect. It is based on institutions that are created to further interests of particular actors by binding others to certain obligations that may be to their detriment. Structural power captures the social relations aspect of power. Structure defines the social relationship between different actors, which is shaped by power. Productive power refers to the ability to give meanings of concepts and their relative significance. It is a more general form of power than structural power because it shapes interests and identities by defining meanings and significance for an overall system of interactions, rather than the development of identities through direct interaction evidenced by structural power.

Institutions, in addition to power, are an integral part of international politics according to constructivists. Finnemore (1996) argues that international organizations are independent actors that socialize states to accept new norms and values. In this way, these organizations act as teachers. In her study on the United Nations Educational, Scientific, and Cultural Organization (UNESCO), she finds that the organization was able to effectively promote its science policy among its member states (Finnemore 1993). Instead of UNESCO acting as an agent to promote cooperation, it performed as an autonomous actor that actively, and successfully, convinced states of the importance of adopting a science bureaucracy regardless of its level of development. In this role, institutions may help to shape, and even change, a state's interests.

MARXISM AND NEO-MARXISM

The roots of Marxist theories of international relations can be traced to the work of Karl Marx and Friedrich Engels during the nineteenth century. They believed that economics was the driving force behind politics and social relationships. Society was based upon a conflict between the capitalist class, who owned the means of economic production, and a proletarian class whose labor would be exploited by the capitalist class for its economic gain. The relationship between the two classes was conflictual and would eventually lead to a social revolution that would undermine the capitalist economic system. These aspects of class conflict, structured around the capitalist economic system, were incorporated into Marxist perspectives on the nature of international politics. All politics, whether international or domestic, occurred under the umbrella of a capitalist global economy. For the most part, Marx did not address international relations as part of his analysis. John Hobson and Vladimir Lenin, however, expanded Marxist analysis to demonstrate how capitalism served as a motivation for imperialism and exploitation.

One influential variation of Marxism was dependency theory. It extended a Marxist view on class to international affairs. This theory, largely coming out of Latin American scholarship, assumed that global capitalism creates a linkage between rich states and poor states where the rich states exploited the resources of poor states to enrich their economic production. The poor states were constrained in their development by this relationship because their resources were being used to benefit the wealthier states to their detriment. Cardoso and Faletto (1979) believed that foreign capital created a dependency for Latin American states on wealthier countries. They also argued, however, that some domestic groups in poorer states form coalitions with foreign capitalists in order to advance their own interests, as well as that of foreign capital, through the policies of their state.

Similarly, world systems theory also provides a class-based analysis of the international system. This approach views the system as based on an international division of labor divided among different classes of states: a core, a periphery, and a semi-periphery (Wallerstein 1974). The core states are at the center of global capitalism. They are developed states that provide most of the world's capital and have a highly skilled labor force. These states drive and maintain the global capitalist economic system. The peripheral states are poor, developing countries that provide raw materials and cheap, unskilled labor to the global economy. The semi-peripheral states are those that are moderate in both their economic development and skill of their workforce. They could be declining members of the core, or more economically advanced peripheral states. Wallerstein (1974), considered the primary proponent of world systems theory, finds that the modern international system, which originated in sixteenth-century Europe, is structured around global capitalism. The system functions to benefit the economic development and growth of the core to the detriment of the peripheral states, and to a lesser extent, the semi-peripheral states of the world.

Dependency and world systems theories are state-centric approaches rooted in Marxism. Another theoretical variation based on this philosophy comes from the work of Antonio Gramsci, who brought more political analysis into the Marxist approach. According to Gramsci, political elites maintain control of lower classes based upon ideological hegemony (Simon 1982). Hegemony, in this view, is based on ideas rather than material power. These elites, often associated with the capitalist class, socialize other classes into accepting and consenting to their values and rule. A major implication of this process, of course, is that class consciousness for the proletariat will be more difficult to achieve, which renders the prospects for a social revolution to be much less likely.

Neo-Gramscian theorists have made major contributions in the study of international relations. Teschke (2008: 173) argues that neo-Gramscian theory "presents the most influential Marxist theory in contemporary international relations discourse." Cox (1987) is a major contributor to this approach. Cox argues that production provides structure for human society and power derives from it, which determines how production is organized. He divided these modes of production into twelve different types: subsistence, peasant-lord, primitive labor market, household, self-employment, enterprise labor market, bipartism, enterprise corporatism, tripartism, state corporatism, communal, and central planning. Each mode provides expected social behaviors to bind workers to value that particular mode of production. The state provides the primary determinant of the mode of production, and it is influenced by historic blocs, which is "the term applied to the particular configuration of social classes and ideology that give context to a historical state" (Cox 1987: 409). These historic blocs function at the state level through the dominant social class, as well as internationally through a hegemonic state, interests of a hegemonic class, and transnational agents, such as international organizations. Cox finds that the post-1945 neoliberal economic order is based on a historical bloc promoting neoliberal ideology of the dominant class; U.S. hegemony supporting such a perspective; and actors such as the IMF, World Bank, and multinational corporations as transnational agents diffusing the interests of the historic bloc on a global scale. Ideas, state power, and transactional agents act in concert to structure global relations.

INTERNATIONAL RELATIONS THEORY AND GLOBAL HEALTH GOVERNANCE

As with globalization, global governance is a concept that gained momentum after the end of the Cold War. They are also similar in that they are both difficult to define. In 1995, the Commission on Global Governance issued an early report on the concept, which defined global governance as the following:

> Governance is the sum of the many ways individuals and institutions, public and private, manage their common affairs. It is a continuing process through which conflicting or diverse interests may be accommodated and cooperative action may be taken. It includes formal institutions and regimes empowered to enforce compliance, as well as informal arrangements that people and institutions have agreed to or perceive to be in their interest. (Commission on Global Governance 1995: 2)

In the context of global health governance, David Fidler (2010: 3) defines it as:

> the use of formal and informal institutions, rules, and processes by states, intergovernmental organizations, and nonstate actors to deal with challenges to health that require cross-border collective action to address effectively.

Although Fidler's definition of global health governance is more concise than the Commission on Global Governance's definition of the general concept, it still indicates the complexity of the system. Governance is not designed in a formal, hierarchical manner with regulatory authority like a government. It is system where a multitude of actors interact with one another to resolve various transnational health issues. These interactions may be shaped by formal rules, but they may also be based on informal understandings. The roles of the individual actors may not necessarily be clearly defined due to the element of informality that is present in a governance system. To further add to the complexity, global health governance includes a "variety of policies—some complementary, some disjointed or even conflicting—which are made in multiple sites and at multiple levels of global governance" (McInnes et al. 2014: 96)

As a means to give more structure to global health governance to address some of its ambiguity, Gostin (2007) proposed a Framework Convention on Global Health (FCGH). This legal agreement would be based on several broad principles. These principles include coordination of actions between state and non-state actors, obligatory funding requirements for global health, data gathering and reporting, scientific analysis, and enforcement mechanisms for non-compliance. After reaching an agreement that embodies these principles, national governments then would agree to negotiate separate protocols designed to be more detailed and more specific in addressing the objectives of the convention. Gostin argues that the FCGH would be a way to develop an international regime for health effectively by making it a process including many different actors involved in global health governance and allowing them incrementally to build the regime after developing a convention based on broad details. Consensus building and the development of a community of actors who want to improve global health for all will be necessary for the regime to be effective.

In response to the FCGH proposal, Hoffman and Røttingen (2013) suggest that while it is an admirable idea from a social justice perspective, it has some significant limitations in regard to its practicality. One point that they make is that in addition to duplicating other treaties and institutions that already cover areas that would be included, a strong legal response would have to set priorities of some areas of health over others. In terms of implementation, dispute resolution, or interpretation of the convention, powerful states would have inherent advantages over poor states and non-state actors in a legalized process. Such legal obligations might also pressure poor states to allocate resources to improve global health over their internal needs. They suggest that a more disaggregated form of governance, such as the current system, might be more effective to enabling flexibility through multiple channels of interaction and a variety of forums for negotiation. This flexibility, in contrast to a relatively rigid legalized system, would have the advantage of reducing the potential of negotiation impasses or political stalemates to block health reforms.

As these different views on a FCGH indicate, the nature of global governance and its preferred form are rooted in various perspectives of international politics. Theories of international relations can help provide greater context in understanding a complex concept, such as global governance, by interpreting and assessing its fundamental assumptions. Gostin's view is based on a liberal perspective, where international problems can be resolved through cooperation based on institutions and rules. Hoffman and Røttingen are more influenced by realism in their analysis, as they note how the differences in power among various actors in global health governance will contribute to the ineffectiveness of a legalized system.

The basic concept of global governance does present a challenge to traditional theories of international relations, particularly realism, due to their emphasis on international anarchy and interstate interactions as structuring forces of global politics. In fact, the idea of global governance emerged within the study of international relations as a reaction against the inadequacies of realism and liberal institutionalism in explaining the rise of non-state actors (Weiss 2000). The numerous actors involved in the process and the variety of interactions among them make global governance a complex phenomenon that Murphy (2000) has described as "poorly understood."

Because realism focuses on anarchy as a structuring principle of international politics, realists tend to be skeptical about the concept of global governance. Gilpin (2002), for instance, explains that while governance may be qualitatively different from government in terms of its type of authority, governance still requires power to function effectively. Despite the growth of globalization, the state still has a monopoly on power, and as a result, effective global governance will be dependent on the role and the interests of the most powerful states. Similarly, Krasner (2004) and Sterling-Folker (2005) suggest that a system of global governance will not be sustainable without powerful states willing to support it. Powerful states have developed the structure and context of global governance that have allowed non-state actors and transnational interactions to become growing features of the international landscape. Krasner (2004) argues that the process of globalization occurs due to the state's role in providing a legal and institutional framework for non-state actors to operate, in protecting its citizens from the negative impacts of the process, and in setting the rules of international transactions, which are determined by states, particularly the most powerful.

The realist view of the dependence of global governance on state power indicates that global governance will be structured on the basis of state interests, which realists believe to be national security. According to realists, cooperation and international order are most problematic in the area of security, where issues of sovereignty costs, distribution of power, and relative gains are most pronounced. Although health is certainly related to security in that poor health can contribute to the diminution of human and economic resources that could weaken the power and the security of the state, the realist perspective on security has been based upon the protection of sovereignty and territorial integrity of the state, largely from external threats. Traditionally, international health institutions, such as the WHO, have been regarded as welfare or humanitarian institutions rather than security related. As Youde (2016) notes, even with greater political attention paid to global health since 2000, it is unlikely to become on par with security as an area of "high politics." Consequently, health is seen by realists as an area of "low politics," meaning that it is more of an individual or group concern rather than one of national interest. Despite this tendency by realists to mitigate health as an international policy issue, a viable system of global health governance could still be compatible with realism. Relative gains concerns in this area are not major barriers to cooperation, and so forming a functional system of global governance may be possible. The realist expectation, however, would be that such a system of governance would be structured around the health-related preferences of the most powerful states and dependent on their support.

Much of the early neoliberal institutionalist analysis on global governance was based on the concept of regimes. Institutions and regimes are closely related. In fact, Goertz (2003) views institutions and regimes as being synonymous. He offers a minimal conception of institutions in stating that "an institution (or equivalently a regime) is a structure of norms and rules" (Goertz 2003: 15). The regime approach to cooperation went beyond "hard" international law with its emphasis on authoritative rules and enforcement mechanisms to also include the role of "softer" measures such as norms and customs as means to contribute to more structured cooperation. Krasner's (1982: 186) widely accepted definition of regimes refers to them as "sets of implicit or explicit principles, norms, rules, and decision-making procedures around which actors' expectations converge in a given issue area." Institutions play a key role in maintaining regimes after they have been created. Their role is to reinforce patterns of cooperation by helping resolve Prisoner's Dilemma problems by providing information and also facilitating linking of issues (Keohane 1984).

The relationship between international regimes and global governance is a close one. Young (1999) views regimes as a source of governance. As such, they perform different tasks: regulatory, procedural, programmatic, and generative. The first two tasks center around most neoliberal institutionalist views regarding regimes, specifically, the role of the regime in the management of collective action through mutually agreed-upon rules. The programmatic task differs in that it addresses the coordination of behavior-based shaping practice, rather than promoting rule-based behavior. The generative task fits more with a social constructivist view in that it addresses the role of the regime in facilitating learning among regime participants and the emergence of new norms as a result of interactions within the regime. The central task of a regime would depend on its particular character. In terms of regime analysis, Young (2001) distinguishes between collective action and social practice models for understanding the nature of regimes. Collective action models focus on the regulatory nature of regimes and the development of policies in regimes that induce compliance. Social practice models pay attention to the normative and social learning aspects of cooperation that can be promoted through regimes.

The literature on regimes has incorporated social practice and collective models in analyzing the effectiveness of regimes on state behavior. Chayes and Chayes (1995) view regimes as regulatory instruments. In their view, however, compliance with regimes is not based on coercive enforcement measures. Rather, states tend to comply with regimes due to the attraction of the efficiency and norms of the regimes, as well as a means to promote their self-interest. Regimes serve to manage compliance rather than enforcement. Mitchell (1994, 1998), however, emphasizes the regulative aspect of regimes and suggests that the design of the regime does matter. Regimes that can effectively promote transparency, by increasing incentives for reporting and enhancing monitoring, will be more successful in promoting compliance.

While regime theory could be considered a neoliberal interpretation of global governance, the concepts of regimes and governance do have some differences. The concept of regimes has been criticized due to its overemphasis on rational choice and the role of the state and formal institutions in managing cooperation, as well as its tendency to view the maintenance of order, rather than justice, as the function of the regime (Volger 2003). From this perspective, the global governance concept implies that international cooperation lacks formality and order, and that the authority of governance is diffused among a variety of multilevel actors.

A neoliberal institutional approach to global health governance would view the provision of health as a collective action problem, where good health would benefit all states. Accordingly, as a collective good, the expectation is that quality health on a global level would be undersupplied due to the anarchic structure of the international system and the egoism of the individual states. This problem of undersupply, however, may be mitigated by the creation of institutions and regimes that could help provide global health through their rules, norms, and decision-making procedures.

In the area of health, the key institution is the WHO. It serves as a forum for international negotiations on health policy and a resource for information on health, and it also plays a leadership role in health due the technical expertise of its personnel. The WHO has a close connection to states through six regional offices and over a hundred national offices. Over 190 states are members of the WHO, and they have accepted its constitution as a legal obligation, making it a foundational document for global health. Within the WHO, the World Health Assembly (WHA) is the supreme decision-making body. Delegates from member states participate in the WHA to determine the policies of the organization. Another important institution in global health governance is the World Bank. It has emerged as another significant actor in global health, especially in regard to its funding assistance programs.

Neoliberals would assume that the provision of good health will be based on effective cooperation among national governments. Institutions, including both international organizations and international law, can facilitate cooperation. The effectiveness of these institutions, however, will be based on a couple of factors: institutional design and the authority delegated to the institution. Those institutions lacking these features will be more limited in enabling states to reach mutually beneficial outcomes. For global health governance to be effective in improving the world's health, health-related institutions and international law need to be sufficiently viable to resolve cooperation, collaboration, and coordination problems among states.

Because constructivism is more about process rather than a unified theory, it is more limited in its predictive power-drawing hypotheses about global health governance compared to realism and neoliberal institutionalism. Hopf (1998), however, believes that constructivism does have the potential for prediction. In the area of international cooperation, he points out that rather than viewing cooperation as based on either narrow or enlightened self-interest, constructivists would assess the strength of cooperation to be based on whether social practices and norms have developed a mutually constituted identity among relative actors. Determining causation would be based on the nature and durability of the shared identity. A constructivist approach would suggest that the effectiveness of global governance in health would be dependent on the social structure in global health and how that it shapes identities, norms, and practices.

Using a constructive approach to global health governance, a couple of hypotheses can be derived. The first would concern the development of a constitutive norm. If such a norm associated with health were to strengthen over time, it would be expected that it would become a greater part of the identities and interests of states, as well contribute to growth in related institutions. The second hypotheses would involve a regulative norm. This norm would constrain states from acting in a particular manner rather than become part of their identity. Its process could be based on coercion through sanction or threat of sanction, a positive incentive for compliance, or it could be based on social pressure by way of its widely accepted legitimacy. A regulative health norm would be expected to influence the behavior and policy of states to be in alignment with that norm.

In regard to global health, however, McInnes and Lee (2012) point out that emerging norms face a challenge in that they may be in competition with other norms. They identify five competing frames in which global health may be constructed. These frames include (1) evidence-based medicine, which emphasizes health as a science; (2) human rights, which identifies health as a legal right for all people; (3) economism, which views health as a commodity subject to market forces; (4) security, which views health primarily as a public good that needs protection from outside threats; and (5) development, which considers global health issues to be more associated with developing countries that bear a great majority of the world's health problems. Social discourse and interaction would provide the process to decide which global health norms become a greater part of the identity of the actors in global health governance. The stronger norms will be more influential in the designing and implementation of global health policies.

From a neo-Marxist perspective on global governance, Murphy (1994) argues that international organizations play a key role in the spread of global capitalism. They assist in establishing infrastructures of communication, information, and expertise to promote acceptance of neoliberal ideology. Contemporary globalization, however, has also been associated with the rise of non-state actors. The global movement toward neoliberalism has contributed to a trend of IGOs contracting their traditional services to non-governmental organizations (NGOs) due to their efficiency, or perhaps because they can perform these tasks more inexpensively. Regardless of the reason, according to Murphy (2000: 795), NGOs are "playing a further essential role in international governance." In his view, institutions act to promote ideology. Even if an international class analysis would not fully capture the nature of global governance, Murphy (2000: 799) suggests that "it may be more accurate, or least less controversial to argue that contemporary global governance remains a predictable institutional response not to the interests of a fully formed class, but to the overall logic of industrial capitalism." Supranational governance will be desired as markets continue to go beyond the management of the state.

In applying such a perspective to health, Navarro (1976) argues that the health care system of a capitalist economy is based on the neoliberal ideology of the capitalist class. For example, in discussing the relatively poor health of Americans living in rural Appalachia, he argues that it is not due to a lack of material resources in the region but results from "the absence of power and control that people have over the resources they produce" (Navarro 1976: 73). Globally, the dominance of the neoliberal ideology in both developed and developing countries has led to growing inequalities in the quality of health both between and within states. The power of this ideology is such that even the WHO, an international institution that has an objective of achieving the highest level of health for all people, has become biased toward endorsing neoliberal solutions to health policy problems (Navarro 2002). In order to more adequately address inequalities in health, global health governance needs to overcome the power of the neoliberal ideology and support policies more favorable to distributing greater benefits to poor populations. In a study of developed countries from 1945 to 1980, Navarro and Shi (2001) found that countries largely influenced by political parties that favored redistributive economic and social policies, as well as full employment policies, witnessed greater improvements in population health.

The different expectations about global health governance of these four theories can be found in table 1.2. Taken together, the assumptions of these theories illustrate the obstacles and opportunities for effective policy-making in global health governance. In terms of obstacles, realists can point to the difficulties for successful cooperation on transnational issues due to anarchy, concern over the loss of state sovereignty, and the motivation of states to be competing for power. Marxists and neo-Marxist perspectives note how economic inequality, the embeddedness of capitalism in political institutions, and the power of profit-maximizing business elites constrain the provision of

Table 1.2. International Relations Theory and Expectations about Global Health Governance

Realism/Neorealism—Policies of global health governance will largely be dictated by the interests of the world's most powerful states. The governance system should be most responsive to global health interests when powerful states face a possibility of a health threat to their security. Health-related issues that primarily burden weaker states will get less attention and support.

Liberalism/Neoliberalism—All states can benefit from quality global health as a collective good. Global health governance can help provide better health by encouraging national governments to work together through rules, norms, and decision-making procedures. While international institutions may serve this purpose, the legal design of these institutions and the extent of authority delegated to them by national governments will influence their effectiveness.

Constructivism—The salience of global health as an international political issue is dependent on how the concept is framed and the strength of social norms regarding global health issues. The effectiveness of global health governance will be based on the strength and general acceptance of a particular norm. The more that a global health norm becomes accepted as part of a state's identity, the easier it will be for the implementation of global health policies.

Marxism/Neo-Marxism—Global health issues are subordinate to the profit-maximizing motives of the capitalist class. Social class division leads to health inequality between and within states with economically poorer population receiving a much greater proportion of ill health. Global health often becomes framed in terms of neoliberal ideology. As a result, health becomes a commodity whose provision is dictated by market forces. Global health governance acts to perpetuate this system.

quality health on a global scale. For opportunities, liberals offer the prospect of international organizations and agreements to facilitate cooperation and cultivate effective collective efforts to address the problems of global health. Constructvists can look to the framing of issues, norm diffusion, and socialization as a means to improve the policies of global health governance. The political obstacles to providing quality global health are certainly present. Whether the opportunities to overcome them are sufficient to resolve or even mitigate them will be examined throughout this book.

PLAN OF THE BOOK

This book will address three different themes regarding the relationship between global governance and health. This first theme will address the obstacles and opportunities that confront global health governance. In all of these chapters, the different theories of international relations will be used to offer different explanations for the politics of global health governance. Insights from these theories can inform us about the prospects for successful policy solutions to global health problems and what obstacles and opportunities must be addressed in effective decision-making and implementation.

The second theme is the growing role of IGOs and non-state actors to promote cooperation and assist independent states to improve public health. This theme will be specifically considered in chapter 2 on IGOs and chapter 3 on non-state actors that focus on the role of these actors in global health actors. The efforts of these actors will also be addressed in the five issue areas in chapters 4–8.

The third theme is the utility of international law and political agreements to resolve the problems in global health. This theme will be examined in chapters 4–8. Chapter 4 will address global efforts at controlling infectious or communicable diseases, with a focus on malaria, tuberculosis, and HIV/AIDS. Chapter 5 will examine global health security, in particular, the efforts of global health governance in protecting individuals from the spread of emerging infectious diseases and biological weapons. Chapter 6 will examine global cooperation in addressing chronic or non-communicable diseases, with a focus on significant risk factors linked to these diseases, tobacco, obesity, and alcohol. Chapter 7 will consider the issue of health as a human right. The strengths and weaknesses of global health governance in addressing this principle will be a focus. Chapter 8 will cover the relationship between global health and the environment. Much of the harm posed to human health is related to environmental factors. Because environmental protection supersedes state sovereignty, the measures taken by global governance will be critical in improving the quality environment and reducing its burden on global health.

DISCUSSION QUESTIONS

1. What are the United Nation's Sustainable Development Goals (SDGs)? How do these goals address global health? Are the health-related SDG goals likely to be met by 2030? What are potential obstacles and opportunities?
2. Compare classical realist and neorealist views on international politics. What do these approaches suggest about global health governance?
3. Explain why neoliberal institutionalists would assume that strong institutions would be important for effective global health governance? How does this view compare with that of realism?
4. How does constructivism differ from realism and liberalism? What are different frames in which global health may be socially constructed?
5. What are some assumptions of Marxist and neo-Marxist perspectives on politics, and how do these views relate to global health governance?

SUGGESTED READINGS

Cox, Robert W. 1987. *Production, Power, and World Order*. New York: Columbia University Press.

A seminal analysis of the modes of the social relations of production, the state, the international system, and their interrelationship.

Keohane, Robert O. 1984. *After Hegemony: Cooperation and Discord in the World Political Economy*. Princeton, NJ: Princeton University Press.

Demonstration of how rational choice leads to international cooperation.

McInnes, Colin, Adam Kamradt-Scott, Kelley Lee, Anne Roemer-Mahler, Simon Rushton, and Owain David Williams. 2014. *The Transformation of Global Health Governance*. New York: Palgrave Macmillan.

A detailed analysis of global health governance.

McInnes, Colin, and Kelley Lee. 2012. *Global Health and International Relations*. Cambridge, UK: Polity.

Illustrates a constructivist view on the connection between health and international relations.

Waltz, Kenneth. 1979. *Theory of International Politics*. Reading, MA: Addison-Wesley.

A seminal work on neorealism as a fundamental theory of international relations.

Wendt, Alexander. 1992. "Anarchy is what states make of it: The social construction of power politics." *International Organization* 46 (2): 391–425.

Provides a constructivist explanation of the international system.

Chapter 2

Intergovernmental Organizations and Global Health Governance

This chapter will analyze the role of the World Health Organization (WHO), World Bank, World Trade Organization (WTO), and the International Monetary Fund (IMF), which have emerged as important actors in global health. In addition to describing the structure and function of these intergovernmental organizations (IGOs), their influence on key aspects of global health will be explored. As noted in chapter 1, global health governance is not a new phenomenon. Its origins can be traced to the concerns of European powers about the transmission of infectious disease emanating from the Middle East and Asia during the nineteenth century. The standard practice of European states at this time was to conduct quarantines preventing infectious diseases from spreading. Quarantines prevented persons, animals, and goods believed to be infected from entering the territory of a state. Historically, these measures were taken unilaterally. That is, the decision to institute a quarantine was the sole discretion of an individual state. A state was under no obligation to coordinate its efforts with other states. As a result, quarantines could contribute to interstate friction as they created significant burdens on travel and commerce. Quarantines also tended to be ineffective, and the measures taken against individuals suspected of carrying a disease could be harsh and oppressive. Consequently, international cooperation appeared to be a more efficient strategy for protecting people from the spread of disease across national borders.

INTERNATIONAL SANITARY CONVENTIONS

The introduction of cholera into Europe during the first half of the nineteenth century provided the impetus to reevaluate the practice of unilateral quarantines. Cholera contributed to the deaths of thousands of individuals across

Europe during this time. Scientists knew very little about the disease and how it spread. France had sought to convene an international conference a few years after the cholera pandemic had begun in Europe during the 1830s. Political support for such a conference, however, was lacking until 1851 when thirteen states agreed to meet to discuss a multilateral solution to the problem. The expectation was that the first International Sanitary Conference would culminate in a treaty to effectively control cholera in Europe through a coordinated response.

Negotiations at the conference, however, revealed some significant conflict of interests. Britain, due to its position as the world's major trading power at this time, was opposed to an agreement to coordinate quarantine standards. The British believed that quarantines were harmful to Britain's commercial interests. Additionally, the ineffectiveness of quarantines in containing cholera made them very skeptical as to the utility of a coordinated response. To reinforce its position, the British delegation also argued that cholera was caused by natural conditions, and so improved water and soil quality, not quarantines, were the appropriate means to combat the disease. Other parties to the conference, especially states located around the Mediterranean had different beliefs. They were convinced that cholera was transferred by human contact. Quarantine procedures needed to be improved, but the quarantine was necessary to prevent human infections. A draft treaty was developed, but it did not receive a sufficient number of ratifications, which effectively rendered international cholera control to be moot (Howard-Jones 1975).

Despite the failed result of the first International Sanitary Conference, the event did mark the first time that states tried to formulate an international response to a health issue. Several states still wanted to pursue a treaty-based solution to the cholera pandemic as their unilateral quarantine measures continued to be ineffective. Additional conferences took place over the next four decades as Europe continued to experience cholera pandemics. Finally, in 1892, the first International Sanitary Convention was concluded. The only disease covered by the agreement, however, was cholera. A major factor in influencing this successful negotiation was a scientific breakthrough by German scientist Robert Koch whose work in bacteriology led to the discovery of the bacillus for anthrax in 1876, tuberculosis in 1882, and cholera in 1883. He discovered that the cholera pathogen was transferred by humans, mostly by the consumption of food and water that had been contaminated by infected fecal matter. Koch's finding took place years before the 1892 treaty. It was only until further studies supported his conclusion that states reached a consensus and were willing to commit to an international standard for controlling cholera.

Once the first International Sanitary Convention was established, others soon followed in 1893, 1894, and 1897. The most significant change during this time was the addition of the plague to join cholera as a contagious disease covered by an international agreement. The inclusion of the plague rather than other diseases was an example of how international standards for infectious disease control were shaped by the interests of European powers at the beginning of the twentieth century. The United States advocated the inclusion of yellow fever in the conventions. Because yellow fever was much more of a problem in the Western Hemisphere than in Europe, the conference delegates, who were mostly representing European countries, rejected this proposal (Howard-Jones 1975). In response, the United States and other states in the Americas elected to form the first IGO devoted to health, the International Sanitary Bureau, in 1902. This organization became the Pan-American Sanitary Bureau in 1923 to reflect its regional orientation.

The fifth International Sanitary Convention in 1903 was notable for a couple of achievements. First, it consolidated the four previous treaties into a single document. Second, member states agreed to follow the example of the Americas and establish an international health organization to supplement the convention. The Office International d'Hygiène Publique (OIHP) came into existence in 1907. After the devastation of World War I, the League of Nations was formed with the task of providing international peace and security and preventing another global conflict from reoccurring. Even though the League of Nations was primarily a security organization, its foundation was based on liberal principles of human welfare. As a result, health was part of its agenda. The League of Nations initially intended to take control over the OIHP and establish a new health organization as an affiliate (Howard-Jones 1978). This new organization would have a much more comprehensive program than the OIHP, which was primarily focused on data collection and information sharing. The United States objected to this plan because it was not a member of the League of Nations, and due to an overall lack of political support the OIHP remained an independent organization. The League decided to continue with its efforts and formed the Health Organization of the League of Nations (HOLN) in 1923.

More International Sanitary Conventions were concluded in 1912 and 1926. These agreements did not substantially change earlier commitments, but they served to expand the coverage of diseases to include yellow fever, smallpox, and typhus. As with all forms of international governance in the early twentieth century, however, global health required reconstruction following World War II. The League of Nations was disbanded and replaced by the United Nations (UN). HOLN also expired as an organization, and the OIHP was absorbed into a new institution, the WHO. This organization was designed to be a more powerful influence in global health than its predecessors. The previous international agreements on global health were placed under its purview.

POST–WORLD WAR II DEVELOPMENTS

In the post–World War era, the WHO was expected to be the lead actor in developing a global public policy for the management of health. Over time, the WHO has been joined by the World Bank, the WTO, and IMF as highly influential IGOs in global health. Of these organizations, only the WHO focuses exclusively on health. The WHO was formed as a UN specialized agency to facilitate international cooperation in health. It still continues to play a leading role in global health governance due to its connection to national health ministries, through their participation in the World Health Assembly (WHA), and the medical expertise of its staff members. The WHO's leadership role in global health started to be challenged in the 1980s as the World Bank moved to integrate health development into its lending policy. By 1990, the Bank's health loans began to exceed the regular budget of the WHO (Buse and Gwin 1998). While health is not covered in the IMF's mandate, its lending practices and policy guidance may influence health outcomes in some states. The WTO is more of a newcomer to global health governance. Its role demonstrates blurring of lines between health and other global policy areas. While the WTO is not a funding agency like the World Bank and IMF, it does oversee significant international trade agreements in goods and services.

The WHO, World Bank, WTO, and IMF are cornerstone organizations of global health governance. Although important, however, their relative influence in health policy vis-à-vis other actors, is debatable. Key questions regarding these IGOs include the following: What is the extent of their influence in global health? Are some of these organizations more influential organizations than others? Are these organizations, in fact, autonomous actors? The different perspectives of international relations outlined in chapter 1, as well as theories focusing on organizational dynamics, can provide some guidance in answering these questions.

THE WORLD HEALTH ORGANIZATION

Despite the consistent attention that international politics had paid to global health during the previous century, it was not an issue on the agenda at the San Francisco conference in 1945 to complete negotiations for the UN charter. Brazil and China objected to this omission, as they argued that good health was an important part of international peace. Delegates from these states submitted a declaration calling for a new international health organization to be associated with the UN and effectively replacing the roles served by OIHP and HOLN. After unanimous acceptance of this declaration, several states began preparations to offer their support for the new organization. In the following year, the UN's Economic and Social Council (ECOSOC) passed a resolution calling for a special committee of health experts to develop proposals for the organization and to submit these proposals to an international health conference to be conducted in New York in June 1946 (Shimkin 1946).

The International Health Conference of 1946 was the first conference of the UN. While member states strongly supported the principle of an international health organization, some areas of contention were manifested at the conference. One area had primarily to do with significant philosophical differences between the United States and the Soviet Union. The United States desired the new health organization to follow a similar role of its predecessors and focus its attention on surveillance and control of infectious diseases. The Soviet Union, in contrast, wanted to broaden this organization's mandate to include the social determinants of health as part of its mission. The Soviet position was based upon the belief that good health was not only a result of biomedical science, but it was also rooted in the social consequences of poverty and economic inequality (Lee 2009). The United States was not supportive of this view. It found a social medical approach to effectively operate as a criticism of capitalism. The fact that it was advocated by its geopolitical rival increased the intransigence of the U.S. position. Additionally, the United States wanted to maintain the existence and independence of the Pan American Health Organization (PAHO). The United States found that the health interests of the Americas, mainly yellow fever, were mostly discounted by the Eurocentric International Sanitary Conferences. It did have concerns that the new organization may not be sufficiently sensitive to regional needs. The United States also had substantial influence in PAHO. If it were to be absorbed into the new international health organization, the United States would lose some of its power over regional health issues.

Notwithstanding this political conflict, the strong international consensus to create a new organization devoted to health and a severe cholera outbreak in Egypt spurred momentum for the draft constitution for the WHO to be ratified by sufficient number of states to go into effect in April 1948. Although the WHO was successfully launched, the issues surrounding its birth continued to plague the organization for decades. It consistently was caught in the middle of Cold War politics, which contributed to its relative passivity as an international actor until the 1990s. As a compromise, the PAHO continued to exist as one of the WHO's regional offices with some autonomy. The independence of these regional offices, however, has also posed a problem for the WHO in policy implementation. Over time, a de facto two-tiered system has been developed for the WHO as the regional states, rather than the WHO, decided the staffing of these offices. Godlee (1998: 296), for example, has criticized the training and resources of these offices, and has referred to them as "one of the weakest links in the WHO's chain of influence."

The WHO Constitution revealed the elements of both social and biomedical approaches to global health. The preamble defines health as "a state of complete physical, mental and social well-being and not merely the absence of disease or infirmity" (Constitution of the World Health Organization 1946). It also equates health with human rights with another provision in the preamble: "The enjoyment of the highest attainable standard of health is one of the fundamental rights of every human being without distinction of race, religion, political belief, economic or social condition" (Constitution of the World Health Organization 1946). While the preamble was not intended to be legally binding per se, it sets out the specific objectives of the organization. In fact, Orgad (2010) has found that increasingly national courts have found the language of constitutional preambles to create legal rights that are not explicitly stated in other sections of the constitution. Under this interpretation, the WHO Constitution would be a legal source of health as a human right. This provision alone goes far beyond the previous international health regime centered on the biomedical purposes of OIHP, HOLN, and the International Sanitary Conventions.

The WHO Constitution specifies that the goal of the organization is "the attainment of by all peoples of the highest possible level of health" (Constitution of the World Health Organization 1946). To accomplish this objective, the WHO has been given twenty-two functions. These functions center around the WHO's role to promote cooperation in health among various actors, enhance the availability and dissemination of information on health, and accomplish administrative and technical tasks to promote global health. The Constitution also establishes the membership requirements, the structure, budget, decision-making and dispute settlement procedures of the organization.

Structure of the World Health Organization

The structure of the WHO has not changed since the Constitution went into effect in 1948. Article 9 provides the establishment of three different organs for the WHO: the WHA, the Executive Board, and the Secretariat. The WHA is the primary decision-making body. All member states of the WHO have at least one delegate in the WHA. These delegates must be among the highest qualified medical professionals in their state. The WHA typically meets every year in May at the WHO's headquarters in Geneva, Switzerland. It may also have additional meetings for special sessions. The main function of the WHA is to decide the general policies for the WHO. Its additional duties include the appointment of the WHO's Director-General, manage the organization's budget, and consider recommendations on health from other organizations such as the UN General Assembly. The most potential legal power for the WHA (as well as the WHO as a whole) is found in Article 19 of the Constitution. Under this article, the WHA has the power to "adopt conventions or agreements with respect to any matter within the competence of the Organization" (Constitution of the World Health Organization 1946). This provision is the WHO's treaty-making power. It was not used by the WHA until 2003 with the Framework Convention on Tobacco Control (FCTC). Prior to this point, the WHA had not seriously considered the adoption of an international treaty for a health issue. Because the WHO has now adopted such a treaty under Article 19, it was speculated that the organization be more inclined to support additional treaties in the future. Over a decade after the FCTC, however, no other treaties have been adopted by the WHO despite calls for similar responses to obesity and alcohol. At this point in time, it appears that tobacco may have been an exceptional case, and the WHA may just be very reluctant to invoke its authority under Article 19.

The WHA was also given the authority under Article 21 to adopt regulations regarding quarantine and sanitary measures; nomenclatures for diseases and causes of death; and standards regarding safety, advertising, and labeling for biological and pharmaceutical products used in international trade. Article 22 served to increase the significance of this provision by stating that the regulations adopted by the WHA would be binding for all member states. The most significant aspect of this provision concerned the International Sanitary Conventions. In 1951, the WHA adopted the International Sanitary Regulations (ISR) to replace the earlier conventions. These conventions and the entire regime for infectious disease control had been deemed unsuccessful. According to Fidler (2005: 332), "formulating rules by ad hoc treaty negotiations proved cumbersome, slow and resistant to amendments needed to account for changes in scientific knowledge and the speed, scope, volume and patterns of international trade." Even though the ISR was to serve as a replacement for the International Sanitary Conventions, its rules were not substantially different. Only cholera, plague, yellow fever, smallpox, typhus, and relapsing fever were covered by the ISR. The most significant change was the inclusion of the WHO as the manager of the regulations. States were now obligated to notify and report information regarding the covered diseases to the WHO rather than each other. The WHO would then coordinate the global dissemination of disease-related information to national governments.

In addition to its regulatory power provided in Articles 21 and 22 of the WHO Constitution, the WHA was also given authority to make recommendations to member states on any issues related to health. All WHO member states have one vote in the WHA. Decisions made by the WHA are determined by a majority vote unless the WHA considers the decision to be an important question, in which case, a two-thirds vote would be required. The decisions made by the WHA are non-binding, unless they are regulations covered by

Article 21. Even in this case, member states do have the opportunity to reject or make reservations to these regulations, if they notify the Director-General within a time period established by the WHA.

While the WHA serves as the organization's decision-maker, the responsibility for implementing these decisions lies with the Executive Board. This organ is a much smaller body than the WHA with only thirty-four members. These individuals are elected by the WHA, which must take into account an equitable geographic distribution in its selections. Members of the Executive Board should also be experts in health. The Executive Board is required to meet two times a year. These meetings usually take place in January and May. Article 28 of the Constitution provides nine functions for the Board. Most significant is its function to serve as the executive body of the WHO. It also has the authority to provide advice or proposals to the WHA. In addition to its designated functions, the WHA may also decide to delegate other functions to the Board.

The Secretariat serves as the bureaucracy of the WHO. It is composed of a Director-General and technical and administrative staff members. The Director-General is the head of the WHO, even though the WHA is the chief decision-maker. This individual is nominated by the Executive Board and then appointed by the WHA. The duties of Director-General specified in the Constitution include preparation of reports on the organization's financial status and appointment of the WHO's staff. A key aspect of this office, as well as the entire Secretariat, is neutrality. Unlike the WHA, members of the Secretariat owe their allegiance to the organization, not their home state. They may not receive instructions from any national governments in the course of their duties. Although the Constitution establishes the Director-General as a lead bureaucrat, the informal power of this position has made it much more powerful in practice. This informal power emanates from the neutrality and prestige of the office. The Director-General can be very persuasive in influencing Executive Board and WHA policies. These bodies have often supported his or her initiatives even though they have no legal obligation to do so. A list of the WHO's Directors-General can be found in table 2.1.

World Health Organization's Programs and Politics

The early years of the WHO were focused on technical issues (Davies 2010). In particular, the WHO emphasized a biomedical approach, concentrating on vertical health programs, which were programs aimed to control specific diseases. The WHO took this approach even though its first Directors-General, Brock Chisholm of Canada, was more inclined toward social medicine. As was the case with negotiations for the WHO Constitution, the driving force

Table 2.1. World Health Organization Directors-General

Director General	*Nationality*	*Term of Office*
Brock Chisholm	Canada	1948–1953
Marcolino Gomes Candau	Brazil	1953–1973
Halfdan Mahler	Denmark	1973–1988
Hiroshi Nakajima	Japan	1988–1998
Gro Harlem Brundtland	Norway	1998–2003
Lee Jong-wook	South Korea	2003–2006
Anders Nordström	Sweden	2006–2007
Margaret Chan	China	2007–2017
Tedros Adhanom Ghebreyesus	Ethiopia	2017–present

behind biomedicine was the United States. When the Soviet Union elected to boycott the UN due to that organization's refusal to recognize the People's Republic of China as a sovereign state, it effectively diminished its role in the entire UN system, including the WHO. The United States took advantage of this situation to push its agenda in the WHO (Brown, Cueto, and Free 2006).

The first major vertical health program supported by the WHO was directed at the eradication of malaria in 1955. This program was a very popular one for the WHO for a couple of reasons. First, the successful use of dichloro-diphenyl-trichloroethane (DDT) to combat the disease during World War II created a great sense of optimism that the malaria problem could be effectively "solved" by an extensive DDT campaign on a global scale. A favorable outcome of this campaign would go far in increasing the credibility and prestige of the young organization in world politics. Second, the United States had a compelling national interest in the program. If it was successful, the United States could benefit from the opening of more foreign markets to American goods, and the United States could also use a victory over malaria as a tool in its fight against the spread of communist ideology (Packard 1997).

The malaria eradication program, for the most part, proved to be unsuccessful. The WHO decided to end the program in 1969 as mosquitoes began to develop resistance to DDT, and the program was proving to be too costly based upon its results. Developed countries were able to successfully eradicate the disease during the campaign, but developing countries, with the exception of Caribbean islands, did not achieve much of a benefit. Packard (2007) has argued that the campaign largely failed because it was focused too much on biomedical science and ignored important social and economic practices of the countries where DDT was employed, such as agricultural activity, deforestation, and the quality of its health infrastructure.

As the Soviet Union returned to the UN system, its interest in the WHO was to advocate for an eradication campaign against smallpox. The United States decided to offer its support in 1965 as the malaria program was in decline (Brown, Cueto, and Free 2006). With such a strong consensus, the WHO launched a smallpox eradication program in 1967. This venture proved to be much more successful than the malaria eradication program. By focusing on vaccinations and surveillance of the disease, a sustained effort led to the eradication of smallpox by 1977. The success of the smallpox eradication program enhanced the political profile of the WHO, especially in light of the failure of malaria program in the 1960s. It also increased confidence in the effectiveness of vertical programs for disease control.

The landscape of international politics underwent some significant changes in the 1970s, which in turn affected the WHO. The Soviet Union and the United States began to improve their relationship, and the United States began to open itself to diplomatic relations with the People's Republic of China. Even more significant for the UN system was the emergence of former European colonies as independent states. As more of these new states joined the UN and the WHO in the 1960s and 1970s, they brought a political agenda supporting economic development. The increasing numbers and corresponding voting power of these states posed a challenge to the United States and its support of an open global economy and biomedical and technological solutions to global health problems. Doubts about vertical health programs remained despite the highly successful outcome of the smallpox eradication program. Smallpox was seen as an unusual case because of the availability of a vaccine and limited training requirements for workers in the field to carry out the campaign (Greene et al. 2013). Most diseases, particularly in developing countries, were not as amenable to such a tactic. The most significant problem was that even though smallpox was eradicated, the health infrastructure of many of the newly independent states remained weak and underdeveloped.

The change in global governance that developing states desired manifested itself in the UN. Because the UN General Assembly also had a decision-making system like the WHA, developing countries in Africa, Asia, and Latin America were able to assemble a strong coalition with majority voting power. In 1974, the coalition exercised its power in UN General Assembly to persuade that body to adopt a resolution for a New International Economic Order (NIEO). The primary objective of the NIEO was economic development. To achieve this goal, these states wanted to be able to regulate the activities of multinational corporations, control over their natural resources, economic assistance and debt relief from developed states, more favorable treatment in international trade, and greater access to science and technology from developed states. The WHO's Director-General at this time, Halfdan Mahler of

Denmark, was supportive of NIEO's principles. He was also wary, however, that developed states did not agree with this agenda, and so he attempted to be careful about incorporating NIEO's principles into the WHO (Chorev 2012). Mahler decided to choose a new direction for the WHO based on a plan called "Health for All by the Year 2000." The WHA passed resolution WHA30.43 in 1977, which defined this objective as "the main social target of governments and the WHO in the coming two decades should be the attainment by all citizens of the world by the year 2000 of a level of health that will permit them to lead a socially and economically productive life." The adoption of the Health for All strategy signaled an end to the vertical health programs that dominated the WHO's agenda during the 1950s and 1960s. Mahler viewed it as moving the WHO closer to the NIEO's principles while also providing greater adherence to the WHO Constitution's goal of the highest possible level of health (Chorev 2012).

The next step was for an international health conference to be held in the Soviet Union at Alma-Ata in the Republic of Kazakhstan in 1978 to discuss a global strategy to achieve the health for all objective. The conference produced the Alma-Ata Declaration, which endorsed primary health care as the means to provide global health. The declaration also included a very broad definition of what would constitute primary health. According to Cueto (2004: 1867), the declaration promoting the primary health care approach was based on three themes: "appropriate technology, opposition to medical elitism, and the concept of health as a tool for socioeconomic development." Appropriate technology referred to the importance of using technology that could be effectively employed to poor and rural areas of developing countries. The opposition to medical elitism meant that a much greater need was present in developing countries for general health practitioners instead of specialized personnel. Working with local communities to address health needs rather than top-down directives from the WHO was part of the primary health care plan. Health as a tool for development stressed the connection between these two concepts.

The WHA adopted the Alma-Ata Declaration in 1979, but many concerns quickly developed as to whether it was a feasible strategy. Walsh and Walsh (1979) published an influential paper advocating the concept of selective primary health care to serve as an interim strategy to lead up to the standards of the Alma-Ata declaration. This approach emphasized growth monitoring of infants, oral rehydration, breastfeeding, and immunization, especially for young children (also known as the GOBI interventions). Selective primary health care was very attractive to health donors and agencies because it was much less expensive than the primary health care strategy, and its goals were much easier to measure and evaluate (Cueto 2004). The United Nations Children's Fund (UNICEF) endorsed selective primary health care much more strongly than the WHO due to the plan's emphasis on children. As selective primary care gained more and more acceptance, UNICEF's profile as an actor in global health began to increase at the expense of the WHO, especially after the World Bank also endorsed the approach (Basilico et al. 2013). As debates between the merits of primary health care versus those of selective primary health care continued, the relationship between the WHO and UNICEF became increasingly strained during the early 1980s (Cueto 2004).

As with the NIEO movement, the WHO became caught in another shift in global politics during the 1980s. The elections of Margaret Thatcher in 1979 and Ronald Reagan in 1980 as leaders of the United Kingdom and the United States, respectively, were a first step in a major transformation of the global economy. Both Thatcher and Reagan were strong proponents of neoliberal economic policy, which emphasized a limited role of the state in favor of the market. Not only did the United Kingdom and the United States adopt these economic policies, but also they used their power in global economic institutions such as the World Bank and the IMF to encourage other states to open their economies to free trade, investment, and privatization. The philosophy behind neoliberalism was that the market was much more efficient at allocating goods and services and in turn, better equipped than the state to meet health needs. This position served as a direct challenge to the NIEO and the primary health care movements as neoliberalism began to frame health as a commodity rather than a human right (Basilico et al. 2013).

Neoliberalism began to influence developing states with the foreign debt crisis of 1982. These states had adopted protectionist trade policies in the 1960s and 1970s to reduce their economic dependence on developed countries. This policy did promote industrialization in developing states, but these states also struggled with economic growth. Developed states were more reluctant to buy their exports, because of the trade barriers imposed by the developing economies. To maintain their protectionist trade policies, developing states sought loans from foreign lenders to make up their lack of growth from international trade. Due to rising interest rates during the 1970s, their debt began to increase. In 1982, Mexico announced it was unable to service its foreign debt. Soon after, several developing states, mostly in Latin America, also had great difficulty in paying their debt. The United States was willing to assist states such as Mexico in restoring their financial solvency but on the condition that these states made significant reforms to their economic policy. Specifically, the adoption of neoliberal economic policies in return for World Bank and IMF loans. Due to their precarious financial situations, developing states opened their economies to developed countries and multinational corporations, which began to effectively undermine the NIEO movement.

The shift toward neoliberalism adversely affected the WHO in the 1980s and early 1990s. Chorev (2012) notes that the WHO experienced financial, authority, and leadership crises during this period of time. States began to increasingly withhold their funding contributions to the WHO, which put a significant strain on its budget. The WHO, however, was able to receive some compensation for the shortfall by means of extrabudgetary funds (EBFs). These funds are voluntary contributions by member states that are not part of the monies they are obligated to pay the WHO. Beginning in the 1980s, the WHO's total budget increasingly was composed of EBFs. In 1975, EBFS constituted 29 percent of the WHO's budget. By 1985 EBFs became 50 percent of the budget, and in 2007 they rose to 72 percent (Lee 2009: 40). Most of the EBFs were contributed by developed states. As the WHO became more dependent on EBFs, developed states began to gain more influence in the organization, even though developing states had more voting power in the WHA (Chorev 2012). The WHO's role as the leader in global health governance was also challenged during this time. The World Bank began to develop an interest in health, and its embrace of neoliberal principles, along with its capacity to provide funds gave it a distinct advantage over the WHO in shaping global health policy. A loss of confidence in the WHO was most pronounced with the removal of HIV/AIDS eradication programs from the WHO, and putting it under the authority of a new organization, the Joint United Nations Programme on HIV/AIDS (UNAIDS) (Chorev 2012). Leadership in the WHO, itself, also became a problem. After Halfdan Mahler left the position of Director-General in 1988, Hiroshi Nakajima of Japan was chosen as his successor. His selection was unpopular with developed states, and his leadership of the organization became further eroded by his poor relationship with the WHO staff (Chorev 2012).

The WHO sought change in the late 1990s with the election of Gro Harlem Brundtland of Norway in 1998. As neoliberalism became even a stronger norm after the Cold War, Brundtland decided that the WHO needed to become more supportive of this philosophy and adopt an approach to health based more on economism. For instance, Brundtland established the Commission on Macroeconomics and Health (CMH) to research and advise national governments on health and its relationship to national economic policies. This approach made the WHO much more popular with developed states along with the World Bank. The WHO began to follow the Bank's lead and view health more in economic terms such as the *cost-effectiveness* of particular health interventions and frame the improvement of health as linked more to economic development and productivity rather than as a human right. Brundtland even went further to pursue partnerships for the WHO with other organizations. For example, the WHO's Roll Back Malaria campaign was performed in partnership with the World Bank, UNICEF, and the United

Nations Development Programme. Additionally, Brundtland brought legal innovation to the WHO as, under her tenure, the FCTC became the first international treaty adopted by the WHO.

Lee Jong-wook replaced Brundtland as Director-General in 2003. Although he served in this position only for a couple of years until his death in 2006, the WHO began some important initiatives during that time. He is mostly associated with the WHO's 3 by 5 initiative to work in cooperative arrangement with other actors in global health, such as UNAIDS, to provide antiretroviral treatment to 3 million people infected with HIV/AIDS by 2005. Although the initiative failed to reach its goal, the number of people in developing states receiving this treatment increased from 400,000 in December 2003 to 1 million by June 2005 (World Health Organization 2005).

Another significant development during this time was the revision of the International Health Regulations (IHR). The International Sanitary Regulations that the WHO adopted in 1951 remained largely unchanged until 1969 when they were renamed as the IHR. The obligations and coverage under the IHR, however, were mostly the same as the 1951 regulations. The IHR added provisions for cholera in 1973 and removed smallpox from the regulations after it had been deemed as successfully eradicated in 1981. Both the ISR and IHR were considered to be failures as policy instruments (Fidler 2005). Not only was compliance with these regulations a problem, but they were primarily based on a nineteenth-century perspective of global health. The movement to revise the IHR really gained momentum due to the evolution of new infectious diseases such as HIV/AIDS, as well as an outbreak of the plague in India in 1994, which led to states placing restrictions on that country that did not adhere to the IHR. The WHA passed a resolution in 1995 requesting that Director-General Nakajima begin to prepare the process for a revision of the IHR. It took three years for a provisional draft to be submitted to the WHA, and it was not until 2005 when revised IHR were approved. The WHO had strongly supported a revision, but the process took a long time due to working out various technical and political difficulties. The event that spurred the passage of IHR 2005 was the severe acute respiratory syndrome (SARS) pandemic of 2003. The sudden global impact of a new disease was convincing enough to generate sufficient political will in the WHA to adopt the agreement.

IHR 2005 was significantly different from IHR 1969. Instead of specifically naming the diseases to be covered under the agreement, IHR 2005 was much more flexible. Diseases that were to be reported by national governments to the WHO were "all events which may constitute a public health emergency of international concern within its territory" (World Health Organization 2016a: 12). The qualification standard for a public health emergency of international concern (PHEIC) was determined by an algorithm included as part of the IHR. It required that outbreaks of certain diseases (smallpox, poliomyelitis, new subtypes of human influenza, and SARS) must be reported to the WHO. Another category of diseases (cholera, pneumonic plague, yellow fever, West Nile fever, and viral hemorrhagic fevers) would be applied to the algorithm, if these outbreaks were "serious," "unusual," or posed "significant risks" to international commerce or travel. The IHR 2005 also left open the possibility of other diseases that may be subject to the algorithm in the future. Additionally, the revised IHR placed greater obligations on states to provide effective surveillance and response for infectious diseases. The WHO was also given more authority to control infectious diseases than it had under IHR 1969. It was allowed to use non-governmental sources of information in monitoring diseases and could share this information with other states without the need of any government's consent. The WHO's Director-General was also given the authority to determine whether a disease qualified as a PHEIC. According to Fidler and Gostin's (2006: 90) analysis, the IHR 2005's "information and verification provisions privilege global governance over state sovereignty."

With Lee Jong-wook's unfortunate death, the WHO's leadership took somewhat of a turn with the election of Margaret Chan of China as the Director-General in 2006. The selection of Chan indicated a move away from neoliberalism and more toward the primary health care movement of the 1970s (Chorev 2012). The 2008 WHO World Health report was entitled *Primary Health Care: Now More than Ever*. It called for a return to the principles of Alma-Ata, and placed an emphasis on health inequalities. Chan was also a strong supporter of the social determinants of health approach rather than biomedicine to promote global health (Davies 2010). Although this approach differs from the emphasis on neoliberalism that WHO supported in the 1990s and early 2000s, it did fit with a growing discontentment globally with neoliberalism in the wake of the global financial crisis of 2008. Chan's reelection to a second term as WHO's Director-General in 2012 indicated international approval of the direction she had taken with the organization.

Much of the WHO's credibility as an effective IGO was, however, compromised by the widespread criticism of its slow response to the Ebola outbreak of 2014. Kamradt-Scott (2016) suggested that three different factors contributed to the WHO's inadequate response. The first factor was a lack of staff. Due to funding cuts, the WHO significantly reduced the number of its staff members in the Secretariat in the year prior to the outbreak. These cuts included a 51 percent reduction in the WHO's "outbreak and crisis response" budget for 2014–2015 (Kamradt-Scott 2016: 408). Another factor had to do with the WHO's bureaucratic culture. The organization was unwilling to challenge country reports from the affected West African countries that understated the impact of the disease. Its concern that it might have been criticized as acting too aggressively by its member states contributed to a relatively passive response in the early stages of the outbreak. A third factor was the link between the WHO Secretariat in Geneva and its regional office in Africa. The WHO had expected its regional offices to carry more of the burden due to its budget cuts. Poor communication and coordination between the two offices constrained the WHO's capacity to respond.

In May 2017, the WHA elected Tedros Adhanom Ghebreyesus, former minister of Health and minister of Foreign Affairs of Ethiopia, to succeed Chan. He is the WHO's first Director-General from Africa. Among his priorities, Ghebreyesus has mentioned promoting universal health coverage, access to medicines, health security, and the health effects of climate change. He also has indicated a sense of urgency in improving the WHO's capacity to respond more rapidly to global health emergencies in light of the Ebola crisis (Horton and Samarasekera 2016).

Using a constructivist analysis, McInnes (2015) argues that in the context of global governance, the WHO had been identified as an organization with expert and delegated authority and not one with capacity-based authority. The WHO accepted this identification and its image as an organization that was based on technical support and expert advice, rather than one that is operationally engaged in a crisis situation. In this sense, the role created for the WHO in global governance was not suitable to respond quickly and decisively to a major international health crisis. In order to respond more effectively to such crises in the future, the WHO must shift its identification from an expert and delegated model to a capacity model. Whether the WHO moves in this direction, however, depends on if the WHO and other actors accept such an identification for the WHO in a post-Ebola world.

THE WORLD BANK

The World Bank, although not a health organization, has become quite possibly the most powerful actor in global health governance. The World Bank is a group of five different institutions. The first institution of the World Bank, the International Bank for Reconstruction and Development (IBRD) was founded, along with the IMF at the Bretton Woods conference in 1944. The IBRD remained as the only institution of the World Bank until the International Finance Corporation (IFC) was established in 1956. The failure of the reconstruction of global governance after World War I contributed to a global economic depression in the 1930s, which was followed by an even more catastrophic world war in the 1940s. In order to provide for future stability in the global economy once World War II concluded, the United Kingdom and the United States recognized the importance of international institutions to promote economic cooperation among states. Although over forty states participated at the Bretton Woods conference, the United Kingdom and the United States dominated the negotiations (Eichengreen and Kenen 1994). An international monetary policy was viewed by both to be a critical area to develop and maintain a robust global economy. The IMF was established to fulfill this purpose.

The American and British negotiators had a much easier time in agreeing on monetary policy compared to trade. Negotiations for an IGO for trade were unsuccessful. The parties did accept a framework on trade, the General Agreement on Tariffs and Trade (GATT), which was expected to serve as a placeholder source of international trade rules until an agreement for an international trade organization could be reached. The World Bank proposal was not nearly as a significant issue at Bretton Woods as monetary and trade relations (Eichengreen and Kenen 1994). It was designed to assist in financing post-war reconstruction and economic development.

Structure of the World Bank

The organizational structure of the World Bank is quite different from that of the WHO. Instead of a "one country, one vote system" of decision-making, the World Bank uses a weighted voting system, where voting is based on the financial contribution that each state makes to the World Bank. These financial contributions are based on the economic strength of each state, so developed states provide more capital than developing countries, but they also have much more voting power in the organization. The World Bank's Board of Governors is its primary decision-making body, but it only meets annually. Much of the responsibility for managing the policies of the organizations is in the hands of the Bank's Executive Board of twenty-five members. The five largest shareholders in the World Bank each select one executive director, while the others are elected by the Bank's membership. Both the Board of Governors and the Executive Board use the weighted voting systems, effectively giving states such as the United States in particular power as the Bank's largest shareholder, but also the United Kingdom, France, Germany, China, and Japan substantial decision-making power in setting the Bank's policies. Even though national governments provide funds to the Bank, most of the funds of the IBRD come from financial markets (Cohn 2016). This feature does grant World Bank officials more autonomy than their WHO counterparts. This autonomy is particularly apparent in regard to developing countries due to the organization's voting system.

World Bank's Programs and Policies

After the success of the financial aid to Europe through the Marshall Plan, the Bank turned its attention to development in the 1950s. Its first loan for development went to Chile in 1949 for power plant equipment and agricultural machinery (Asher and Mason 1973). Soon after, it made a series of loans for power projects in Mexico, Brazil, El Salvador, and Colombia. This pattern of lending was very typical for the World Bank in its first decade. Over 95 percent of its loans to developing states between 1948 and 1961 were for power, transportation, industry, and telecommunications (Ruger 2005). Loans for infrastructure were very attractive to the World Bank because their connection to economic development was clear, and the direct results from the loan were tangible and measurable. As a result, loans for sanitation, health, and education were not in the Bank's interests because they lacked these qualities (Asher and Mason 1973).

The World Bank's approach to lending was reevaluated with the selection of Robert McNamara, the former secretary of Defense for the United States, as its president in 1968. McNamara wanted to move away from the Bank's traditional focus on financial investments on infrastructure to attacking the problem of poverty. It took time but the Bank's gradual change toward poverty reduction programs served as an admission that the poor were not benefiting from its financing policies (Kapur, Lewis, and Webb 1997). McNamara's first plan was addressed at population control, which was soon followed by the Bank's first loan for family planning to Jamaica in 1970. Malnutrition was also an important item for McNamara's policy reduction program. Health became addressed by the World Bank for the first time with the creation of the Onchocerciasis Control Program to eradicate the disease of river blindness in eleven West African states. The success of this program contributed to enhanced support for health-related projects by the Bank. In 1979, the Bank created a department for health, nutrition, and population control, and in 1980 in the Bank's world development report, malnutrition and poor health were established as leading causes of global poverty and major constraints on economic growth in developing states (Ruger 2005).

Although the World Bank had begun lending for health, it also modified its general lending policies during the 1980s. The Bank began adoption of structural adjustment programs (SAPs). These programs were based on conditional lending by the Bank. In order to receive loans from the Bank, the receipt state would agree to reform their economic policies along the lines of neoliberalism. More specifically, the Bank would typically require national governments to open their economy to foreign trade and investment, encourage privatization, limit government intervention in the economy, reduce government spending, and shrink public debt. SAPs emerged as a result of the neoliberal turn in international politics in the early 1980s. The World Bank's incorporation of SAPs was influenced by a report written by Elliott Berg in 1981, which claimed that extensive government intervention in the economies of Sub-Saharan Africa was responsible for the lack of economic growth in that region (Basilico et al. 2013). This approach oriented the Bank's policy toward health to be based on privatization. In 1987, the Bank published a report titled *Financing Health Services in Developing Countries: An Agenda for Reform.* This report advocated a policy of user fees to improve health in these states. A charge for health services would serve to provide a financial boost to health services as well as reduce the burden on the health care system by encouraging patients to seek less expensive treatment options (Akin, Birdsall, and Ferranti 1987). The user fees issue along with Bank's support for the reduction of government spending, including in the health care sector, stood in stark contrast to the WHO and its "health for all" principles. Nevertheless, the Bank armed its funding power and support from developed states and began its ascendancy in global health governance during this decade. At the beginning of the 1990s, the lending that the Bank had provided for global health was greater than the entire budget of the WHO (Brown, Cueto, and Free 2006).

The World Bank began to surpass the WHO as the most influential actor in global health with its publication of *World Development Report 1993: Investing in Health* (Abbasi 1999). This report supported two significant changes to the global health: a more equitable distribution of health resources and an emphasis on cost-effectiveness as a guiding principle for health care management (Basilico et al. 2013). To measure cost-effectiveness, the *World Development Report 1993* (World Bank 1993) developed the unit of disability-adjusted life year (DALY). DALY provided an assessment of the number of years that the economic productivity of an individual could be lost from a disability caused by a disease. Using this measure, the report found that services such as breastfeeding, immunizations, and reduction of smoking were cost-effective health interventions, while treatment for chronic diseases and cancer were not (Chorev 2012). This highly influential report served to assert economism as a means to assess health care policies and programs.

The 1990s also witnessed the World Bank's reassessment of neoliberalism as its guiding principle in SAPs. These programs were criticized by UNICEF for negatively affecting health and education in developing states. The World Bank examined this issue in sub-Saharan Africa and produced a report finding that SAPs were not as effective among states in this region as the Bank had anticipated. The problem, according to the report, was not SAPs per se but the weak governmental institutions in these states (Demmers, Fernandez Jilberto, and Hogenboom 2004). In response, the report suggested that good governance was the appropriate remedy for economic development. These states required more efficient governments with little corruption that were staffed with capable bureaucrats.

Once these institutions were established, then SAPs would be a much more productive response to economic development. The World Bank elected to adopt good governance as its primary strategy with the selection of James Wolfensohn as its president in 1995. Wolfensohn supported a focus on good governance to help deflect some of the criticisms of the Bank's lending policies (Harman 2010). With the good governance approach, the Bank would reward states who, in the Bank's judgment, instituted "good" economic, social, and political policies rather than just reward states that adopted neoliberal economic reforms (Harrison 2004). Good governance served as a compromise between neoliberals, who wanted states to become more capitalistic, and developing states, who wanted a more enhanced role for the state.

One key health program that emerged from the Bank's good governance approach was the Multicountry HIV/AIDS program (MAP) in 2000. Initially directed at sub-Saharan Africa, MAP provided loans to states with high incidences of HIV/AIDS. These loans were designed to encourage collaboration between government and civil society in combating the disease. The Bank would provide monies to non-state actors to support their projects. The government would manage the process and work with these actors to support their project. Civil society was an important component of the MAP program. In order for states to receive funding, the Bank required 40–60 percent of the funds to be distributed to non-governmental organizations (NGOs) (Harman 2010). Such a substantial role for civil society in the program fits with the Bank's vision of good governance. Rather than putting all the control of the program in the hands of weak governments with significant levels of corruption, a power-sharing arrangement between the state and NGOs would enhance the prospects of the funds being used for their intended purpose. States were also required to develop a national strategy for combating HIV/AIDS and establish a coordinating body to administer the program that was not located in the national health ministry (Harman 2010).

The World Bank's next strategy for health was established in its 2007 report, *Healthy Development: The World Bank Strategy for Health, Nutrition, and Population Results*. Its four strategic objectives were (1) improve important outcomes for health, nutrition, and population; (2) provide financial protection to prevent poverty due to disease; (3) improve the financial condition of areas related to health, nutrition, and population; and (4) improve governance in the health sector (World Bank 2007). The growing connection between the World Bank and health was further developed by the appointment of American Jim Yong Kim as president in 2012. Kim was a global health expert, who had previously served as a director of the WHO's HIV/AIDS department. Under Kim's leadership, the Bank has been pursuing the goals of eradicating extreme poverty and promote shared prosperity by 2030. In terms of health, the Bank has emphasized universal health coverage, defined as "ensuring that people have access to the health care they need without suffering financial hardship" (World Bank 2017).

The two themes of the Bank's policies are the importance of demonstrable improvements in health-related outcomes for the Bank's lending programs and continuing the good governance approach adopted by the Bank in the mid-1990s. Harman (2009) argues that the Bank's approach to economic conditionality is softer than that of the IMF and the WTO in that its good governance approach encourages the state and civil society actors to collaborate with the Bank in devising strategies to improve health in their countries. The Bank's policies, however, are still shaped by neoliberal proclivities, and the Bank wants the reform of health care systems to align with its interests. Although the Bank may have moved away from its top-down position in its lending decisions with client states since the 1980s, the process is still not entirely collaborative.

THE INTERNATIONAL MONETARY FUND

The IMF is the sister institution of the World Bank. In addition to also being a product of the Bretton Woods conference in 1944, the World Bank required that states that wished to become members of the Bank must first join the IMF. The mandate of the IMF is to promote international monetary cooperation. Its primary duty is to ensure the stability of the world's monetary system. To address this task, the IMF provides advice to its member states on macroeconomic and financial policies to enhance their economic performance and stability. Like the World Bank, the IMF is also a funding institution. IMF lending, however, is based upon assisting states in alleviating balance of payments problems rather than more general economic development. These problems refer to a financial situation in a particular country, where the state has difficulty in meeting its obligations for international payments. If a state finds itself in such an instance, its currency could begin to depreciate, which could lead to a disruption in both its financial and employment sectors. IMF funds help to maintain currency stability, but these loans have significant conditions. States must agree to implement economic reforms recommended by the organization to receive IMF funds.

Organizationally, the IMF is structurally the same as the World Bank. Its primary decision-making body is the Board of Governors. Every IMF member has one governor to represent their interests on the Board, but the voting system is weighted based upon each member's financial contributions to the IMF. The IMF also has an Executive Board of twenty-four directors who manage the daily affairs of the IMF, because the Board of Governors meets only once a year. The Executive Board is led by a managing director, who serves the head of staff and chief executive of the organization. While the World Bank's president has always been an American national, the managing director of the IMF has always been from a European country.

While the IMF shares many similarities with the World Bank, it is not nearly as significant as an actor in global health governance. It does not have a health-related department, nor does it financially support any health programs. Its effect on global health is much more indirect. The conditions that the IMF places on its loans are designed to promote economic reforms in a borrowing state, but they have tangential impact on the state's health policy. As with the case of the World Bank, the IMF adopted SAPs based upon neoliberal economic principles. The IMF's support of market-friendly policies and privatization influenced borrowing states to move more toward this direction in its health sector.

A major factor regarding SAPs and developing states is that these programs often mandate a reduction in public spending. As a result, social services such as health and education are under pressure to be cut in order to meet the requirements necessary for IMF funding. When states receive IMF funds, they are encouraged to place those funds in their central bank's international reserves to lower inflation, maintain financial stability, and protect against economic problems. In response, states were encouraged to increasingly privatize their health care sector. Among countries in Latin America, Chile, Colombia, and Brazil were the only states to at least partially privatize their health services during the 1990s, while other Latin American governments have made more limited reforms to move toward privatization. The results do not seem to be positive for health care. A study by Homedes and Ugalde (2005), for example, found that after a decade or more of instituting neoliberal economic reforms, these states have had to put more resources into health care without improving the overall efficiency of health services. Another study on SAPs in Latin America and the Caribbean by Franco-Giraldo, Palma, and Alvarez-Dardet (2006) found that during the 1980s and 1990s, neoliberal economic reforms negatively impacted health conditions in those countries. In a wider study conducted by Stuckler, Basu, and McKee (2011), researchers discovered that states that were borrowing funds from the IMF from 1996 to 2006 were putting less of their international financial aid into health systems than states who did not borrow from the IMF. While the researchers acknowledge that these results could be due to financial mismanagement, they speculate that aid may be diverted away from health to other areas to satisfy the IMF's loans conditions. This finding was consistent with another study of sixteen West African states from 1995 to 2014, which found that IMF policy reforms reduced government health expenditures by 0.25 percent per capita (Stubbs et al. 2017). The Ebola crisis of 2014–2015, however, demonstrated how the IMF can also be a positive agent for global health as the IMF provided US$130 million in emergency funding to the West African countries most affected by the outbreak (International Monetary Fund 2018).

Like the World Bank, the IMF moved away from strict neoliberalism to the good governance model in the 1990s. Even with this shift, however, the IMF maintains a strong commitment to neoliberal principles in its funding decisions. Due to its mandate, area of operations, and expertise of its staff, health is not a central concern of the IMF per se. Its priority is to assist states in achieving financial stability. Once states have accomplished that goal, then they should be in better position economically to improve the quality of their health systems. Although some evidence has indicated that neoliberal macroeconomic reforms have had some negative influences on health, the number of other external and internal variables relevant to the relationship between economics and health make it difficult to determine the direct impact of the IMF on global health with any great specificity. Its role, however, should be considered when evaluating the potential obstacles and opportunities for global health governance.

THE WORLD TRADE ORGANIZATION

The WTO is a much newer organization than the World Bank and the IMF. It does share a similar experience, however, in that its origins are rooted in the Bretton Woods conference of 1944. During the negotiations, the participants agreed in principle that an international trade organization was necessary to complement the World Bank and IMF in managing global economic relations. A conference for the International Trade Organization (ITO) was scheduled to take place in Havana, Cuba, in 1947. At the same time, twenty-three states entered into GATT to reduce tariff barriers. It was expected that the GATT agreement would be later incorporated into the ITO framework, but the Havana Charter failed to receive a sufficient number of ratifications by national governments, and so the ITO was never established (Cohn 2016). GATT was a much narrower and informal agreement than the Havana Charter. With the failure of the proposed ITO, GATT became the de facto rules for international trade. GATT proved to be highly successful during its first round of trade negotiations in 1947 where the twenty-three parties to the agreement, who accounted for a great majority of world trade at that time, significantly reduced their tariffs on imported goods. After a period of stagnation during the 1950s, the Kennedy negotiation round of the 1960s and the Tokyo round of the 1970s led to significant reductions in both tariff levels and non-tariff barriers to trade (Irwin 1995).

Despite its success, GATT was always viewed as a temporary measure to facilitate global trade, and a few unsuccessful attempts were made to transform it into a conventional organization during the 1950s and 1960s (Hoekman and Kostecki 2001). The international community became much more amenable to creating a trade organization during the 1980s. In addition to the ideological shift toward neoliberalism and the foreign debt crisis arising from protectionist trade policies during this decade, GATT was becoming increasingly unsuitable for the realities of the global economy in the late twentieth century. Its omission of trade in agriculture and textiles, as well as its lack of coverage for trade in services and protections for intellectual property, became the main focus of GATT's Uruguay Round of negotiations, which lasted from 1986 to 1994. Until that time, the Uruguay Round had the most participating states and lasted longer than any previous round of international trade negotiations. It concluded with an agreement to establish and the WTO as the lead global institution for international trade. GATT, however, did survive. A revised version of the GATT agreement was included as the WTO's treaty for the international trade of goods. The Agreements on Technical Barriers to Trade (TBT), Sanitary and Phytosanitary Measures (SPS), Trade-Related Aspects of Intellectual Property Rights (TRIPS), and Trade in Services (GATS) were also included as agreements covered by the umbrella of the WTO.

Structure of the World Trade Organization

The WTO is led by a Ministerial Conference, which consists of representatives from all member states. Although the Ministerial Conference is the WTO's highest decision-making body, it usually meets only once in every two years. The General Council, which is located at the WTO's headquarters in Geneva, Switzerland, serves as the primary manager for carrying out the functions of the WTO. The General Council also meets as the organization's Dispute Settlement Body (DSB) to adjudicate trade disputes and as the Trade Policy Review Body (TPRB), to examine trade policies of member states. Three specialized councils, the Council for Trade in Goods, the Council for Trade-Related Aspects of Intellectual Property, and the Council for Trade in Services serve under the General Council. The WTO is also supported by a secretariat to provide support for the daily operations of the organization. The Director-General leads the Secretariat and acts as the WTO's chief administrative officer. As is the case with the WHO, the Director-General has little formal power. He or she cannot institute a complaint against any member state for possible trade violations, nor provide any authoritative interpretations of the WTO agreements (Hoekman and Kostecki 2001).

The decision-making rules are substantially different in the WTO compared to the IMF and World Bank. Ever since GATT, it has been based on the practice of obtaining a consensus. Rather than formal vote counting, a consensus decision means that a decision will be accepted by the WTO as long as no member state manifests a strong objection to the decision. The WTO rules do allow for a formal vote, if an agreement is not sufficient for a consensus. At this point, the WTO relies on the "one country, one vote system." If a vote is taken, the threshold for decision to be adopted by the WHO depends on the issue at stake. The WTO's rules have procedures that vary from a unanimous voting requirement to a simple majority. Nevertheless, consensus decision-making is the dominant practice of the WTO (Ehlermann and Ehring 2005).

Agreements of the World Trade Organization and Global Health

As a trade organization, the WTO does not directly regulate global health issues, nor does it provide funding for any health-related programs like the World Bank. International trade policies, however, often have implications for the quality of health. Trade and health are disparate norms in international politics. While the two are not essentially conflictual, a policy that is optimal for trade may not necessarily be good for public health. The fundamental principles of the WTO are non-discrimination and national treatment. *Non-discrimination* refers to the policy that a WTO member state must offer the same terms of trade to all other WTO member states. *National treatment* means that any imported goods must be regulated in the same manner as products that are produced domestically. These principles are included in the GATT and GATS agreements. These agreements, however, also recognize the right of states to protect health. Article XX (b) in GATT allows member states to place restrictions on imported goods if they pose a health risk to humans, animals, or plants. GATS, in Article XIV, also allows restrictions on services if a particular service also poses a health risk. These provisions are subject to the non-discrimination principle. So, if a WTO member restricts imports on a particular product on health grounds, it must maintain the same restrictions on that product for every WTO member that is exporting that product.

In addition to the requirement that a health-related restriction on trade be non-discriminatory, it must also be legitimate. The question of whether the legitimacy of the health claim must be supported by scientific evidence was addressed by the Appellate Body of the WTO's DSB in a 2001 decision. This case originated with the adoption of a ban by France in 1996 on the import of products that contained asbestos. Canada brought the case against France in the DSB claiming that France's prohibition on importing Canada's chrysotile asbestos fibers was an unfair restriction on trade. The Appellate Body supported France's position and found that France could ban imports of these products as long as it was based on some scientific evidence that it was harmful. The result of this decision indicates that a national government will receive a fair amount of deference on making a health exception claim under GATT's XX (b). At the same time, this claim may still be challenged, and it must have "some" scientific merit to qualify as a trade exception (Saspin et al. 2003). In interpreting the health exception to all WTO agreements, to be valid, the restriction on trade must also be necessary.

The WTO recognizes the high importance of health, but it will also consider whether the measure will be effective to protect health interests, or if its impact on trade will be overly burdensome (World Health Organization and World Trade Organization 2002). In the 2001 asbestos case, France's ban was found to meet the standard of necessity. Although this situation demonstrates that the WTO is receptive to trade protectionism on health grounds, one concern about the determination of health risk in such disputes is that the decision is primarily made by trade experts rather than individuals with a background in health (Lee and Koivusalo 2005).

While GATT and its health exception to trade can be traced back to the original agreement in 1947, GATS is a much newer agreement that went into effect at the end of the Uruguay Round in 1995. GATS has a number of different implications for the provision of health. It can involve the provision of medical treatment across borders, the movement of individuals who travel to other states to seek such treatment, and foreign ownership of health care facilities. States are not obligated to make a commitment to any health-related services under GATS. If, however, a national government elects to make a commitment to health services under GATS, it must also assume market access obligations in addition to subscribing to the principles of non-discrimination and national treatment in the provision of these services by foreign companies and workers. The major concerns regarding GATS in the area of health services are that the agreement may act to undermine a national government's ability to design its health care policy and the possibility that foreign competition may adversely impact domestic health care providers that are supported by the government. Although these concerns have merit, as Belsky et al. (2004) point out, governments can regulate health care services by foreign providers as long as the regulations are non-discriminatory and meet the standard of being necessary for ensuring the quality of the services. The capacity to effectively manage foreign health services does, however, vary among different states. According to Woodward (2005), developing states tend to be more tempted to make commitments to GATS in the area of health services to attract foreign investment and to serve as a bargaining tool to negotiate better trade concessions from developed economies. Developing states may be more willing to risk losing autonomy over their health care system, especially in serving their low-income populations, to promote economic benefits primarily for business and political elites (Woodward 2005: 530).

Other WTO agreements that address protections for health include the TBT and the SPS. TBT originally came into force in 1980 and then was revised as part of the Uruguay Round of negotiations in 1995. The agreement does allow for states to place restrictions on trade for legitimate reasons, including the health of humans, animals, or plants. As with GATT, for these restrictions to be valid, they must meet the non-discrimination and necessity standards. In a 2010 case before the WTO's DSB's panel, Indonesia claimed that a 2009 U.S. law, which banned the sale of clove cigarettes, violated GATT and several provisions of the TBT agreement by acting as an unfair restriction on trade. In interpreting the TBT in regard to Indonesia's complaint, the dispute settlement panel found that the American regulation was necessary and not unduly restrictive for the protection of health. The panel also found, however, that the United States did not meet the national treatment standard because clove cigarettes imported from Indonesia received more restrictive treatment than menthol cigarettes primarily produced in the United States, which the panel found to be a similar product. As Voon (2013) argues, the panel's decision indicates that states may use the TBT agreement to place restrictions on products that they deem to be harmful to human health, including tobacco, as long as the regulations are applied in the same manner to comparable foreign and domestic products.

The SPS agreement addresses rules for states to protect human, animal, and plant life from unsafe food and disease-carrying organisms, while not unduly restricting international trade. SPS covers a narrower category of health risks than TBT because it focuses on contaminants in food and beverages and the importation on animals or plants that may have diseases. Harmful products such as tobacco and alcohol would fit under the TBT because they do not meet the standard for coverage for SPS. In addition to coverage, SPS and TBT differ in that the SPS requires scientific data to support a claim, while the TBT standard is based on the legitimacy of the measure, which does not necessarily hinge on such information (World Health Organization and World Trade Organization 2002). A major issue in the WTO regarding SPS has been genetically modified foods. The first case under SPS was brought by the United States against the European Community prohibiting the importation of hormone-fed cattle which was an unfair trade restriction in 1996. The WTO panel sided with the United States due to insufficient scientific evidence that consumption of the beef was harmful to human health. A similar case reached the WTO in 2003 when the United States, Canada, and Argentina brought a claim against the European Community for its regulation of genetically modified organisms, and argued it was effectively discriminating against imports of foods with these organisms in favor of "like" products that did not have genetically modified organisms. In this case, the WTO also found that the health risk justifying the restrictions on imports of these foods by the European Community was not adequately supported by scientific evidence.

While the GATT, GATS, TBT, and SPS agreements create issues for states in protecting themselves from potentially harmful products and services in the course of international commerce, the main issue with the TRIPS agreement has to do with its capacity to offer adequate health treatments. Specifically, access to essential medicines. As mentioned, TRIPS was another agreement arising out of the Uruguay Round that went into force along with the WTO's formation in 1995. TRIPS relates to the protection of intellectual property rights such as patents, trademarks, industrial designs, and copyrights. It was an agreement that was particularly desired by the United States and also supported by the European Union, two actors that dominate the global ownership of intellectual property. Developing states did not wish to be a part of this agreement, but they were pressured into accepting it by developed states. Before TRIPS, several states such as Brazil and India did not allow for the patenting of medicines, while other states such as Canada allowed the production of generic versions of a particular drug (Heywood 2002). TRIPS made it much more difficult for states to continue these practices even for antiretroviral drugs (ARVs) to treat HIV/AIDS. The enhanced protection of international intellectual property made ARVs and other drugs much more expensive for developing states.

Pharmaceutical companies were major beneficiaries of TRIPS because they could maintain higher prices due to reduced competition by producers of generic drugs (Abbott 2002: 18). The TRIPS agreement, however, did not ignore the implications of health in strengthening the international regime for intellectual property rights. Article 8 in the agreement provides states with a right to make regulations to protect public health as long as they are applied to be consistent with their duty to protect intellectual property rights. The problem, however, is even with the recognition to protect health, developing states would still be subject to fighting legal battles over interpretations over TRIPS with developed states (Heywood 2002: 226).

Developing states were not pleased with TRIPS and its impact on access to medicines from the outset and launched several challenges based on a potential loophole in Article 31 of TRIPS, which gave WTO members the right to issue a compulsory license, which meant they could license a producer to make a patented product without the patent holder's permission. This right, however, was subject to some important conditions: an attempt should first be made to receive the patent holder's permission, the license would be non-exclusive, the license would only be valid until during the time necessary to fill the need for the product, and the product must be mostly produced for the domestic market. Brazil, for example, passed a law in 1996 permitting compulsory licensing of any patents for products that were not manufactured in

Brazil. The passage of this law led to a dispute with the United States, which filed a complaint with the WTO (Lanoszka 2003). The most significant challenge occurred in South Africa. In 1997, the South African government permitted the compulsory licensing of ARVs to significantly lower the cost of treating HIV/AIDS in that country. In response, forty drug companies initiated a lawsuit against the government claiming that its Medicines Amendment Act not only contravened TRIPS but was even unconstitutional due to the authority it provided to the Minister of Health to supersede national patent laws (Lanoszka 2003). The lawsuit, however, never came to fruition. A number of NGOs and civil society organizations protested against it, and the drug companies decided to drop the suit due to the backlash that it generated against the pharmaceutical industry.

As a result of the controversy, a revision of TRIPS was a major topic of discussion at WTO ministerial meeting that took place in Doha, Qatar, in 2001. During negotiations, the WTO adopted the Declaration on the TRIPS Agreement and Public Health, also known as the Doha Declaration. The declaration affirmed that WTO member states had a right to promote and provide public access to medicines. In addition, the declaration granted each member state the right to issue compulsory licenses and the right to determine the conditions for issuing these licenses as well as those for a national emergency. The most significant source of disagreement at Doha was in regard to the TRIPS provision that the production of goods under a compulsory license must be primarily aimed for domestic use. A compromise on this issue was reached in 2003, in which compulsory licenses for production of drugs for export could be permitted to eligible states suffering from public health problems. Eligible states would include the poorest of the developing states. Other developing states could also become eligible for acquiring exports of these generic pharmaceuticals as long as they complied a series of procedures that were mostly designed to show their transparency in these transactions with the WHO (Abbott 2005).

The Doha Declaration clearly represented a victory for developing states on the issue of access of medicines. Of course why did the United States and other developed states decide to agree to these terms after strongly contesting the position of the developing states? One explanation has to do with the influence of NGOs. These organizations launched a major campaign against TRIPS due to the limitations it placed on access to medicines. This campaign was based on disseminating information regarding how TRIPS was contributing to making medical treatment prohibitively expensive for the world's poor and on grafting this issue as a human rights concern. NGOs worked together to pressure developed states to soften their stance on TRIPS, as well as assisting in the efforts to bring developing states together to form a stronger coalition to challenge the world's great economic powers. Although Drezner

(2007) believes that the NGO movement accelerated the agreement at Doha, he finds this to be an incomplete explanation. Instead, he argues that it was actually the security concerns of the United States about the spread of HIV/AIDS that motivated it to become more amenable to the position of developing states. After the terrorist attacks of September 11, 2001, the United States became more sensitive about political instability in the developing world. Fear of how HIV/AIDS could contribute to state failure and refugee problems played an important role in the change in the American position. This position was indicated at Doha as the United States proved to be much more willing to enhance access to essential medicines for the weakest states, particularly those in sub-Saharan Africa, than for all developing states.

BOX 2.1 FREE TRADE AGREEMENTS (FTAs): CHALLENGING THE WTO AND THE DOHA DECLARATION THROUGH TRIPS-PLUS?

TRIPS-plus refers to the practice of developed states to utilize bilateral and regional free trade agreements (FTAs) outside of the WTO framework to achieve greater protections for intellectual property than those offered by TRIPS. As Abbott (2005) notes, this strategy shifted the forum of trade negotiations away from the WTO to a bilateral setting where developing countries have not been as effective. Negotiating thorough the WTO offers certain protections to smaller states such as working with coalitions of similar states to increase bargaining power and the possibility of resolving conflict through a dispute settlement mechanism. These states may become much more vulnerable to the interests of larger states in trade negotiations, especially bilateral, that occur outside of the WTO and lack these safeguards.

Although developing states are free to choose whether or not they wish to enter into an FTA, they are often willing to accept increased protection for intellectual property in free trade agreement in exchange for anticipated benefits for commerce (Correa 2006). In terms of potential influence of FTAs, evidence indicates a significant decline in the issuance of compulsory licensing for the production of generic drugs after 2006 (Beall and Kuhn 2012). Son and Lee (2017), however, have noted a resurgence of compulsory licensing in 2012 and 2014, which they credit to a growing global justice movement by civil society. Whether TRIPS-plus or this global justice movement will be more influential in the development of compulsory licensing will be an interesting issue in the future.

The WTO operates differently than other IGOs involved in global health governance. Rather than impacting health directly or indirectly through bureaucratic initiatives and financing, the WTO primarily affects health through the interpretation of international trade agreements. This interpretation is developed by the organization's dispute settlement body. Even though this body is composed of trade experts, and not health experts, the WTO treaties and past decisions by WTO panels have made it clear that health is a protected right. What remains unclear, however, is exactly what is the extent of that right? The WTO is certainly an influential factor in attempting to answer that question.

INTERGOVERNMENTAL ORGANIZATIONS AS ACTORS IN GLOBAL HEALTH

The WHO, World Bank, IMF, and WTO along with the UN and various UN-affiliated agencies such as UNICEF are among the most significant actors in global health governance. The extent of their role, however, varies based upon their organizational mandates and objectives. The various theoretical perspectives of international relations also differ in their view as to how influential these organizations are in their impact on global health. Realists, due to their state-centric focus, do not tend to find these organizations to be particularly significant in their own right. Mearsheimer (1994/1995), for example, has made the case that international institutions are generally ineffective actors. Correspondingly, IGOs serve as a reflection of the distribution of power in the international system rather than as an autonomous entity. IGOs' actions are based on the calculations of the interests of their most powerful member states. Drezner's (2007) examination of the WTO's TRIPS agreement is supportive of this view even though the Doha Declaration was deemed as advancing the interests of developing states. The concessions made on TRIPS by developed states were based on the national security interests of great powers. During the 1990s, the Clinton administration in the United States became increasingly concerned that HIV/AIDS epidemic in the developing world would contribute to the economic and social instability of weaker states, military conflicts, and a refugee crisis. Security officials in the United States were becoming aware of this connection before civil society's backlash against TRIPS (Drezner 2007: 186). The Bush administration concurred with this view, and so the United States became more amenable. In addition, the shift in the American position on TRIPS could also be viewed as a concession to developing states to move the Doha round of trade negotiations further.

The analysis of the WHO, World Bank, and IMF also provide evidence to support the realist assumption that IGOs are in fact marginal actors in global health governance. The WHO has historically struggled when it has supported policies contrary to the interests of major powers. This outcome was most apparent when the WHO elected to support the primary health care agenda. In response major powers, led by the United States, constrained funding to the WHO, which in turn, increasingly accepted EBFs to reduce its funding shortfall. They were also able to effectively shift the forum for global health governance from the WHO to the World Bank, where they had more control. In the 1990s, the WHO moved more toward economism to accommodate the change desired by major powers in global health governance. Even though the WHO may align philosophically more with developing states, realists would certainly argue that by political necessity it requires the support of developed states to effectively implement policy. The influence of powerful states is even more direct in the World Bank and IMF based on the design of those organizations. The weighted voting system helps to ensure that those institutions will act in their favor.

As covered in chapter 1, neoliberal institutionalists assume that states are more cooperative actors than realists suggest. IGOs help to facilitate cooperation by providing a forum to enhance the prospects for successful negotiation and collective action. In this manner, neoliberal institutionalists would support the proposition that the WHO, IMF, World Bank, and WTO are, in fact, effective actors in global governance. Evidence indicates that the WHO has effectively framed issues and promoted consensus-building on a number of different health issues. The FCTC serves as a compelling example of how the WHO has been able to establish an accepted set of rules for global health. IHR 2005 and the powers that it delegates to the WHO indicate an acknowledgment by states that the WHO is the key focal point for effective infectious disease control. The World Bank has provided funding for health care programs such as MAP. Despite criticisms regarding SAPs sponsored by the World Bank and the IMF, these programs have been instituted with the intention of improving the long-term economic stability of states suffering from financial difficulties. Neoliberals believe that once the economy of these states improves, then these states will be able to provide higher quality care. Although the extent of protection may be unclear, the rules of the WTO also address the need to protect health. From a broader view, neoliberal institutionalists would also claim that the improvements in global health since 2000 can be associated with the expansion of IGO activity and proliferation of international agreements addressing health during this time.

Social constructuctivists also view IGOs as influential actors in international politics. They serve as agents of change by socializing other actors into accepting international norms. The WHO has been a lead agent in promoting global health during its existence. In addition to establishing a number of health standards and guidelines that have influenced health care practices in several states, the WHO has also successfully influenced states to support its various health campaigns over the years ranging from its malaria and tuberculosis programs to its anti-tobacco initiative. According to McInnes (2015), the WHO is traditionally identified by the international community as having expert and delegated authority. The implication of this social identity is that the WHO has been in a role "in which it is more important to be correct than prompt, and in which its normative power arises in no small part from the quality of the advice it provides" (McInnes 2015: 1307). While the WHO's image as an expert authority may be beneficial to promoting norm diffusion, the Ebola outbreak of 2014 also indicated that this image was not conducive to responding to a major health crises.

The World Bank has also socialized states to adopt certain health initiatives. When the World Bank elected to support health-related projects, its actions and research transferred the perspective of states on health into economic terms. Interventions in health became to be viewed not just as beneficial for humanitarian and ethical reasons but also cost effective as well. Developed states began to increasingly support efforts at improving global health as they began to realize how they could also benefit economically from improved health in developing countries. While the WTO has not been nearly as an active agent in the socialization of global health standards as the WHO and the World Bank, its rules and decisions by its dispute settlement panels do have an influence. They serve as an acknowledgment to the international community that protection of health remains an important principle in the context of free and open commerce.

Marxists and neo-Marxists, however, would find that the efforts of IGOs in global health governance are effectively compromised by the forces of capitalism. In this view, the World Bank and IMF are major keystones of the global economy. Their priority is to promote and maintain the capitalist economic system and the interests of the capitalist class. According to the neo-Gramscian perspective, health support offered by the World Bank is utilized as a means to convince developing countries and poorer populations to accept capitalist economic practices. Marxists would also tend to view the policies of the WTO as a detriment to global health. The rules of the WTO make it more difficult for states to regulate their imports from abroad, and TRIPS acts to make essential medicines prohibitively expensive for much of the world's poor. Marxists would argue that the health protection standards in the WTO are illusory in practice. The WTO has not been supportive of health claims in its decision-making proceedings. Additionally, the FCTC does not address the possibility of restrictions on the importation of tobacco on the basis of protection of health. Even with the Doha Declaration, Marxists could point to the TRIPS-plus provisions as another indicator of how the WTO principles prioritize the interests of multinational corporations and the world's core capitalist economies over global health. While Marxists would likely agree that the WHO has been a much more genuine supporter of global health, over time it has been consistently constrained by agents of global capitalism when it has sought to align itself with the interests of developing states. The policy shift by the WHO toward economism in the 1990s was designed to restore the WHO's relevancy as an actor in global health. Although the WHO may continue to philosophically support the "health for all" standard, its policies are still constrained by an international system that is dominated by capitalists' norms and interests.

While the major theories of international relations, in particular, realism and neoliberal institutionalism, provide useful insights in understanding the dynamics of interstate relations in the context of international organizations, they do not provide quite as much guidance in explaining how internal factors may affect the preferences and behavior of these organizations as actors in their own right. Analyses utilizing rational choice and constructivist perspectives, however, have devoted more attention to examining these issues. Much of the rational choice perspective has been based on viewing the relationship between the member states and the organization as an interaction between a principal and an agent. The states serve as the principals in this relationship by defining their preferences and delegating authority to the organization, their agent, to implement the states' desired policy. The principal has incentives to delegate such authority because the agent may have some special knowledge or expertise, may be able to further facilitate cooperation by providing services for monitoring, sharing of information, and agenda-setting. Agents can also make commitments by member states more credible if they are delegated some power for enforcement or settling disputes (Hawkins et al. 2006). The key issue of course has to do with how much independent authority is the principal willing to grant the delegate to perform these tasks?

A study by Cortell and Peterson (2006) evaluated the principal-agent relationship in the case of two major organizations in global health, the WHO and the WTO. They argue that the grant of authority to both these organizations is relatively high. This claim is based upon two factors: (1) both have large international staffs that are hired based on their expertise and serve to represent the organization rather than a particular member state and (2) decision-making rules that make it difficult for a limited number of states to effectively impose their specific preferences on the organization as a whole. In their analysis, Cortell and Peterson (2006) find that despite a significant delegation of authority, staff members usually did not attempt to exhibit too much independence from the preferences of member states. The potential loss of legitimacy for the organization, as well as financing, seemed to constrain bureaucrats in the WHO. For members of the WTO's Appellate Body of its DSB, concerns regarding the perception of legitimacy of their decisions by member states also seemed to inhibit their autonomy as an agent. These findings fit with observations of both organizations in that the WHO has generally been cautious and reluctant to challenge great powers, with the exception of the SARS, on major global health policies. In the WTO case, it indicates how difficult it might be for trade officials to accept a broad view of the health exception as an acceptable restraint on trade without clearer guidance from member states on the appropriate standard.

The constructivist perspective focus more on international organizations as bureaucracies rather than agents per se. In addition to delegated authority from principals, bureaucracies also gain authority from morality, such as health and human rights purposes, and their expertise. Using these forms of authority, IGOs can be powerful actors by shaping understandings of issues and problems and developing new norms (Barnett and Finnemore 2004). Rather than acting simply as agents, these organizations may, in fact, be able to shape the preferences of member states. As bureaucracies, however, IGOs may be geared toward decision-making based upon standard operating procedures and organizational culture rather than rationalism. This perspective suggests that the WHO, as the most significant IGO in global governance that is primarily dedicated to health, would have a significant capacity to operate autonomously due to its moral and expert authority. The anti-tobacco campaign, in particular, demonstrates how the WHO was able to influence the preferences of member states to an extent necessary to create the FCTC. At the same time, this perspective also indicates how the preferences of the WHO may be based on the outcome of negotiating a clash between biomedical and economism cultures within the organization, rather than promoting a rational-based interest.

A similar view has been suggested by Chorev (2012). She agrees with the principal-agent and constructivist perspectives in that IGOs act as autonomous actors, but she does not find that these perspectives sufficiently explain the outcome when the interests of these organizations directly conflict with that of member states. Under this circumstance, she proposes that IGOs respond either passively, where they will accept the preferences of the member states because they do not wish to be sanctioned for non-compliance, or they will respond strategically, in which case they will try to change the meaning of the preferences to fit with the organization's objectives. In her study of the WHO, Chorev argues that the organization frequently asserts its autonomy vis-à-vis member states by responding strategically to their interests. For example, when neoliberalism became an established norm in the 1990s and 2000s, the WHO was still able to launch its anti-tobacco initiative by framing the issue to emphasize the economic costs that tobacco use posed on member states. In doing so, the WHO was successful in achieving its interest by convincing states that tobacco control was, in fact, not inconsistent with principles of neoliberalism.

According to Chorev, a key factor as to whether an IGO will act passively or strategically has to do with its leadership. Those leaders of the WHO, such as Mahler and Brundtland, who could skillfully adapt the interests of the organization to the prevailing norms of international politics, were able to effectively promote the independence of the organization. Less effective leaders would either respond passively or would not have the interests of their organization accommodated by member states. In this manner, even though IGOs are constrained as actors due to their dependence on member states for resources and political legitimacy, with effective leadership they may be able to still "game" the system to assert some degree of autonomy in shaping global health policy.

CONCLUSION

The WHO was established to be the world's leading IGO for global health in the post–World War II era. As health issues, however, became more connected to economic policy over time, other IGOs such as the IMF, WTO, and especially the World Bank have become increasingly involved in global health politics even though health was not a part of their original mandate. While the WHO does have an advantage in shaping global health policy due to its health-based mandate and the expertise of its bureaucracy, the World Bank has become, perhaps, an even more powerful actor in global health governance due to its capacity to provide funding to health-based initiatives. The influences of the IMF and the WTO are more indirect, but their decisions regarding structural adjustment programs and global trade law and policy, respectively, have impacted how national governments can address health issues.

Different theories of international relations provide important insights as to the role and relative influence of IGOs in global health. Due to its assumption that states are dominant actors in international politics, realism suggests that IGOs have a rather limited role. Global health policies largely require the support of great powers to be effective. Neoliberal institutionalists, however, are much more optimistic. In their view, these organizations facilitate cooperation and consensus-building among member states. Constructivists also tend to view IGOs as important actors but see them as most valuable in promoting norms and socializing states and individuals into accepting particular policies as suitable practices in addressing global health. Marxist-based perspectives, however, emphasize how capitalism has compromised the ability of IGOs, especially the WHO, in their ability to provide quality health for all people. Organizational theories such as principal-agent and strategic response can also provide enhanced understanding of how IGOs might influence policies on global health. A common link among all these perspectives is that IGOs do exhibit some potential for improving global health. Even realists might find that states may be more willing on health-based initiatives than other international issues because these initiatives could create a collective good with a minimal cost to state sovereignty. Another lesson than can be learned from these perspectives, however, is that IGOs have a number of obstacles to overcome to develop effective global health policies, and skillful management of its relations with state and non-state actors are prerequisites for doing so.

DISCUSSION QUESTIONS

1. What is the structure of the World Health Organization (WHO), and what are its main principles based on its constitution?
2. What was the significance of the Alma-Ata Declaration? Is the declaration relevant today?
3. Explain the significance of reforms that the WHO has made over time.
4. How may international economic institutions such as the World Bank, International Monetary Fund, and World Trade Organization be considered important actors in global health?
5. Based on principal-agent and constructivist approaches, are intergovernmental organizations in global health autonomous actors? Why or Why not?

SUGGESTED READINGS

Chorev, Nitsan. 2012. *The World Health Organization between North and South*. Ithaca, NY: Cornell University Press.

Excellent account of the relationship between the World Health Organization's bureaucracy and its member states.

Harman, Sophie. 2010. *The World Bank and HIV/AIDS*. London: Routledge.

Examines the process of the World Bank's activity in global health governance with a focus on HIV/AIDS.

Hawkins, Darren G., David A. Lake, Daniel L. Nielson, and Michael J. Tierney. 2006. *Delegation and Agency in International Organizations*. Cambridge, UK: Cambridge University Press.

Insightful overview of the relationship between states and intergovernmental organizations based on principal-agent theory.

Howard-Jones, Norman. 1975. *The Scientific Background to the International Sanitary Conferences 1851–1938*. Geneva: World Health Organization.

Comprehensive account of international cooperation and health before World War II.

Lee, Kelley. 2009. *The World Health Organization (WHO)*. New York: Routledge.

Comprehensive overview and analysis of the World Health Organization's structure and policies.

Chapter 3

Non-State Actors and Global Health Governance

Non-state actors are also important players in global health governance. During the quarantines of the nineteenth century and early twentieth century, transnational commercial interests encouraged national governments to come to an agreement on uniform quarantine controls to reduce the burden that different national standards had on trade (Fidler 2001). Among non-governmental organizations (NGOs) involved in global health prior to World War II, the most significant was the Rockefeller Foundation established in 1913 by business tycoon and philanthropist John D. Rockefeller. After initiating a successful program against hookworm diseases, the Rockefeller Foundation established an International Health Board, which became the International Health Division (IHD) in 1927 (Birn and Free 2013). The IHD had operations all over the world. It provided valuable funding and expertise in sustaining campaigns against yellow fever and malaria in addition to hookworm disease. It also served as a major donor to the Health Organization of the League of Nations, and its former staff members continued to play influential roles in global health after the IHD dissolved following the establishment of the World Health Organization (WHO) in 1948 (Birn and Free 2013).

Until the mid-twentieth century, the role of non-state actors had been very constrained in world politics due to the historical domination of the power of national governments. The Rockefeller Foundation was clearly an exception resulting from its substantial base of funding. As globalization accelerated since the end of the Cold War, however, non-state actors became prominent in world politics both in terms of numbers and influence. Business enterprises have evolved into multinational corporations (MNCs) that own economic assets in multiple states and can transfer goods and services much more easily around the world. While private foundations continue to be significant actors in global health governance, other NGOs that primarily offer health services and policy advocacy have also become active participants. The management challenge that globalization provided to the states has, simultaneously, presented a greater opportunity for non-state actors.

In the area of health, MNCs operate in many different ways. Their practices in regard to price and access to pharmaceuticals can impact how disease-combating drugs are distributed around the world. Some MNCs, such as those in the tobacco, alcohol, and food industry, provide global distribution of products that may prove harmful to human health. In other areas, MNCs' preferences in regard to labor and environmental policies may also act to affect the health of populations of countries hosting their operations. Because MNCs are largely unregulated at the global level, institutions of global governance must find creative and effective ways to interact with these actors to develop productive policies to promote health.

NGOs are similar to MNCs in that they are also private actors who are not directly connected to national governments. They can be distinguished from MNCs in that their purpose tends to support a particular economic, political, or social cause rather than the pursuit of profits. The number and role of NGOs in world politics grew significantly after World War II. With the negotiations taking place for reconstruction of the world order at the end of the war, NGOs lobbied to be included as a formal partner in global governance to coincide with the founding of the United Nations (UN) (Charnovitz 2006).

Bartsch and Kohlmorgen (2007: 93) argue that NGOs are more prominent in health than in other areas of global politics. They base this claim on the long history of non-state actors' participation in global health issues and the current difficulties for intergovernmental organizations (IGOs) in assisting developing states with all of their health-related needs. Ethical obligations to assist people in less developed countries suffering from poor health also contribute to the political support of these NGOs. Functions for NGOs involved in health include political, operational, and self-empowerment dimensions (Bartsch and Kohlmorgen 2007). In terms of political activities these organizations have organized campaigns promoting particular causes such as access to pharmaceuticals, protective measures for HIV/AIDS, and risks associated with tobacco consumption. Operationally, NGOs can provide the delivery of health service and medical care, as well as offer financial support for health projects. For self-empowerment, these organizations can provide a voice in the political arena for affected populations, the vast majority of whom lack access to policy-makers in national governments or IGOs.

In assessing the role of non-state actors, whether they are MNCs or NGOs, in global governance it is apparent that their emergence is connected to globalization. As markets have opened and technology has connected people and culture more closely than ever before, states may be losing power, and non-state actors could be rising to fill in gaps that were previously dominated by national governments. Mathews (1997) has made the case that the end of the Cold War has led to a decline in the power of states and a corresponding rise in the power of non-state actors. She points that this is largely due to the political and social consequences of computer and telecommunication technology. Already constrained by territorial borders, national governments can no longer control information and efficiently address the problems posed by globalization. NGOs can conduct operations transnationally and create communities of like-minded individuals who are not bound by national loyalties. MNCs, she argues, are detaching themselves from their home states, and are attempting to avoid national regulations based on the mobility of their enterprises. In this view, the international system is shifting away from states as the global center of power. Realists, of course, would not concur. They may acknowledge that interactions are becoming more transnational at the end of the Cold War, and perhaps are even more challenging for states to regulate. But they would emphasize that the ultimate power in world politics is still entrenched in national interests.

This chapter will further analyze these differing perspectives on non-state actors in global health. A list of selected non-state actors can be found in table 3.1. Key questions to be considered are do non-state actors play an influential role in global health? How exactly might non-state actors have a meaningful impact on global health policy? Is there a difference between the impact of MNCs and NGOs? To approach these questions, the next section of the chapter will review four different types of non-state actors and their role in global health governance. The actors include MNCs, NGOs, private foundations, and an organizational hybrid between state and non-state actors known as public-private partnerships (PPPs). Various theories specific to these non-state actors, as well as more general approaches to international

Table 3.1. Selected Types of Non-State Actors in Global Governance

Actor	*Characterization*
Multinational corporations	Business enterprises that own economic assets in more than one state and seek to maximize profits.
Non-governmental organizations	Private organizations that tend to support a particular economic, political, or social cause.
Private foundations	Non-profit organizations that primarily focus on providing donations for public goods.
Public-private partnerships	Hybrid actor based on a collaborative relationship among a variety of public and private actors.

relations such as realism, neoliberal institutionalism, Marxism, and constructivism, will be utilized to help provide an assessment of how these actors fit in global health governance.

MULTINATIONAL CORPORATIONS

MNCs are non-state actors that conduct activities in many countries around the world. What distinguishes MNCs from most other non-state actors is that their main purpose is to produce profits. MNCs have capital and technological resources that states covet. As Gilpin (2001) notes, MNCs have become key actors in global politics because their decisions and activities impact trade flows and the location of industry. Roach (2005) describes a number of ways that MNCs can exercise power. Due to their ability to transfer their operations from one state to another fairly easily, they can be very persuasive in convincing national governments to offer them favorable tax incentives and corporate-friendly environmental regulations. The promise of jobs and income provides another source of leverage that MNCs may exercise in bargaining with states. Political lobbying and campaign financing may also serve as influential tools for MNCs. As the global economy has become increasingly deregulated, states have often found themselves competing against one another and willing to alter their policies to attract the services of MNCs. International trade agreements may empower MNCs as well, as they may include provisions that protect them from some forms of national regulations.

Although MNCs are potentially powerful actors in global governance due to their economic clout, they have not received much scholarly attention in this role. A major reason for this outcome is that the two most influential theories in international relations, realism and neoliberal institutionalism, are state-centric approaches that assume MNCs are not primary actors. Realists, in particular, hold that MNCs act mostly as agents of member states. For example, a study by Doremus et al. (1998) of American, German, and Japanese firms found that MNCs are very much tied to their home states. Strategic decision-making in areas such as investment and research and development is often influenced by the political, social, and cultural environment of their home and not just the function of profit maximization. As a result, they argue that corporations act differently depending on where their base of operations is located.

Liberals have made greater strides to incorporating MNCs, in addition to NGOs, as actors through international regime analysis. The concept of regimes, however, is fairly vague and most analysis utilizing the concept focuses on how various forms of institutions may constrain state behavior. It does not provide specificity as to the role and function that MNCs play in a regime. As noted by Davis (2013) among theories of international relations, neo-Marxism provides the greatest emphasis on MNCs as an actor in world politics. These approaches have often viewed corporate interests as serving the interests of developed states. MNCs have also been seen as the main vehicles in the promotion of international capitalism and establishment of an international division of labor, which constrains the potential economic development of poorer states.

Some studies have attempted to establish a framework for understanding the place of MNCs in global governance. Levy and Prakash (2003), for instance, developed a typology for analyzing international regimes from the position of the MNC. They propose that, in terms of regimes, MNCs focus on the purpose and the authority of the regime. In terms of purpose, MNCs are interested in whether the regime is one that promotes market liberalization, such as the WTO and the various agreements related to international trade such as GATT and TRIPS, or if its purpose is to constrain international commerce in some manner. The variables that shape the authority of a regime are its mechanisms for monitoring and enforcement of the regime's rules. Specifically, whether this authority is situated at the national or regional level, it generally can be expected that most MNCs, especially if they are efficient producers, will favor market liberalization while opposing regulatory regimes. The position of an MNC on the particular purpose of a regime will largely hinge on whether the regime will enhance or detract from the MNC's competiveness. Levy and Prakash (2003) cite the example of the automobile industry in North America as an example of a group of MNCs who would like to see some regulation in order to assist them in becoming more competitive with foreign companies. In terms of authority, MNCs tend to prefer compliance mechanisms at the international level for economic issues while favoring national level regulations for environmental and social issues. These preferences, however, conflict with most NGOs who would prefer the opposite (Levy and Prakash 2003). They do note in their study that although MNCs are more supportive of global governance on economic issues, they also suggest that the position of MNCs is also affected by its relative power compared to other actors in the regime and the cost of bargaining in any attempts to modify the regime. As a result, they argue that the interests and the power of MNCs vary depending on the issue and the relative strength of other parties involved in negotiations of governance.

Fuchs (2007) also offers a theoretical framework for understanding the role of MNCs in global governance. Her framework is based upon different types of power that MNCs can utilize in global governance, especially in their relationships with national governments. These types of power are instrumental, structural, and discursive. *Instrumental power* refers to the influence that the MNC may have through lobbying and financing political candidates.

Structural power is based on the corporation's ability to influence the agenda and rules of global governance, mostly through public-private partnerships (PPPs) and self-regulation. The third type of power, *discursive*, results from the influence that corporations may have of shaping norms and ideas surrounding political issues. The norm that MNCs attempt to promote, of course, is privatization. By utilizing these three powers, she finds that corporations are significant actors in shaping global governance. Fuchs (2007) does, however, point out that corporations are still constrained as actors largely due to their lack of a formal legal role in the system of governance. As a consequence, corporations need to count on the support of states and civil society actors. Without such support, corporations may lose legitimacy, which could in turn undermine all bases of their power.

Another analytical framework by Detomasi (2007) examines the relationship among states, MNCs, and civil society through what he refers to as Global Public Policy Networks (GPPN). These networks bring this group of actors together to solve collective action problems by joining the expertise of non-state actors with the legitimacy and legal power of states. MNCs benefit by constructing a dialogue with the other actors to identify the expected standards for their behavior in areas such as labor, working conditions, and the environment. He proposes that GPPN potentially enhances the efficiency of global governance by providing a forum for negotiation, greater information-sharing, an increased legitimacy of decision-making and establishing codes of conduct, as well as more effective resolution of disputes. As an example of a significant GPPN, Detomasi (2007) cites the UN's Global Compact program. This initiative requests MNCs to be responsible actors acknowledging the problems of economic development and collaborate with governments and non-state actors in improving human rights, labor, and environmental standards as part of their business practice. The Global Compact has over 12,000 corporate partners, and the UN has referred to it as the "largest voluntary corporate initiative in the world" (United Nations 2013).

These frameworks stand in contrast to the neo-Gramscian variation of Marxism, which views MNCs as part of a transnational historical bloc that has used its power to promote neoliberal norms and social class division on a global scale (Cox 1987). Alternatively, the approaches by Levy and Prakash (2003), Fuchs (2007), and Detomasi (2007) view the world in a more state-centric manner. A common theme across these three frameworks has to do with the relational power on MNCs. While they all agree that MNCs can be powerful actors in global governance, they also find that the influence of MNCs does have some dependency on whether or not their preferences are going to find support among other actors in global governance. To understand the role of MNCs in global health governance, these frameworks will be applied to MNC activity in the areas of access to pharmaceuticals and the distribution of tobacco and unhealthy products.

Access to Pharmaceuticals

The issue of access to pharmaceuticals in global health governance is largely shaped by the World Trade Organization's (WTO) Agreement on Trade-Related Aspects of Intellectual Property Rights (TRIPS), which is covered in greater detail in chapter 2. As previously discussed, the purpose of the TRIPS agreement is to protect intellectual property rights. This agreement supports MNCs involved in the production of pharmaceutical products in that they can invest funds in research and development for drugs while having their innovations protected from copying by others. As noted in chapter 2, the controversy is that these drugs, which can produce significant health benefits, can be prohibitively expensive to the poor. TRIPS agreement does not completely prohibit the production of cheaper, generic substitutes for these drugs. It allows WTO members the right to grant a compulsory license to produce or import a patented product without the consent of the company holding the patent rights. The grant of a compulsory license, however, was difficult to provide under the terms of the agreement. The issue created a divide between MNCs and developed states, which are home to most of these MNCs, and NGOs and developing states, which claimed that the TRIPS agreement effectively promoted the interests of the market over human health. As Abbott (2005: 323) points outs, the pharmaceutical industry is highly concentrated. Control is dominated by companies located in only a few developed states, such as the United States, United Kingdom, Germany, Japan, and Switzerland. These states, especially the United States, which hosted most of the pharmaceutical companies holding patents, were the strongest supporters of patent protection (Abbott 2005). According to the NGO Oxfam, however, the trade association of pharmaceutical industries in the United States, the Pharmaceutical Research and Manufacturers of America (PhRMA), has a close and influential relationship with the Office of the United States Trade Representative (USTR) (Lanoszka 2003: 191).

The most significant action taken by MNCs to protect their patent rights was the decision of forty of these companies to initiate a lawsuit against the South African government in 1998 to prevent it from implementing legislation that would reduce the price of pharmaceuticals in that country. This lawsuit occurred after PhRMA had requested the USTR to respond against South Africa's legislation as a violation against TRIPS. Even though the USTR put pressure on South Africa, several pharmaceutical companies decided to go through with the lawsuit (Lanoszka 2003). As South Africa had one of the world's largest populations of victims of HIV/AIDS in the world, a coalition of NGOs began a global campaign through various forms of media including the Internet against these corporations. This coalition, known as the Treatment Access Campaign (TAC), was also permitted by South Africa's highest court to submit evidence of the pharmaceutical companies' research and development costs for drugs treating HIV/AIDS, as well as their expenses for marketing these drugs (Barnard 2002). In response to the growing negative publicity regarding the lawsuit, some pharmaceutical companies began to offer price discounts in South Africa. In fact, the cost of the triple-drug antiretroviral treatment per patient dropped by over 60 percent from 2000 to 2001 (Barnard 2002). Soon after, however, the pharmaceutical companies decided to dismiss the lawsuit.

As also noted in chapter 2, the momentum generated by TAC regarding the ethical dilemma of the TRIPS agreement and the fight against HIV/AIDS led to the adoption of the Doha Declaration, which in addition to affirming the rights of states to issue compulsory licenses for drug production allowed exports of the drugs to poorer states that do not have the capacity to produce such drugs on their own. Although the Doha Declaration served as a strike against the interests of pharmaceutical companies, the inclusion of TRIPS-plus provision in bilateral free trade agreements continued to allow them some intellectual property protection. Sell (2007) suggests that the close ties between PhRMA and the USTR has promoted a practice where the United States has aggressively pursued strong intellectual property rights protection as a condition for greater access to the American market. These provisions include such terms as prohibitions on use of test data; prohibition of parallel importation, which means that a U.S. patent holder would need to approve imports of generic versions of a drug from another country; more restrictive standards for granting compulsory licenses; and extensions for the term of patents beyond TRIPS agreement's twenty-year limit. According to Sell (2007: 60) many of these provisions were developed by major pharmaceutical companies. Because the TRIPS agreement allows agreements that provide more extensive intellectual property rights, the inclusion of these additional protections in free trade agreements are consistent with the TRIPS agreement, even though they may violate the spirit of the Doha Declaration. The result is that these agreements serve to reduce access to pharmaceuticals by making the production and distribution of generic drugs more difficult (Correa 2006). Because the pharmaceutical industry was still able to gain the support of the U.S. government, and to a significant extent, the European Union (EU) as well, they have been able to shield themselves against attempts by NGOs and developing states to counter their influence over drug prices.

Response to Tobacco Control

While the controversy over access to pharmaceuticals involves corporations trying to use the obligations in an international treaty to protect their interests, in the area of tobacco control, corporations are acting to weaken the implementation of a treaty, the Framework Convention on Tobacco Control (FCTC).

The development and the provisions of the FCTC, which was adopted by the WHO in 2003, are covered in more detail in chapter 6. The tobacco industry had long been a target of control since the mid-twentieth century due to the unhealthy nature of its product. Gostin (2014) describes these waves of lawsuits against tobacco companies in the United States. The first wave was from 1954 to 1973. The subject of this litigation focused on the relationship between the use of tobacco and lung cancer with the tobacco industry challenging the scientific findings that had established such a connection. The next wave of litigation was from 1983 to 1992. As scientific evidence linking tobacco use and poor health became more robust during this time, the tobacco industry began to rely more on the defense that smokers had assumed the risk of these problems by using tobacco products in these lawsuits. The third and current wave of litigation began in 1998 with the settlement of a lawsuit between the four largest tobacco companies in the United States with attorneys general from forty-six American states that required a release of confidential documents. Information in these documents revealed that these companies had knowingly acted to conceal the dangers of tobacco use to public and had used measures of deceit to challenge scientific findings that established a connection between tobacco use and ill health (Yach et al. 2007).

Three years prior to the third wave of litigation, the WHO had begun the initiation of an international treaty for tobacco control. The settlement of the lawsuit in 1998 and the release of the tobacco industry's internal documents proved to be quite damaging to the reputation of the industry. In 1999, the World Bank published a report finding that tobacco control would actually be economically beneficial, rather than harmful, for many countries. The combination of these events generated increased political will to support the WHO's proposal for the FCTC.

The tobacco industry, however, vociferously fought against this movement. Weishaar et al. (2012) discovered a comprehensive global campaign utilized by multinational tobacco corporations to undermine the FCTC negotiations. In their analysis, they divided the campaign by the multinational corporations into two parts: framing and tactics. Framing refers to how the tobacco industry wanted other actors to perceive the issue of tobacco control. The key frames used by the tobacco companies included (1) economic costs that would result from the FCTC; (2) tobacco control as an interest of rich countries that would be to the economic detriment of poorer states; (3) the FCTC as a conflicting standard with international trade; (4) the infringement that the FCTC, as adopted by the WHO, would pose on state sovereignty; and (5) corporate social responsibility and voluntary measures by the tobacco industry as a more effective alternative to tobacco control. To promote the adoption of these frames, multinational tobacco corporations invoked a number of different tactics. For instance, they targeted states such as Germany, Russia,

Turkey, and Spain, which they believed may be supportive of their position. They also hired scientists to promote their position and counter the report by the World Bank; recruited allies in other industries that could be adversely affected, such as the hospitality industry; invested more in advertising; and used the media, especially members who were strong advocates of free market practices in efforts to take a stand against the FCTC (Weishaar et al. 2012). Additionally, tobacco MNCs Philip Morris and R. J. Reynolds hired a public relations firm to gather intelligence and advise them on how to weaken civil society organizations promoting tobacco control (Carter 2002).

In recognition of the potential threat that the FCTC presented to profits of the sale of tobacco products, three of the world's largest tobacco corporations, British American Tobacco, Philip Morris, and Japan Tobacco International, began to develop an alternative regulatory scheme called Project Cerberus (Mamudu, Hammond, and Glantz 2008). This project was to promote voluntary standards for the industry in marketing tobacco, known as the International Tobacco Products Marketing Standards (ITPMS), which was announced in 2001. The motivation for Project Cerberus was to improve the public image of the tobacco industry, as well as to have a voice in process of global governance for tobacco control (Mamudu, Hammond, and Glantz 2008). The ITPMS developed by the tobacco industry included standards mostly aimed at preventing exposure of tobacco marketing to young people. Such restrictions included prohibitions on direct marketing to youth; prohibitions on marketing by television, radio, or in movie theaters; and enforcement of minimum age restrictions for the sale of tobacco products. Despite this announcement, officials at both the WHO and World Bank expressed skepticism as to the prospect of the tobacco industry being capable of self-regulation and rejected the ITPMS (Mamudu, Hammond, and Glantz 2008).

Despite the failure of the ITPMS and the adoption of the FCTC, the tobacco industry still managed to find ways to thwart the influence of international tobacco control. In particular, the tobacco industry has become more aggressive in challenging national tobacco control policies by the means of bilateral investment treaties (BITs). These agreements, which are negotiated between national governments, are designed to offer protection for foreign investment. BITs usually provide that subsidiaries of MNCs will receive the same treatment as national firms, they also tend to prohibit national requirements for restricting how MNCs can export or purchase goods, and they provide a means for dispute resolution between MNCs and their host state (Cohn 2016). Traditionally MNCs had utilized provisions of GATT/WTO as protection against efforts by national governments for tobacco control (Mamudu 2014). To use GATT/WTO rules to their advantage, their interests had to be supported by a national government on the basis that such control policies placed an undue burden on international trade.

After an unfavorable ruling from a GATT dispute settlement panel in 1990, tobacco corporations began to look to BITs as an alternative means to combat tobacco control (Mamudu 2014). The first use of a BIT was not until 2010, however, as Philip Morris International elected to directly challenge the tobacco control policy of Uruguay by filing a claim against the government of that country in the World Bank's International Center for Settlement of Investment Disputes (ICSID). Philip Morris, a Swiss MNC, argued that Uruguay's anti-tobacco legislation violated the 1998 BIT between Switzerland and Uruguay and harmed its investment in that country.

The next legal challenge for tobacco MNCs was Australia's plain packaging law, which was the first in the world to require tobacco products to be sold in undecorated packages with the inclusion of a graphic health warning. After a massive media campaign against the law by Big Tobacco, the "big five" largest global tobacco industry companies, some MNCs filed an unsuccessful lawsuit in the High Court of Australia claiming that the plain packaging law was unconstitutional (Gostin 2014). Big Tobacco was also able to convince Cuba, the Dominican Republic, Honduras, Indonesia, and Ukraine to file a complaint against Australia in the WTO on the grounds that plain packaging law violated TRIPS by preventing these MNCs from using their trademarks on their products. In 2011, Philip Morris Asia used the 1993 Hong Kong-Australia BIT to file a claim against Australia in the UN Commission on International Trade Law (UNCITRAL) on the grounds that the plain packaging law violated the BIT. Philip Morris Asia, in fact, moved its headquarters to Hong Kong to specifically challenge the Australian law in an international arbitration panel (Mamudu 2014). Australia successfully prevailed in the UNCITRAL dispute. (The WTO ruled in favor of Australia in June 2018.) This use of BITs, however, demonstrates the creativity and resilience of MNCs to continue to "game" the system of global governance and potentially combat international efforts at tobacco control despite international norms, the support of powerful IGOs (WHO and World Bank), and the majority of national governments to reduce the consumption of harmful tobacco products.

BOX 3.1 REGULATING THE FOOD INDUSTRY: HAS IT LEARNED LESSONS FROM TOBACCO?

The food industry has sought to avoid international regulation using many of the same tactics as the tobacco industry. Ken (2014) has argued that corporations have used tactics similar to social movement organizations in addressing the problem of childhood obesity. In particular, they emphasized framing the issue to fit their interest, a key tactic of NGOs, as a means to influence public discourse and behavior. When the food industry saw the anti-obesity movement as a potential threat to its profits, it has strategically turned to corporate social responsibility as a response. As Ken (2014: 132) states, these corporations have "skillfully positioned themselves as not as humble and contrite contributors to the problem but as saviors necessary for delivering Americans out of the prisons of their own bad choices." To maintain a positive public image the food industry has sought to legitimate itself by seeking to align itself with responsible stakeholders in the process such as health educators, schools, and doctors as part of a larger community fighting the obesity epidemic, particularly with children. In this manner they are seeking to avoid culpability for growth in obesity, while still focusing on maximizing profits by selling more "low-calorie," "reduced sugar," or "healthier" versions of certain foods rather than reducing their sales of those food products to the public (Ken 2014).

MNCs and Global Health Governance

The approaches offered by Levy and Prakash (2003), Fuchs (2007), and Detomasi (2007) all can account for the behavior of MNCs in the areas of access to pharmaceuticals and tobacco control. In both of these cases, the international community has developed agreements in the form of the Doha Declaration on the TRIPS Agreement and the FCTC, to address health concerns, which in turn, would negatively affect the profits of MNCs producing goods in these areas. Even as MNCs have objected to these agreements, a common response has been to frame themselves as "good" partners in the process and not as adversaries to public health. In the case of pharmaceuticals, MNC s have made the claim that their patents must be protected because these companies need to make some money from the sale of pharmaceuticals in order to further advance research and development to produce new and better drugs. For the sale of tobacco, MNCs have emphasized the economic benefits to national economies from their investments. They have also depicted themselves as socially responsible actors who can more effectively manage the consumption of tobacco through self-regulation rather than rules set by national governments.

Another common strategy of MNCs in these areas is to align themselves with other actors, most notably powerful states, to assist them in protecting against the loss of profits. These allies are susceptible to the interests of MNCs because they have been persuaded that the loss of profits by MNCs will also be economically detrimental to them as well. For example, bilateral trade and investment treaties have been used by MNCs to counter the effects of the Doha Declaration. Additionally, the tobacco industry has successfully lobbied the U.S. government to support its interests in the negotiations on the FCTC. Associating its business activities with strong neoliberal norms has been the most successful means for MNCs to fend off movements for international regulations to promote health.

In applying Levy and Prakash's (2003) framework, MNCs in these health-related areas clearly favor a global health regime that fits with market liberalization. They have utilized all the international legal tools that promote free markets, such as the WTO and various bilateral trade and investment agreements to maintain a place for free markets in global health. As Levy and Prakash (2003) and Fuchs (2007) note, however, the power of MNCs is constrained by that of other actors. MNCs have had to make some concessions, but their ability to receive some support from national governments has also helped in limiting the international community's efforts at regulating them, even for the cause of better global health. MNCs have been effective in using political lobbying and framing to influence other actors in global health governance to reconcile policy with corporate interests. Detomasi (2007) makes the case that collective action problems, such as global health, may be more effectively addressed with corporate participation. This may be true as MNCs have incentives to participate in global governance. It seems, however, that such involvement depends on whether corporations are willing to be genuine stakeholders in improving health, or whether their partnership is more of a facade to promote perceptions of their legitimacy. The effectiveness of this partnership may depend on the issue area. Past MNC behavior does lead to skepticism that corporations can be such genuine stakeholders, especially in the area of tobacco control where consumption of the product is inherently harmful.

NON-GOVERNMENTAL ORGANIZATIONS

The number of NGOs active in global politics has increased substantially. This is indicated by the growth in NGOs that have been granted consultative status with the UN's Economic and Social Council (ECOSOC). The UN granted such status to forty-one organizations in 1946. That number increased to over 3,500 by 2003 (Nowotny 2011). Currently well over 4,000 NGOs enjoy consultative status (NGO Branch, Office for ECOSOC Support and Coordination, and UN Department of Economic and Social Affairs 2018). The 1980s and 1990s, in particular, witnessed a substantial rise in the number of international NGOs.

An important question, of course, is what can account for this rising presence of NGOs in global governance? Reimann (2006) argues that three important trends in international politics since the 1980s explain the rapid expansion of NGOs: an increase in international political opportunities; pro-NGO norms; and the development of functional interdependence among NGOs, IGOs, and the states. In terms of political opportunities, she finds that in addition to more funding given to NGOs, IGOs have increasingly given access to NGOs as more policy issues have taken a transnational character. The expansion of the number of international treaties over the past thirty to forty years has created a greater need for IGOs to look to NGOs for support in governance. Since the 1990s, for example, the UN has made it easier for NGOs to attend the meetings of its General Assembly. Increases in the number of UN-sponsored conferences along with rules allowing greater NGO participation has also developed since the 1970s (Reimann 2006). Along with greater opportunity is the pro-NGO norms. According to this concept, the global shift toward neoliberal economic policy in the 1980s was accompanied by the idea that NGOs were part of the free market process. Even though NGOs are generally non-profit actors, in the post–Cold War era it became increasingly accepted that a strong civil society was necessary for democracy and open markets to be successful. The UN and financial institutions such as the World Bank were important actors in promoting this norm to national governments, particularly those in the developing world.

A broader view of the emergence of NGOs over time has been offered by Heins (2008). He argues that NGOs are the result of a causality of ultimate, intermediate, and proximate conditions. The ultimate conditions for the development of NGO are liberal states and suitable communications and transportation technologies. They are the most important factors for NGOs to function effectively. Historically, these conditions have been the strongest in the post–Cold War era. Democratic government and liberalism have been strengthening as norms in international politics since the 1990s. The technological revolution in the 1990s with the dissemination of Internet and wireless technology has made communication far easier and cheaper than at any point in human history. Both of these factors can be associated with the growth in the number of NGOs. In terms of intermediate conditions, he identifies the decline of the national interest and the rise of the moral public, both of which have also been more prevalent after the Cold War. He argues that over time, as states have become more developed they have become less interested in expanding their power and more interested in providing for the welfare of their people. Simultaneously, morality has been a rising norm as well as publics' expectations of greater protections for health, welfare, and values from their national government. The proximate conditions refer to the role of IGOs and the states. For IGOs, collaboration with NGOs can enhance the perception that they are moral, neutral, and expert actors. This perception may give them an advantage over states in promoting policies. States have a couple of different reasons to support NGOs. First, weaker states may need the assistance of NGOs to provide particular services to their population they may not be able to adequately supply. Second, more powerful states, especially liberal ones, see benefits in working with NGOs as they have encountered more pressure from their populations to solve social problems outside of their borders.

One issue in understanding the role of NGOs in global health governance is defining exactly what kind of actor qualifies as a NGO. While the UN Charter may have first used the term "non-governmental organization" in a legal sense, it did not define its meaning. In his survey of various definitions of NGOs used by other IGOs, Willetts (2011) finds some commonalities. These include the recognition that NGOs are independent from governments, and they are not engaged in making profits or commercial activities. They also must have some sort of a formal organizational structure.

Kaldor (2003: 79) identifies NGOs as a specific type of actor in the global civil society, which she defines as "the global process through which individuals debate, influence and negotiate an ongoing social contract or set of contracts with the centres of political and economic authority." Her first two types of global civil society actors are what she refers to as "old" and "new" social movements. These actors are more loosely organized than NGOs. The "old" social movements included a variety of organizations, groups, and individuals who favor more traditional causes such as worker's rights and self-determination. They also rely on tactics such as demonstrations and strikes. The "new" social movements differ in that they focus on more on social issues post-1970s, such as human rights and the environment. They rely more on the media to support their cause. Another type of actor is transnational civic networks. These networks connect NGOs, individuals, groups, and social movements to a particular issue. What distinguishes the NGO as a civil society actor is that it is structured on an organizational framework and has a more defined social role than social movements and civic networks.

The distinctive nature of the NGO as an actor in world politics is emphasized by Heins (2008) in constructing a definition of these organizations. He finds that three aspects of international NGOs, in particular, stand out in understanding their role. First, not only are NGOs independent from states, but they also do not wish to compete or share power with states. Their goal is to influence the preferences of the states so that they will be congruent with the NGO's interest. Second, NGOs speak for all individuals affected by a particular issue, not just members of the organization. Third, their interests are not constrained by borders but are universal in scope. Although he acknowledges that NGOs are similar to social movements, they differ in that NGOs provide a specific access point for individuals to support a particular cause.

In applying these different conceptualizations to understanding the role of NGOs in global governance, a common theme is that these actors are, by their very nature, much weaker than national governments. Due to their inherent weakness, perhaps the most important question regarding NGOs in global governance is can they make a difference? and if so how? Keck and Sikkink (1998) consider this question by examining NGOs as a central part of a transnational advocacy network. They suggest that such networks can potentially be effective at policy agenda-setting, persuading commitments from actors involved in policy-making, affecting policy outcomes at the national and international levels, and creating behavioral change. Whether or not such networks may be effective is dependent on certain variables. The variables revolve around characteristics of the source (e.g., network) and the target (e.g., the states). In terms of the source, the strength of the network and the nature of the issue are the most important factors. To affect behavioral change, networks must be able to convince states that its values fit with their interests. In particular, they refer to human rights issues, especially those involving physical harm, as having universal appeal. They must be able to frame an issue so that it fits a particular culture and belief system of the people of their target state. If the network lacks the strength to carry this out, or if the issue cannot adequately find a place in a belief system, then the network will most likely be unsuccessful. For the target, the two main factors are its political openness and its susceptibility to material and moral leverage. Even if a network is strong and its interests are culturally congruent with the people of a particular target state, if that state has restrictive policies for political expression and is not sensitive to how it perceived by others (e.g., North Korea) then the network will also be likely to be ineffective.

Both Heins (2008) and Sending and Neumann (2006) suggest that in conceptualizing the role of NGOs in global governance, it is important to take into account that NGOs are not seeking to directly challenge the power of national governments. They both do not find the basis of their political relationship to be a zero-sum game for policy outcomes. Heins uses the metaphor of a "parasitism" to explain how NGOs relate to states and IGOs. By this term, he means that NGOs serve to "infect" these more powerful actors with their beliefs (Heins 2008: 38). In this manner, they are attempting to change the behavior of the actors that make and implement policy. Sending and Neumann (2008) similarly argue that NGOs do not choose to challenge the power of the states. They are much more subtle actors. Their increasing influence in post–Cold War politics is due to how they have become not just objects but also subjects of government. This conceptualization means that governments are now acting through NGOs, not just exercising their political power over them. The activities of NGOs, whether they are providing information, providing policy advocacy, or mobilizing public opinion are part of, rather than in competition with, the state's governability of its people. Put another way, civil society and the government have become interconnected in the process of governing contemporary society. Governments need to collaborate with NGOs to assist in providing services and support their legitimacy. As Sending and Neumann (2008) note in their study of the international campaign to ban landmines, government officials in Norway found the expertise and the passion of NGOs to be valuable in formulating the national policy on the issue.

To further explore NGOs in the area of global health, two different types of NGOs will be analyzed. These NGOs are considered to be among the most powerful in global health. The first type will be multinational NGOs that are involved in health projects in developing states, Médecins Sans Frontières (MSF) and Oxfam International. The other type of NGO is the private foundation. In this case, the focus will be on the world's largest foundation for global health, the Bill and Melinda Gates Foundation. This analysis will examine the purposes and activities of these NGOs and consider their role and relative influence as actors in global health governance.

Médecins Sans Frontières (Doctors Without Borders)

Médecins Sans Frontières (Doctors Without Borders) is a multinational NGO that was founded in Paris in 1971 by a group of doctors inspired by their experiences in the Biafra War that took place in Nigeria during the late 1960s. These doctors wanted to create an independent organization that would provide medical aid to all persons regardless of their national boundaries. According to the MSF Charter, the organization adheres to five principles. These include medical ethics, independence of the organization from national governments and IGOs, neutrality, bearing witness or the right to speak out against undue suffering, and accountability (Médecins Sans Frontières 2014). While MSF was influenced by the neutrality of the International Committee of the Red Cross (ICRC) in providing medical care, it differed in that it also included a right to speak out against the practices of national governments. This right included the use of the media, if these governments contributed to undue suffering. In fact, the genesis of MSF can be traced to French Red Cross volunteers who publicly voiced objection to genocidal practices during the Biafra War (Davey 2011). MSF, however, also established itself as a human rights organization that would be ideologically neutral and would not be critical of governments or other organizations unless their policies were directly contributing to health hazards.

Although MSF declared itself to be a neutral organization, its principle of bearing witness was a challenge for an apolitical orientation. In 1979, its first president Bernard Kouchner supported a project to charter a boat to be used to rescue Vietnamese refugees who were fleeing their country through the South China Sea. Kouchner's expedition included members of the media to enhance its publicity. This venture developed into a schism within MSF over the interpretation of the Charter's provision for bearing witness. Kouchner believed that the promotion of symbolic actions such as the rescue of the Vietnamese "boat people" were part of "bearing witness." Most MSF members, especially younger members, disagreed with this view and believed that the organization's focus should be on the provision of medical services, and not more general humanitarian concerns. They believed MSF's function of bearing witness should be more constrained, and not used to promote media events. Kouchner and his supporters left MSF due to this disagreement and founded another organization known as Médecins du Monde (Doctors of the World) (Fox 2014).

Another political conflict occurred within MSF with its creation of the Liberté Sans Frontières Foundation (LSF) in 1984. Although the foundation was established to be a politically neutral research center for issues of human rights and development, in practice, LSF took an ideological stand against leftist ideology, communism, as well as authoritarian practices in third world countries (Davey 2011). This position by the LSF led to a dispute between MSF France, which was responsible for the creation of the LSF, and the MSF section in Belgium, which claimed that support of the LSF violated the neutrality provision in the MSF Charter. The dispute was intense enough that MSF France brought a lawsuit against MSF Belgium in an unsuccessful attempt to remove the MSF brand name from the Belgium section (Fox 2014). The most significant challenge for MSF's political neutrality, however, was the Ethiopian famine of 1984–1985. While several international humanitarian organizations, including MSF, provided relief assistance in Ethiopia, the Ethiopian government used the presence of these NGOs to legitimize its goal of moving people from northern to southern Ethiopia. Although northern Ethiopia was besieged by the famine, the government was also motivated by an opportunity to weaken opposition in the north (Fox 2014). Many Ethiopians died during the process of this relocation. By 1985 about as many died from this transfer has had died from the famine itself (Davey 2011: 548). MSF publicly spoke out against the Ethiopian government, and its members were expelled from that country soon after. MSF was the only humanitarian organization in Ethiopia to take such a stand against the government's practices during this time (Davey 2011).

The post–Cold War environment created an opportunity for MSF to reassess its balance between its principles of providing urgent medical assistance and speaking out against undue suffering. The experiences during the 1980s with the LSF and Ethiopia had politicized the organization as an anti-communist, anti-totalitarian actor (Fox 2014). In 1996, MSF adopted the Chantilly Agreement to reaffirm the principles of the MSF Charter. It did also, however, clarify that the primary purpose of MSF was to provide emergency medical care. The agreement still included MSF's principle of bearing witness as an important part of its mission. Although, the agreement did further establish that MSF members should refrain from speaking out in cases where their voices could be "manipulated" (Médecins Sans Frontières 1996). One important global health issue of the 1990s that MSF was open to speaking out against was the high cost of pharmaceutical drugs. MSF was one of the NGOs that participated in the TAC campaign opposing the lawsuit by pharmaceutical corporations against the South African government in 1998. While MSF was aligned with the TAC movement, it was still very wary of its independence. For example, MSF did not join TAC as plaintiffs in its lawsuit against the government of South Africa in a 2002 case to make the government approve a drug for prevention of mother-to-child transmission of HIV, although MSF did provide affidavits to support TAC's case (Fox 2014).

MSF was awarded the Nobel Peace Prize in 1999 for its record of humanitarian assistance around the world, further enhancing its status as an actor in global governance. The organization revisited its founding principles and system of operations at a conference in Luxembourg in 2006. MSF's position in regard to HIV/AIDS was particularly notable during the conference. The organization's most aggressive efforts at advocacy had been directed toward the access to essential medicines campaign. These efforts had produced some controversy within the organization because some members were concerned that its association with other NGOs and national governments to promote this cause might compromise the neutrality of MSF (Fox 2014). Despite this concern, MSF stood by its advocacy function for prevention and treatment of AIDS as part of its principle of bearing witness and speaking out against undue suffering. The conference led to the adoption of the La Mancha Agreement, which reaffirmed the MSF Charter and Chantilly Agreement as well as emphasizing that the governance of MSF as an organization would be based on the accountability and transparency of all MSF sections as well as accountability for staff members. In addition to its relief services and humanitarian assistance, in terms of global health governance, MSF is most often associated with international efforts to promote access to pharmaceuticals. Multinational corporations and national governments, however, have not been the only targets of MSF's function of bearing witness. MSF has in the past directed some criticism toward the WHO. Such was the case when MSF claimed that the WHO's tuberculosis control strategy had been inadequate in detecting the number of persons with the disease (Ahmad 2004).

MSF faced one of its greatest challenges with the 2014–2015 Ebola crisis in West Africa. According to Pagano and Poncin (2017), this crisis pushed

MSF to broaden its activities from operational assistance in the treatment of patients to that of a technical advisor, a role that would be expected to be provided by the WHO. Due to dysfunctional healthcare systems and corruption in the affected countries, and the slow response of the WHO to the outbreak, MSF began to play a lead role in coordinating a response with high-level officials in the national governments. This was an unusual role for MSF, but these governments turned to MSF's support because of "the organization's past experience with the virus, WHO technical and political missteps that failed to give direction or coordinate with other actors, and the fact that the epidemic was labeled as a health crisis rather than a humanitarian crisis" (Pagano and Poncin 2017: 43). This case demonstrates how NGOs can play an important role and fill gaps in global health governance, especially when IGOs and states may not be capable of addressing global health problems adequately on their own.

Oxfam International

Oxfam is another multinational humanitarian NGO that has significant involvement in global health. It differs from MSF in that it focuses its attention more on charitable, grant-making activities in addition to relief work. It is also an older organization than MSF, which was born during the political environment of the latter half of the Cold War. Oxfam originated from the events of World War II. A group of individuals in Britain became alarmed at the mounting starvation in Greece after it became occupied by German forces in 1941. Further exacerbating the problem was the refusal by the British government to permit goods to be exported to these occupied areas. In 1942, a national Famine Relief Committee was established by these private individuals to gather information about food supply in German-occupied areas, provide food to these areas, and establish a fund to finance such efforts (Black 1992). Their dilemma, of course, was how to provide famine relief to Greece without violating the British blockade. In October 1942, a branch of the Famine Relief Committee was formed in Oxford, England, as the Oxford Committee for Famine Relief. As the committee had some success in raising funds, its lobbying efforts proved to be unpersuasive in convincing the British government to lift its blockade during the war. After the war, however, the Oxford Committee for Famine Relief accelerated its activities and was a major contributor for relief funds to post-war Europe prior to the assistance from the Marshall Plan in 1948 (Black 1992).

Despite the recovery of Europe in the late 1940s, the committee was determined to continue its work, while other post-war relief agencies decided to end their operations. The organization viewed its next purpose to go beyond Europe and assist with war and disaster relief in other parts of the world. The

Oxford Committee began its first humanitarian operation in a developing country in 1951 with famine relief in Bihar, India. In 1953, the committee provided its first relief efforts for a natural disaster by assisting with the recovery of the Ionian Islands in Greece after they had been struck by an earthquake. By 1970, the Oxford Committee for Famine Relief established its first international office in Canada and changed the official name of the organization to Oxfam.

Oxfam began to move beyond relief work and financial assistance to examining the problem of economic development and poverty in the world to be related to the policies of global economic institutions in the 1980s (Aaronson and Zimmerman 2006). Oxfam grew as an organization and become a more active participant in global health governance in the 1990s with two strategic plans. The first plan was based on consolidating the various sections of Oxfam around the world and building the foundation for Oxfam International, which was established in 1995 as an international secretariat for all of these Oxfam affiliates. Prior to this point, most sections of Oxfam were established independently from the British headquarters and had different perspectives on how to address various global problems (Black 1992). The consolidation mostly benefited Oxfam Great Britain as it was placed as the center organization for Oxfam International in framing global issues (Stroup 2012). The second plan adopted by Oxfam soon thereafter was to address global inequality by focusing political attention on the structural causes of poverty, help individuals exercise their political rights, and to protect poor individuals from the potential harmful effects of free markets (Aaronson and Zimmerman 2006).

One of the major objectives of Oxfam in promoting economic equality was to join with MSF and other NGOs in supporting greater access to pharmaceuticals to the world's poor and participate in the campaign against pharmaceutical MNCs to drop their lawsuit for patent protection in South Africa. Additionally, Oxfam promoted a petition against the TRIPS Agreement and its intellectual property protections that maintained the high cost of drugs. These events led to the promulgation of the Doha Declaration in 2001. Aaronson and Zimmerman (2006: 1015) suggested that "Oxfam's early work in this area shamed and pressured policymakers in other member states to address these concerns and perhaps made these governments more amenable to amending the WTO."

After Doha, Oxfam turned its efforts to focus more on a broader connection between trade policy and economic development. Oxfam promoted reforms such as limits on intellectual property protection, public health as a priority over free trade, and more special protections for developing states under the WTO's rules (Aaronson and Zimmerman 2006). Much of Oxfam's position has been based on its view of "fair trade," meaning the trade needs to be more balanced in that it is essentially controlled by rich states under the current system. Rich states have a number of advantages over poor states under international trade rules, such as utilizing trade rules to open the markets of poor states to their exported goods while not providing the same market access in return (Oxfam International 2014a). This lack of balance in trade relationships contributes to the problem of poverty and its related health issues in developing states.

Agriculture has been a particular sore point for Oxfam, as well as many developing countries, in that rich states continue to provide subsidies to their farmers, which makes it difficult for developing countries, home to 96 percent of the world's farmers, to penetrate their markets (Aaronson and Zimmerman 2006: 1019). Even during its "fair trade" campaign, Oxfam has continued to advocate for reforms on global health issues. In particular, Oxfam has promoted the position that health care is a fundamental right and that more money needs to be spent on public services rather than health care by the private sector (Oxfam International 2014b). In addition, affordable access to pharmaceuticals and treatment and care of individuals with HIV/AIDS continue to be important components of Oxfam's campaign in global health governance.

Bill and Melinda Gates Foundation

Private foundations are non-state actors and part of civil society, but they differ from NGOs such as MSF and Oxfam in that they are exclusively grant-making organizations that are not directly involved in operations or relief work. They also draw their funding from private wealth rather than the receipt of charitable donations. According to Anheier and Daly (2005), foundations serve the purposes of assisting governments or even substituting for governments in providing public goods, preserving traditions and culture, redistributing resources to poorer populations, promoting social change, and investing in risky ventures that may have difficulty in attracting financial capital but may also present the potential for high rewards. Moran and Stevenson (2013) make the case that private foundations serve an important function in global governance in that they can provide resources to help in alleviating the failure of the state and the market to care for disadvantaged populations. In this manner, they can contribute to the efforts of global governance in addressing collective action problems, such as global health, that national governments may have difficulty providing on their own due to lack of resources, political will, or a breakdown in cooperation.

The Bill and Melinda Gates Foundation stands out as the world's most prominent private foundation for global health. In 2016, the Gates Foundation provided over US$3 billion in grants, with US$1.2 billion spent on global health projects (Bill and Melinda Gates Foundation 2016). Within its first decade, the Gates Foundation became a larger donor for global health than all national governments except for the United States and the United Kingdom (McCoy et al. 2009a). The Bill and Melinda Gates Foundation began in 1999 when Bill and Melinda Gates decided to merge the William H. Gates Foundation and the Gates Learning Foundation to provide an even greater philanthropic effort toward global health and education, making it the wealthiest private foundation in the United States (*New York Times* 1999). In early 2000, the Bill and Melinda Gates Foundation became the world's most wealthy private foundation with assets over US$21.8 billion (Forero 2000). It launched its largest global health program toward a single country when in 2002 the foundation pledged to give US$100 million to India to combat HIV/AIDS (Waldman 2002). Even with its considerable wealth, the Gates Foundation received a significant boost in its funds with a pledge of a US$31 billion gift from investor Warren Buffet in 2006, which almost equaled the total wealth of the foundation at that time (McNeil and Lyman 2006). By 2014, the Gates Foundation had more than three times the wealth than any other philanthropic organization in the world, with an endowment of over US$40 billion (Smith 2014). Youde (2013) points out a number of benefits that the Bill and Melinda Gates Foundation has provided to promote global health. These include giving greater publicity to health problems in developing countries, especially neglected diseases that have not received much attention or financial support. Additionally, the foundation's investment in research and technology has contributed to the development of the production of drugs and vaccines needed to combat a variety of global diseases. In addition to making funding providing over for HIV/AIDS as a priority of the foundation, Bill Gates has also called on plans for a global eradication of both malaria and polio.

Despite the substantial funds that the Bill and Melinda Gates Foundation has contributed to global health, concerns have been raised to its role in influencing the global health agenda. Not only is the Gates Foundation the wealthiest philanthropic organization in the world, but it also has members who also sit on the governing bodies of many global health partnerships (McCoy 2009b). The head of the WHO's malaria program wrote a memorandum in 2008, in which he expressed his view that the dominance of the foundation in funding malaria research could contribute to it taking the lead in global health policy toward combating malaria (McNeil 2008). According to McNeil (2008) in regard to the Gates Foundation, "some scientists have said privately that it is creating its own WHO." Additionally, the preference of the Gates Foundation for emphasizing technological solutions to solve health problems over social determinants of health has also raised uneasiness about its influence (Birn 2005; McCoy et al. 2009b). Transparency of the organization may also be an issue. According to McCoy et al. (2009b: 1650),

"Grant making by the Gates Foundation seems to be largely managed through an informal system of personal networks and relationships rather than by a more transparent process based on independent and technical peer review."

These concerns are emblematic of the fact that the Bill and Melinda Gates Foundation has substantially more funds to spend on global health than the WHO, the world's lead IGO for global health. Its substantial wealth and activity provide it with significant influence as an actor in global health governance. In addition to its wealth, the Gates Foundation is also in position to shape global health policy by its ability to finance research and programs that will fit its vision of global health (Eckl 2014). In his study of the Gates Foundation and malaria, Eckl (2014) found that the Gates Foundation was successful in pressuring representatives of the public sector, including the Director-General of the WHO, to follow its lead in calling for the eradication of the disease. Eradication was a strategy that the WHO had abandoned since the 1970s when it began its focus on control of malaria. Eckl (2014) found the influence of the Gates Foundation to be remarkable not only because the organization is not a formal actor in global policy-making, but the feasibility of an eradication program was still highly contested, and other actors failed previously to convince public sector representatives to return to malaria eradication. Nevertheless, the position of the Gates Foundation was given significant weight in both the WHO and the Roll Back Malaria partnership. Because the Gates Foundation is a private actor without direct accountability to any national governments, its growing influence does raise interesting questions as to how much power it will assume in global governance and will solutions for global health problems become driven more by private actors?

Even though it does not seem to be the intention of the Gates Foundation, or any other philanthropic organization, to become such a power in global health policy, it may be an unintended consequence if its funding for global health continues to rise in relation to overall spending by national governments and IGOs. Whether private foundations provide an important role in resolving collective action in global health as suggested by Moran and Stevenson (2013), or whether their increasing influence contributes to more of a "democratic deficit" and elitist decision-making in global health policies, the rise of the Bill and Melinda Gates Foundation in only the last fifteen years has clearly made private foundations important actors in twenty-first century global health.

NGOs and Global Health Governance

In studies of NGOs in international politics, two aspects of NGOs that frequently receive attention are power and independence. As noted by Heins (2008) and Sending and Neumann (2006) NGOs are weaker than states, and as a result, they tend to not directly compete with them for power. The cases of MSF and Oxfam support this view. When these NGOs have exercised their advocacy function, it has been primarily for the purpose of persuading states to align with their interests rather than using coercive measures that they are not equipped to implement. The use of direct power by NGOs is more effective against MNCs. As indicated in the case of access to pharmaceuticals, TAC as a transnational network of NGOs that included MSF and Oxfam, was effective in challenging the efforts of MNCs to use TRIPS and the WTO to maintain the high cost of drugs. A potential problem, of course, that also manifested itself during the campaign is that MNCs can be supported by powerful states, which makes it much more difficult for NGOs and transnational networks to change policy. Because NGOs, even multinational ones such as MSF and Oxfam, lack the economic resources of states and MNCs they must rely on soft power to influence the global health agenda. In this manner, NGOs need to promote themselves as neutral and moral actors to convince states, MNCs, and global populations that their interests are "the right thing to do" to benefit humankind. As a result, NGOs need to be fiercely protective of their image.

The case of MSF indicates how maintaining such legitimacy can be a challenge. MSF has had a long history of balancing its neutral position with its principle of speaking out against undue suffering. At the same time MSF has consistently emphasized its independence, and places advocacy as much less of a priority as Oxfam as it has concentrated on its relief activities as its primary focus (Stroup 2012). Oxfam, as well, has faced a challenge in defending its neutrality. The organization has faced criticisms that despite its anti-free trade position, it is often closely aligned with the British government (Quarmby 2005). Stroup (2012) credits Oxfam's engagement with the government as part of the practice of politics in Britain where the government encourages some collaboration with NGOs as a limited partnership. This practice is not the same in MSF's home base of France where MSF and the French government have not had a particularly cordial relationship. International NGOs are challenged by their relative weakness, uncertain financing, and lack of direct accountability. Maintaining a reputation as independent, "do-gooder" organizations is critical for these organizations to have influence in global governance. MSF and Oxfam serve as examples of NGOs with strong reputations in global health, which greatly contributes to their notable position in its governance.

The factors of power and independence have a different dynamic with the Bill and Melinda Gates Foundation. For a non-commercial, non-state actor, the Gates Foundation is exceptionally powerful in global health. While it does not directly compete with states for power, it provides more funds for global health than any other actor besides the United States. The main limitation of the power of the Gates Foundation is that it does not directly engage in political lobbying and advocacy for specific health policies in the manner of many health-related NGOs such as Oxfam. Its decisions on what health initiatives to fund, however, can be very influential in shaping the global health agenda. As a privately funded actor, the Gates Foundation also has an advantage in maintaining its independence. Even though McCoy et al. (2009b) found the Gates Foundation to be influenced by personal relationships, its exceptional wealth greatly diminishes the prospects that its interests will be entangled with that of a national government.

In addition to having capacity for hard power due to its economic resources, the Gates Foundation also has soft power based upon the moral objectives of its spending. The main weakness of the legitimacy, however, for the Gates Foundation is not its neutrality or morality, rather it is its accountability. Bill and Melinda Gates are two of the three chairs (along with William H. Gates Sr.) of the Gates Foundation. They are also two of its three trustees (along with Warren Buffet). Such an elite group of executive decision-making does lead to concern that the Gates Foundation is dictating policies important to issues in global health without much inclusion of relevant stakeholders. To its credit, the Gates Foundation has addressed this accountability issue by participating in a number of partnership arrangements with representatives of national governments, IGOs, and NGOs. Nevertheless, the Gates Foundation is still an independent actor that does not directly depend on the support of a particular constituency to take action.

GLOBAL HEALTH PUBLIC-PRIVATE PARTNERSHIPS

In addition to distinguishing between MNCs and NGOs, a hybrid actor based on a partnership between the public and private sectors has also become part of global health governance. Global health public-private partnerships (GHPPPs) are relatively new mechanisms having emerged during the mid-1990s. Buse and Walt (2000: 550) define GHPPPs as "a collaborative relationship which transcends national boundaries and brings together at least three parties, among them a corporation (and/or industry association) and an IGO, so as to achieve a shared health-creating goal on the basis of a mutually agreed division of labour." Such collaboration, however, was very limited until the 1980s. The emergence of neoliberalism during this decade was a factor as international organizations, especially the World Bank, became more open to working with private sector actors.

Health, in particular, proved to be a fertile ground for such cooperation due to three factors according to Buse and Walt (2000). First was that public and private sector actors saw great benefits for collaboration. The UN viewed partnering with the private sectors as a means of enhancing its profile in an international system that had a strong norm of free market economics, while the private sector saw the public sector as a means of alleviating potential negative consequences of free market policies on health, such as the manufacturing and sale of pharmaceuticals. Corporate social responsibility can also be considered as part of the motivation for the private sector in these partnerships. Second, a loss of confidence in the UN and its agencies, such as UNICEF, in effectively addressing global health problems was also an incentive for the emergence of GHPPPs. Third, the scope of global health is so broad and involves so many dimensions that it was increasingly viewed as an area that needs participation of a number of different actors to effectively resolve global health problems (Buse and Walt 2000).

GAVI Alliance

Two of the most prominent GHPPPs in global health governance are the GAVI Alliance and the Global Fund to Fight AIDS, Tuberculosis, and Malaria (GFATM). Both GAVI and GFATM are part of the Health Eight (H8) of global health institutions, a group formed in 2007 to help reach the objectives of the UN's Millennium Development Goals. The other institutions that are members of the H8 include UNICEF, the United Nations Population Fund (UNPFA), UNAIDS, and the Bill and Melinda Gates Foundation. The GAVI Alliance, which began as the Global Alliance for Vaccines and Immunizations, was established in 2000 at the World Economic Forum in Davos, Switzerland, after the Gates Foundation pledged US$750 million over five years to join in a partnership with the World Bank, the WHO, and UNICEF to provide vaccines to poor children in developing countries (GAVI Alliance 2018a).

GAVI is currently in phase four of its strategy, which runs from 2016 to 2020, to fulfill its overall mission. In its current phase, GAVI's goals are to (1) increase the use of and coverage of vaccines, (2) improve the delivery of immunizations, (3) improve immunization programs of national governments, and (4) try to influence the market so that vaccines can be readily available at a low cost for the world's poor (GAVI Alliance 2018b). GAVI estimates that in 2016, it has supported the vaccination of 62 million children, and its support has contributed to avoiding the loss of 1.2 million lives in 2016 through its campaigns (GAVI Alliance 2018c). As a GHPPP, GAVI's board includes members of both public and private sectors. In addition to permanent seats given to its original members: World Bank, WHO, UNICEF, and the Gates Foundation, GAVI also has a third of its board from independent individuals who are selected on the basis of their personal skills rather than institutional representation (Lob-Levyt 2011). Another important aspect of GAVI's function is its innovative financing. One of GAVI's funding mechanisms is the International Finance Facility for Immunization (IFFIm), which was based on the sale of bonds that are guaranteed by long-term commitments from donors in private capital markets. Its other innovative funding mechanism is the Advanced Market Commitment (AMC). This mechanism is based on pledges made by donors as a financial incentive for drug manufacturers to invest resources in research and production of vaccines for diseases that are endemic in poorer countries. These mechanisms provide resources for GAVI to offer greater support for the failure of the marketplace to provide global coverage of immunizations against preventable diseases.

The Global Fund for AIDS, Tuberculosis, and Malaria

The Global Fund for AIDS, Tuberculosis, and Malaria (GFATM), which is also highlighted in chapter 4, was established in 2002 as a funding mechanism to combat three of the world's deadliest diseases: AIDS, tuberculosis, and malaria. According to Bartsch (2007), three factors supported the establishment of GFATM. The first was a change in international norms by the late 1990s. The international community, especially developed states, was beginning to realize that neoliberal economic policies were not improving health in the world's poorest countries. The World Bank's study in 1993 that highlighted a connection between health and economic development encouraged states to devote more attention to health on the global agenda. Second was a growing perception that infectious diseases represented a security threat, and third, the interest of states, in particular the United States and Japan, to develop a new institution to address global health that would be outside of the UN and its agencies, in particular the WHO and UNICEF. Effective lobbying by NGOs led to a significant representation of civil society as part of the structure of GFATM (Bartsch 2007).

The governing board of GFATM was designed to include twenty members. Three of these seats went to civil society actors with one member representing an NGO from a developed state; one member representing an NGO from a developing state; and one private individual that is afflicted with AIDS, tuberculosis, or malaria. National governments have fifteen seats, with six seats going to major donors and nine seats divided by geographic regions. The private sector and private foundations have one seat each. All members of the board have one vote. The WHO, World Bank, and UNAIDS are included but as non-voting members. GFATM also has links to civil society through its country coordinating mechanisms (CCMs). These committees are responsible for developing grant proposals to submit to GFATM. CCMs are required to include individuals who have one of the three diseases, and 40 percent of its membership must be from civil society. Despite these attempts at creating a partnership that includes states, civil society, and the private sector, in practice, donor states have had much more influence of the Global Fund's meetings. In fact, according to Brown (2010: 523), "the process no longer resembles a process of mutual understanding and consensus formation, but one of multilateral power politics as usual." Even within several CCMs, government officials tend to be dominant influences over civil society representatives in decision-making (Gostin 2014). In 2012, the Global Fund adopted organizational reforms and approved a new funding model to be more responsive and more financially efficient.

According to GFATM, its efforts have been of significant value in combating AIDS, tuberculosis, and malaria. From its establishment in 2002 until 2016, it provided US$32.6 billion to support programs for HIV, tuberculosis, and malaria. Overall, GFATM claims that it has contributed to saving well over 22 million lives from these diseases since its inception (Global Fund for AIDS, Tuberculosis, and Malaria 2017). Despite its notable achievements, obtaining funding has been challenging for GFATM as it relies on voluntary contributions. In terms of funds, the U.S. government often provides about a third of its donations and not coincidently, tends to take an interest in its decision-making (Clinton and Sridhar 2017). In comparison, GAVI has not had as much difficulty due to its sale of bonds and the fact that it does not require as much funding as GFATM to reach its goals (Gostin 2014). Nevertheless, GAVI relies more on the Bill and Melinda Gates Foundation for financial support than GFATM (Clinton and Sridhar 2017).

Challenges for Global Health Partnerships

Although GHPPPs provide a great opportunity for effective global health governance by bringing together actors from states, corporations, and private foundations, as well as civil society, these relatively new institutions face some significant obstacles. Such issues include weak structures of governance and a lack of transparency and accountability (Baggott 2013). The potential influence of the private sector also raises concerns, especially as to how corporate partners could use their financial power in these partnerships to dictate the global health agenda. Another significant concern is whether corporate partners have genuine intentions to improve global health, or is their participation more selective and driven by corporate social responsibility motives to enhance their public image and commercial appeal.

A study by Buse and Harmer (2007) found several practices by GHPPPs that limit their effectiveness. One is that the priorities of GHPPPs may not be the same as the countries that they are trying to help. GHPPPs have a tendency to desire a fast response to a specific health problem as means to publicly demonstrate their accomplishments. Technological responses that target a particular infectious disease tend to fit this results-oriented approach. This type of response, however, may not necessarily be suitable for the perspective, planning, and budgeting of a particular state's national health ministry. Another problem is that they may not adequately incorporate the interests of the people most affected by a particular health problem. As mentioned previously, GFATM has often been driven by the interests of the donor states rather than the recipients. They also regard the weakening influence of public agencies such as the WHO in favor of the private sector as another negative aspect of some GHPPPs. Inadequate financing and the corresponding heavy reliance on funding from the Bill and Melinda Gates Foundation is also viewed as problematic. Good governance, especially in terms of monitoring and transparency, is a key component to improve the effectiveness of these institutions. More funding and resources, as well as a greater voice in policy-making by major stakeholders (i.e., poor countries and affected populations), are also suggested as actions GHPPPs should take to have a more positive impact on global health.

NON-STATE ACTORS, GLOBAL HEALTH GOVERNANCE, AND INTERNATIONAL RELATIONS THEORY

A variety of entities with different interests and roles such as MNCs, NGOs, private foundations, and GHPPPs fit under a broad umbrella of non-state actors in global health governance. The primary interest of MNCs is to maximize their profits and often promote open markets over state regulation. NGOs, in contrast, are not motivated by generating wealth. Their objective is to promote a special interest, which in global health governance is the provision of health as a public good. To achieve their objectives, NGOs must frequently call upon states to provide regulation over the market because the market leaves many individuals in the world without protection for their health. Private foundations, while not profit-maximizing actors, use corporate wealth to assist states in providing health as a global public good. GHPPPs fill in gaps in global governance and combine corporate wealth and private funding with the advice and expertise of the public sector and civil society. The role and influence of these actors is viewed in different ways by various theories of international relations.

As noted in chapters 1 and 2, the state-centric nature of realism makes that perspective very skeptical as to the influence of any of these non-state actors. Even though this same claim was made in chapter 2 in regard to IGOs, realists tend to pay even less attention to non-state actors because they have much less of an affiliation with national governments. Of these actors, MNCs would seem to be the most prominent to realists because they have some hard power in terms of economic resources. Realists, however, tend to argue that MNCs benefit from a supportive economic system that is established by a hegemonic state, and these firms are not independent actors but are products of their home state (Gilpin 2001). In this view, realists assume that for MNCs to have influence in global health governance, their actions must have some support by powerful states. Because NGOs lack hard power, realists would find their role to be rather insignificant in global health governance. For example, even though NGOs were highly visible in the Access to Medicines Campaign and the successful development of the Doha Declaration, realists would attribute this resolution more to change in the preferences of powerful states, especially the United States and members of the EU, rather than an influential social movement (Drezner 2007). Realists would also point out that the legal gains promoted by civil society actors for both access to pharmaceuticals and tobacco control have been mitigated by states through bilateral trade and investment agreements.

Neoliberal institutionalists are more open to the prospect that non-state actors are key components of global health governance. Their focus on international cooperation, however, is also fairly state-centric. Negotiations by states leading to developments in international law and IGOs would be driving factors in global health through an institutionalist perspective. The regime theory variant of liberalism does allow space for NGOs' contribution to the rules, norms, and principles of global governance by noting that regimes are composed of actors in general, not just state. At the same time, the ambiguity of regime theory does not account for the specific role that non-state actors play in maintaining a regime. Overall, liberal theories of international relations acknowledge that non-state actors are relevant to global health governance. Studies supporting neoliberal institutionalism, however, emphasize states and IGOs as the major actors.

The clarification of the role of non-state actors in global governance has more promise from a constructivist perspective. Non-state actors promote certain norms in their interactions within the context of global health governance. MNCs promote neoliberal values to both state and non-state actors, while NGOs like MSF and Oxfam promote the humanitarian aspects of global health policies. Because constructivists view all aspects of international politics as shaped by norms, identity, and social learning, they would consider that non-state could be significant sources for establishing these features within global health governance. In terms of examples, constructivists could point to NGOs' successful promotion of norms for greater access to pharmaceuticals and tobacco control as significant changes in global health that can be in large part attributed to civil society organizations. Simultaneously, the furtherance of neoliberal norms by MNCs has made it difficult for global health policies to be adopted that may be unduly restrictive on international commerce.

As previously mentioned, Marxism and its variations view non-state actors in the context of an international system based on capitalism and dominated by neoliberal ideology. MNCs are particularly important actors in international politics because they are major vehicles for promoting and sustaining the capitalist economic system. They prioritize profit maximization and open markets over health. To this end, MNCs pressure states to support their objectives, especially when they conflict with the interests of civil society. While NGOs may provide advocacy for populations suffering from poor health conditions, their efforts are constrained by market forces and strong political support for neoliberal economic policies. NGOs may make some minimal progress when MNCs and core capitalist economies believe that improving efforts at global health might help in promoting capitalism, but they will be unable to affect major changes in policy. The FCTC represents such an example. Although its adoption was a political victory for the WHO and civil society organizations, the fact that the treaty did not address trade and that in practice its rules have been circumvented by bilateral trade and investment treaties demonstrates a limitation on using international law to improve global health. Marxists would also tend to be skeptical about GHPPPs. In particular, they would be concerned that these institutions represent an effort by the private sector to assume some of the control over the global health agenda from public institutions such as the WHO and UNICEF.

CONCLUSION

For the most part, non-state actors have not played much of a role in global governance until after World War II. These actors are particularly active in the area of health because many states in the world lack the resources and capacity to provide a good quality of health for all of their people. Multinational corporations, NGOs, private foundations, and global health public-private partnerships (GHPPPs) have taken a much more influential role in global health governance in the post–Cold War era. These actors, however, perform different functions in global health. They also contribute to both the opportunities and obstacles in making the world healthier. MNCs provide research and development for new medicines that can combat some of the world's deadliest diseases. At the same time, the profit motive of MNCs frequently comes into conflict with the interests of civil society and the WHO in providing the best health care for all. NGOs provide much needed relief work and services, as well as a voice in global governance for poor populations. Their efforts, however, are constrained by a lack of resources and limited power.

Since 2000 with the rise of the Bill and Melinda Gates Foundation, private foundations now play an unprecedented role in global health by proving a greater source of financing than ever before. Despite its generous contribution, concerns remain that the Gates Foundation lacks accountability and transparency in its decision-making and may be becoming too powerful an actor in global health. GHPPPs provide an innovative structure to promote cooperation and collaboration between the public and private sector, but they too may be negatively affected by public and corporate interests. For global health governance to be effective, states, IGOs, and these non-state actors must find ways to work collectively and manage their individual deficiencies.

The different theories of international relations have different perspectives on how non-state actors fit within global governance. Realists argue that they are largely irrelevant actors. States, especially the more powerful ones, control the global health agenda. Neoliberal institutionalists believe that non-state actors have an important role. Their analyses, however, tend to reveal that they find that interactions between states and the use of international law and organizations are the driving forces behind global health policy. Constructivism is the most amenable to the prospect that non-state actors are a critical part of global health governance. They can function as norm entrepreneurs and persuade states and individuals that health should be given a higher priority in global politics. Marxist approaches find fault with MNCs and global capitalism as major causes for why health has not been adequately provided to the world's poor. While NGOs may have good intentions in addressing the failure of the market to sufficiently improve health, they are effectively constrained by capitalism both as a structuring force of the international system and as a dominant ideology.

DISCUSSION QUESTIONS

1. How powerful are multinational corporations as actors in global governance? In particular, what role do they play in global health?
2. Why has the number of non-governmental organizations (NGOs) in world politics grown substantially over time? Why have NGOs been so active in global health?
3. What is the role of private foundations in global health governance? Is the Bill and Melinda Gates Foundation a principal actor in global health? Why or why not?
4. What is a public-private partnership? What are the strengths and weaknesses of these actors in global health?
5. Are non-state actors become more powerful relative to states in global health?

SUGGESTED READINGS

Clinton, Chelsea, and Devi Sridhar. 2017. *Governing Global Health: Who Runs the World and Why?* New York: Oxford University Press.

Provides a good analysis of the role of public-private partnerships in global health with a focus on the GAVI Alliance and the Global Fund for AIDS, Tuberculosis, and Malaria.

Fox, Renee. 2014. *Doctors Without Borders: Humanitarian Quests, Impossible Dreams of Médecins Sans Frontières*. Baltimore, MD: Johns Hopkins University Press.

A comprehensive study of the history and culture of Médecins Sans Frontières.

Fuchs, Doris. 2007. *Business Power in Global Governance*. Boulder, CO: Lynne Rienner.

A comprehensive analysis of the role of multinational corporations in global governance.

Heins, Volker. 2008. *Nongovernmental Organizations in International Society: Struggle over Recognition*. New York: Palgrave Macmillan.

Provides a good theoretical and empirical analysis of the role of NGOs in world politics.

Chapter 4

Controlling Infectious Diseases: Malaria, Tuberculosis, and HIV/AIDS

Historically, the main focus of global health governance has been the control of infectious diseases (also known as communicable diseases). This focus remains today as most political attention and funding for global health initiatives are directed toward these diseases, especially the "big three" of malaria, tuberculosis, and HIV/AIDS. These three diseases stand out in discussions of global health because they rank among the leading causes of death worldwide (World Health Organization 2008a). In September 2000, the United Nations (UN) adopted the Millennium Declaration, in which the members of the UN agreed to achieve the objectives of the Millennium Development Goals (MDGs) by 2015. One of the MDGs was directed at infectious diseases, specifically to combat HIV/AIDS, malaria, and other communicable diseases. As their inclusion indicates, the actors involved in global health governance have an especially strong consensus in controlling infectious diseases, especially the "big three." After significant progress in combating infectious disease under the MDG targets, the Sustainable Development Goals (SDGs) succeeded the MDGs with a broader set of goals to be achieved by 2030. In addition to calling for the end of the epidemics of AIDS, tuberculosis, and malaria, a target of the SDGs was to end the epidemic of neglected tropical diseases by 2030 as well. The appropriate policies to accomplish this task and the necessary funding, however, continue to be a challenge.

According to the World Health Organization (WHO), tuberculosis was the ninth leading global cause of death in 2015, contributing to 1.4 million deaths. HIV/AIDS was not among the top ten global causes of death in that year, but it was still responsible for 1.1 million deaths (World Health Organization 2017b). Infectious diseases, along with maternal and prenatal complications, as well as nutrition deficiencies, are a particularly common cause of death in the world's poorest countries. In 2015, 52 percent of deaths in low-income countries were due to these causes compared to only 7 percent in high-income countries (World Health Organization 2017b).

While chronic diseases have significant effects on both developed and developing countries, the burden of infectious diseases is consistently much greater in these low-income countries. This discrepancy contributes to the potential of infectious disease control as a contentious issue in international politics as the states that are most affected by these diseases have the least financial capability to adequately address them (Archibugi and Bizzarri 2005). Despite this challenge, significant progress toward combating the "big three" has been made (United Nations 2015a). Global death rates from malaria declined by 58 percent from 2000 to 2015, while death rates from tuberculosis decreased by 45% from the 1990 rate by the 2015 deadline. Rates of new HIV infections have also declined by 40 percent from 2000 to 2013, but the goal of universal access to antiretroviral drugs (ARVs) by 2015 fell short of the MDG's target with only 36 percent of infected people in developing countries receiving treatment (United Nations 2015b). These data indicate that policies emanating from the process of global health governance are more effective in controlling infectious diseases at the global level more than ever before. Nevertheless, much work still needs to be accomplished as poverty, economic inequality, and newly emerging infectious diseases continue to create obstacles for ensuring adequate health for the world's population.

As noted in chapter 1, some liberal perspectives on international relations tend to view global health as a collective action problem. This classification is especially applicable to infectious diseases. Protection from chronic diseases could also be viewed as a collective good. In this case, everyone could benefit from a reduction in the incidence of chronic disease, and if one person benefits, then others may also share in that benefit. This reduction may be considered as a collective good in that such an overall decline in chronic diseases, especially among younger people, could increase benefits in terms of greater economic productivity and decreasing national health care costs. Control of these particular diseases, however, may also be viewed as an individual, rather than collective, good from a global perspective. If one state successfully lowers its incidence of chronic disease among its population, it does not necessarily directly lead to a reduced threat to other states. The nature of infectious disease, however, creates a different situation. Because these diseases are often spread by human contact, an eradication of a particular infectious disease in one part of the world could, in fact, directly be a health benefit to all.

In addressing infectious disease control as a global public good problem, the key component, of course, is international collective action. Without a world government to discourage free riding on international obligations and facilitate coordination among a disparate group of actors, achieving effective collective action is a difficult task. Neoliberal institutionalism emphasizes the important role of institutions to assist in resolving such problems. As discussed in chapter 2, the only international law covering infectious diseases are the International Health Regulations (IHR), which primarily covers surveillance. With the current lack of hard law in this area, global health governance must also rely on softer approaches to promote collective action among the actors in global governance.

Realism, which has traditionally overlooked global health as an area of "low politics" has taken more notice of global health, particularly infectious diseases, due to their potential as a threat to state security. The view of health as a concern for international security began to emerge in the 1990s. In 1995, the World Health Assembly (WHA) passed a resolution recognizing the international threat posed by emerging infectious diseases. Framing health as a security issue became even more prominent in 2000 when the United Nations Security Council (UNSC) passed Resolution 1308, which recognized that the spread of HIV/AIDS posed a threat to international peace and security. The terrorist attacks of September 11, 2001 on the United States shortly followed by the transmission of anthrax through the American mail system increased awareness of how the spread of infectious diseases could become part of bioterrorism. The SARS pandemic of 2003 also increased fears of the potential of new deadly diseases emerging in the twenty-first century that could threaten human life and economic well-being. Over a decade later, the Ebola outbreak and its spread to developed countries confirmed this apprehension. The worldwide panic created by the epidemic, as well as the UN Security Council's resolution in September 2014 declaring the Ebola outbreak in West Africa as a threat to international peace and security, demonstrated this increased interest. In fact, the 2014 resolution was only the third resolution on a health issue ever passed by the Security Council and was the first resolution that was not based on the HIV/AIDS epidemic.

Constructivist and Marxist approaches also have certain perspectives on an international regime for infectious disease control. Constructivists view international relations as a process, often shaped by the evolution of norms. In the case of infectious diseases, states learned to cooperate in this area due to the ineffectiveness of unilateral quarantine measures. Cooperation among states began to strengthen over time due to lack of effectiveness of existing arrangements and increasing acceptance of a norm of international cooperation to address this problem. The current state of this norm is now embodied in the IHR 2005, which commits states to greater obligations for infectious disease control than ever before. Marxist-based approaches, however, emphasize how this cooperative arrangement is structured around the global capitalist economy. This perspective highlights the fact that infectious diseases have a far more devastating effect on life in the Global South. IHR 2005 does not provide for any requirement of funding from developed states to address this problem in poorer countries. Marxists would also point to the role of multinational corporations (MNCs) and the private sector and how they charge high prices for drugs to treat these diseases in order to maximize profits. These MNCs also rely on core capitalist economies and the World Trade Organization (WTO) to support their practice, which acts to the disadvantage of infected persons in the developing world.

This chapter will examine how these different approaches apply to global governance and its role in controlling infectious diseases. It will focus on two older diseases that still have a major global impact, malaria and tuberculosis, as well as the relatively newer, and the more politically high-profile case of HIV/AIDS. Emerging infectious diseases such as SARS and Ebola haemorrhagic fever will be examined in chapter 5 on global health security. The key questions considered in this chapter are how effective is the current form of global governance in providing control of infectious disease? What needs to be improved? And how politically feasible would it be to implement these improvements? Realism, neoliberal institutionalism, constructivism, and Marxism all offer different insights to assist in addressing these questions.

MALARIA

Malaria is an infectious disease that is transmitted by the bite of female mosquitoes carrying a particular pathogen. The most deadly form is *Plasmodium falciparum*, which is the dominant form of malaria in sub-Saharan Africa. Over 90 percent of infections and deaths caused by malaria globally occur in Africa, although over ninety countries reported transmissions of malaria in 2016. Of these reported cases, however, 80 percent of them were from only fifteen countries, with India as the only one not located in sub-Saharan Africa (WHO 2017c). The WHO estimated that in 2016, 219 million people were infected by malaria, and 445,000 had died due to contracting the disease (WHO 2017c). The MDGs specifically mentioned malaria as one of the diseases, along with HIV/AIDS, that needed to be successfully reduced in terms of prevalence and mortality by 2015.

Malaria has a long history. Literature from ancient civilizations indicates that malaria may have been present as early as 2700 B.C. (Oaks et al. 1991). It was also a global disease that spread across Africa, Asia, Europe, and was even found to have reached the Americas by the time of European exploration of the Western Hemisphere. The discovery of the transmission of malaria did not begin until 1846 when an Italian doctor, Giovanni Rasori, suggested that the disease was transmitted through a parasite. A British physician, Richard

Ross, a British physician and scientist, was the first scientist to demonstrate that the transmission cycle for malaria originated with mosquitoes in 1897, which led to a Nobel Prize in Medicine for his efforts (Oaks et al. 1991).

Effective treatment for malaria, however, was discovered well before Ross's discovery. Indigenous people of South America had found that cinchona bark provided a useful remedy, prior to the arrival of the Europeans. Supplies of this bark were later exported to Europe in the seventeenth century, but it was not until 1820 when it was determined that it was an ingredient within the bark, quinine, that allowed for an effective treatment for malaria (Knell 1991). Despite these breakthroughs, efforts at malaria control were still somewhat limited because it was a disease located primarily in tropical regions, far away from the European powers that had greater resources and capability to control the disease than the territories that were much more affected.

Interest in malaria control grew during the first half of twentieth century due to the expansion of colonization and world war (Harman 2012). The experience of World War II, in particular, contributed to the growing effort. During battles at Bataan, Papua New Guinea, and Guadalcanal, both Allied and Japanese militaries suffered significant losses of personnel due to malaria. These wartime losses spurred the United States to begin a comprehensive anti-malaria campaign. Dichloro-diphenyl-trichloroethane (DDT), which was first synthesized in 1872, was discovered by Paul Müller in 1939 to be a highly effective insecticide. The U.S. Department of Agriculture (USDA) soon after developed aerosol spray also known as the "bug bomb" in 1941 to kill large quantities of mosquitoes quickly and efficiently. In 1942 the U.S. military introduced malaria control units that brought in drugs, insecticides, and mosquito nets to assist in combat, after initially being unprepared to prevent infection from the disease (Joy 1999).

The scientific accomplishments during the war generated a great deal of optimism for the possibility of eliminating malaria. In addition to the war effort, the United States launched its anti-malaria program domestically, which resulted in the almost complete eradication of the disease in the country by 1952 (Oaks et al. 1991). The success of the program in the United States inspired the WHO to promote such a program globally. The Eighth World Health Assembly passed resolution WHA8.30 in 1955, which called for the global eradication of malaria. The use of DDT was a central part of this campaign. It was a relatively cheap product that could efficiently kill mosquitoes over a wide area. The strategy of eradication was based on the indoor residual spraying (IRS) of DDT along with treatment by the drug chloroquine. Advocates for the eradication program had persuasively argued that such an extensive campaign was required before mosquitoes acquired resistance to DDT. Additionally, the promise of eliminating the disease with technologically available means was attractive both in terms of improving global health and reducing long-term economic costs associated with the disease.

The Global Malaria Eradication Program (GMEP) resulted in a heavy use of DDT in affected areas. Over four billion pounds of DDT was employed globally from 1940 to 1973 (Strickman et al. 2009). The overall campaign, however, led to mixed results. In some countries, mostly in Europe and the Americas, GMEP was highly successful, thirty-seven countries had eliminated malaria by 1978. India went from 110 million people infected by malaria in 1955 to under a million by 1968, and Sri Lanka reduced its infected population from 2.8 million in 1946 to only eighteen cases that were reported by 1966 (Mendis et al. 2009). GMEP, however, also encountered some significant problems as well. The assumption that such a blanket campaign would work for all areas of the world turned out to be faulty. The populations of some areas opposed the spraying campaign for cultural and social reasons. Mosquitoes began to develop resistance to DDT, and not only was the use of DDT ineffective in some areas, most notably sub-Saharan Africa, but some areas began to experience a resurgence of malaria after transmission of the disease had halted. Other deficiencies with GMEP included a decline in funding for research on malaria, because it was expected that the disease was on the verge of elimination and the lack of an effective surveillance system to precisely determine the number of malaria cases in some areas (Nájera et al. 2011). Additionally, evidence, as well as public awareness, was beginning to develop over the harmful effects of DDT on human health and the environment (Gunter and Harris 1998). After funding for GMEP began to decrease as well, the WHA began to reconsider the strategy in 1967.

The WHA elected to change its approach from malaria eradication with its approval of resolution WHA22.39 in 1969. While the resolution reaffirmed the eradication strategy, it also suggested that a control strategy based on treatment should be used if eradication efforts were not successful. Although eradication was still the primary goal of the WHO's malaria policy, a series of events in the 1970s transformed it into a de facto control policy. Enthusiasm for the WHO's program waned as it became apparent that global eradication was a much more difficult task than originally envisioned, and more and more states began to ban the use of DDT due to its deleterious impact. The economic recession and oil crisis during that decade decreased funding for malaria and increased the cost of insecticides. The United Nations Children's Fund (UNICEF) also decided to offer more general health programs rather than focus as much attention on malaria as it had previously done (Nájera et al. 2011). States became primarily responsible for their own malaria control efforts as the lack of international funding limited international efforts to eradicate the disease. This overall decline in support, along with increased mosquito resistance to insecticides, contributed to a rise in the incidence of malaria during the 1970s and 1980s in countries like Sri Lanka where the disease was close to eradication.

In the early 1990s, the WHO began to reinvigorate its malaria program. At a 1992 conference in Amsterdam, a Global Strategy for Malaria Control was submitted and endorsed by the conference. It was approved by the WHA in the following year. This strategy was based on four elements: (1) "early diagnosis and prompt treatment," (2) "selective and sustainable protective measures, including vector control," (3) "to detect early, contain, or prevent epidemics," and (4) "to strengthen local capacities in basic and applied research to permit and promote the regular assessment of a country's malaria situation" (World Health Organization 1993). The strategy recognized, however, that international cooperation, especially funding would be necessary for it to be effectively implemented. In addition to the renewed political commitment to international malaria control, three technological innovations were developed during the 1990s to strengthen the effort. First, insecticide-treated bed nets (ITNs) offered better protection to individuals as they served to kill mosquitoes in addition to offering protection. Second, artemisinin-based combination therapy (ACT) emerged in the late 1990s to replace traditional treatment by chloroquine, which had become increasingly less effective since it was introduced in the 1940s. The third innovation was rapid diagnostic tests, which made detection of malaria cheaper and more effective.

The WHO, along with the UNICEF, the United Nations Development Programme (UNDP), and the World Bank, launched the Roll Back Malaria (RBM) Initiative in 1998. The emphasis of this program was on prevention and treatment by improving health services rather than eradication. Its goal was to reduce death from malaria by 50 percent in 2010 and another 50 percent by 2015 (Nabarro and Tayler 1998). To assist RBM and other efforts to combat infectious diseases, the Global Fund to Fight AIDS, Tuberculosis, and Malaria (GFATM) was founded in 2002. GFATM, as discussed in chapter 3, is a public-private partnership for global health designed to increase financing to prevent and treat those three diseases. The members of its Board, who make the final decisions on funding, include representatives from national donor governments; civil society; the private sector; and advisory positions for the WHO, World Bank, and the United Nations Programme on HIV/AIDS (UNAIDS). It is a separate entity from the UN and the WHO, primarily due to the interests of powerful states, such as the United States, Japan, and Italy, which did not want GFATM to be part of the UN system (Kohlmorgen 2007). Grant proposals are developed by states seeking financial assistance through a country coordination mechanism, so that local actors have to work together to design a grant proposal and a plan for implementation. This system recommends and supports the inclusion of non-governmental actors in the grant process. In some cases, however, government officials have largely controlled the coordination mechanism (Brown 2009).

Initially RBM was successful at increasing public awareness and financial commitments for malaria. Its inclusive partnership structure, however, did cause problems. Without an established hierarchy, decision-making and accountability became muddled. Even though RBM was positioned in the WHO, it was not well connected to the organization's departments (*Lancet* 2005). Another challenge had to do with the expensive cost of ACT, which had been established to be a much more effective treatment of malaria than chloroquine. The WHO, however, was reluctant to support the provision of ACT to poor African states due to concerns by governments, such as the United States to use the expensive treatment (McNeil 2002). Similarly, GFATM provided more funding for chloroquine than ACT in 2003, despite the mounting evidence that it was a far inferior drug (Attaran et al. 2004). Much of the criticism of the early years of the RBM was that although funding for malaria was growing, the incidence of malaria was increasing as well.

RBM, however, bounced back in the late 2000s as global deaths from malaria peaked by 2004 and then began to decline (Murray et al. 2012). With this change, international funding for malaria began to grow. International funding to countries suffering from malaria increased from less than US$100 million in 2000 to US$1.7 billion by 2010. In 2016, about US$2.7 billion was used for malaria control and eradication. About 57 percent of the funds in 2016 were through GFATM with the United States providing 38 percent of the international financing (WHO 2017c).

By 2007, the eradication strategy began to be reconsidered in global health governance as Bill and Melinda Gates Foundation announced that it should be the new goal for the global health agenda, and their call was later endorsed by WHO's Director-General Margaret Chan. At this stage, eradication may be more of an aspirational goal than a systematic plan, but it seems to be moving in that direction. The MDGs and RBM's 2008 Global Malaria Action Plan had focused on a significant reduction on incidence and mortality rates from 2000 to 2015. Under the SDGs, however, the target was broadened to end the epidemic of malaria (along with AIDS and tuberculosis) by 2030. A report by the WHO has even identified twenty-one countries in 2016 that could eliminate malaria as soon as 2020 (WHO 2017c).

Opinions on whether or not an eradication strategy is feasible have been mixed. Optimists may point out that the technological means, such as insecticides, ITNs, and ACT, to substantially eliminate the death toll are available. It is just a matter of making these tools available to everyone in affected areas. In addition, measureable progress on reducing the global burden of malaria has been made, as evidenced by the almost 60 percent drop in mortality rates since 2000. Pessimists, however, may point to the weak health care systems in impoverished countries and how these systems have not dramatically improved since the eradication campaigns in the 1950s and the 1960s. They may also point to potential mosquito resistance to ACT that could diminish expected returns from an eradication campaign.

The most significant factor, however, in establishing a feasible campaign is funding. A study by Kiszewski et al. (2007) estimated that it would take US$3.8 billion to US$4.5 billion per year from 2006 to 2015 to meet international targets for malaria control. Financing for this disease is increasing, but it is still not at this level. Although the progress in combating malaria seems to have been sufficient to have reached the MDG target (halt and start reversal) by 2015, eradication is a much more ambitious and costly goal. It may even be more expensive in areas with high rates of malaria transmission, as the development of new tools may be necessary to successfully combat the disease. For example, "In forested areas of Asia and the African savannah where outdoor-resting and outdoor-biting mosquito vectors prevail, the elimination of malaria has not been possible, so far, with existing strategies of ITN and IRS" (Mendis et al. 2009: 7). In addition to requiring a substantial increase in funding, a new global eradication campaign may also be hindered by the fickleness of international donors. If malaria is on the verge of being eliminated, funds may be moved elsewhere. The experience of GMEP, however, has demonstrated that malaria is a resilient disease that may reemerge in an area where eradication is not completed (Sabot et al. 2010). While more research and development may be required to successfully eradicate malaria on a global scale, political will and financial feasibility may be the main obstacles to accomplishing this task.

TUBERCULOSIS

Although tuberculosis was not specifically named in the title of MDG goal number 6, as were HIV/AIDS and malaria, it is one of the world's major diseases and perhaps the most significant of the "other diseases" referred to in the MDGs. It was also specifically included as an epidemic to be eradicated by 2030 in the SDGs. Tuberculosis contributes to more global deaths than any other infectious disease, except possibly HIV/AIDS. In 2016, tuberculosis was responsible for 1.3 million deaths globally. It has a relationship to HIV/AIDS in that many deaths of individuals infected with HIV are due to tuberculosis, and tuberculosis can, in turn, make an individual more susceptible to HIV infection. Of the estimated 10.4 million cases of the disease that year, 45 percent were in Asia and 25 percent in Africa. India, Indonesia, China, the Philippines, and Pakistan accounted for 56 percent of the world's cases of tuberculosis, with India reporting the most (WHO 2017d).

Tuberculosis is caused by an infection of *Mycobacterium tuberculosis*. This pathogen can be transmitted by humans. It is primarily an airborne disease that can be transferred by coughing, sneezing, or speaking by an infected person (Dye and Floyd 2006). Most people exposed to tuberculosis, however, do not acquire the disease. It is estimated that only about 10 percent of infected persons develop tuberculosis (Grange 1999). As with the case of malaria, tuberculosis is not a new disease. Evidence in skeletal remains indicates that it can be traced back to the known beginning of human history. It was a disease that even plagued Ancient Greece when it was known as "phthisis" (Daniel 2006). *Mycobacterium tuberculosis*, however, was not identified as the cause of the disease until Robert Koch's discovery in 1882. This finding spurred more progress on researching the disease, culminating in a development of a vaccine by Albert Calmette and Camille Guerin. This vaccine known as Bacille Calmette-Guerin (BCG) was successfully tested on a newborn infant of a mother suffering from tuberculosis in 1921. Two decades later in 1943, Selman Waksman discovered streptomycin, an antibiotic that could effectively treat and even cure tuberculosis.

With the development of an effective vaccine and treatment, the WHO made tuberculosis control one of its early priorities. The introduction of chemotherapy treatment along with BCG and streptomycin helped to greatly reduce the prevalence of tuberculosis in European and other developed countries, however, the campaign was not effective in developing countries. Similar to the problem with the WHO's malaria eradication program, the weak health care systems in poorer states made the program more difficult to administer. The cost of drugs to treat tuberculosis was also difficult for these countries to afford. By the early 1960s, the WHO realized that a mass global campaign to combat tuberculosis was ineffective in developing states and a new approach was needed to be taken (Raviglione and Pio 2002).

In the mid-1960s, the WHO decided to move from a vertical strategy focusing on tuberculosis control to a horizontal system that would integrate tuberculosis into a general healthcare program. This system would become the standard practice for addressing tuberculosis in most developing countries. This change in strategy, however, was not accompanied by an increase in resources, so the poorest countries did not see improvement in the prevalence of tuberculosis (Raviglione and Pio 2002). As with the campaign for malaria control, the global economic problems of the 1970s contributed to a declining effort in combating tuberculosis. The WHO, national governments, and other relevant actors began to place less emphasis on the disease as part of their agenda. The WHO elected to merge tuberculosis into their respiratory control unit without increasing the unit's resources (Raviglione and Pio 2002). The WHO also reduced the number of staff members specializing in tuberculosis to one person (Walt 1999). Additionally, research and financing for the disease also declined substantially in the 1970s and 1980s. Porter et al. (2002) suggest that the reason for this lack of support had to do with the perception that the disease was losing its impact, largely due to the success of reducing tuberculosis in developed countries during the 1950s. Political rivalries of the Cold War were also a relevant factor.

Even as the global economy began its recovery in the 1980s, the new HIV/AIDS pandemic began to increasingly overshadow tuberculosis even as the global morbidity of tuberculosis was on the rise. HIV was, in fact, contributing to a significant rise of tuberculosis in Africa. The economic decline of the Soviet Union in the late 1980s and the gradual dissolution of that state's basic services led to a health care crisis and a corresponding sharp rise in tuberculosis cases in the Soviet republics (Raviglione and Pio 2002). The disease was also becoming more prevalent in developed states, such as the United States, due to the rise in HIV cases, increasing prevalence of multidrug resistance (MDR) strains, and the impact of an overall decline in tuberculosis funding due to the health care policies of the 1970s and 1980s (Selgelid 2008). The WHO declared tuberculosis to be a "global emergency" in 1993 to promote more attention to the steadily growing burden of the disease. Although the WHO's pronouncement brought greater international attention to the issue, other actors such as the World Bank and global health specialists had actively promoted this change to the international health agenda before the WHO decided to adopt it (Ogden et. al 2003).

In response to the problem, the WHO introduced a new strategy based on directly observed therapy (DOT). This practice was based on establishing a close relationship between health care workers and patients. It was first implemented in 1958 in India by Wallace Fox (Kim et. al 2003). The DOTS strategy was based on five factors: (1) political commitment by national governments to control tuberculosis, (2) case detection by sputum smear microscopy, (3) treatment of individuals testing positive for tuberculosis, (4) maintenance of a sustained supply of tuberculosis drugs, and (5) developing and maintaining a surveillance and reporting program for treatment results (World Health Organization 1998a). This program was also supported by the World Bank, especially due to the relationship between tuberculosis morbidity and poverty. The WHO was quite successful in persuading states to adopt the DOTS program. The number of countries using the strategy increased from less than 10 to 127 from 1990 to 1999, which included the coverage of 80 percent of the incidence of the disease globally (Raviglione and Pio 2002). From 1994 to 2005, over 26 million cases of tuberculosis were discovered and reported globally under the DOTS strategy. Approximately between 77 percent and a little over 80 percent of positively tested patients received successful treatments during this period (Dye and Borgdorff 2008).

Although the DOTS strategy was fairly successful in terms of adoption, case reports, and treatment, it still encountered difficulty in extending coverage to remote areas with a high morbidity of tuberculosis. Many cases of the disease were not reported or treated. The DOTS strategy also experienced the same problems as the malaria control campaigns did in that cultural and social practices in some areas impeded DOTS implementation. Feeble health care systems in some of the poorer countries also created a significant challenge. DOTS' emphasis on service over research and development for new drugs to treat tuberculosis was also a point of criticism (Ogden et. al 2003). In 1998, the WHO decided to modify its approach to DOTS by forming a partnership arrangement with a variety of governmental and non-governmental organizations interested in tuberculosis control. This arrangement was named Stop TB. Its first major activity was assembling a global conference in 2000 that led to the Amsterdam Declaration, where twenty countries with high rates of tuberculosis pledged to expand their coverage of DOTS and detect 70 percent of all cases by 2005.

The political commitment provided by the Amsterdam Declaration contributed to greater support for tuberculosis on the international health agenda. A Global DOTS Expansion Plan (GDEP) was formulated in late 2000 to promote coordination of different agencies within different national health programs and push for more specialized care for individuals with MDR strains of tuberculosis. Stop TB followed by putting forward a Global Plan to Stop TB in 2001, which established research and implementation goals to be reached by 2005. Global funding for tuberculosis control also began to accelerate at this point with the expansion of bilateral aid, along with the establishment of GFATM. Despite these efforts and the improvements in tuberculosis control, the international community's goals were not met by 2005. The DOTS program continued to face a number of challenges. Elzinga et al. (2004) identified three main constraints for effective tuberculosis control: quality of health care, access to the DOTS strategy, and non-adoption of the DOTS strategy by some countries and some health care providers. Even if these areas improve, it has been argued that the development of drugs for treatment needs to be greatly improved (Ma et al. 2010). Until recently, no new classes of drugs for first-line treatment had been developed since the 1960s. Innovation in drug treatment is particularly needed for those individuals who have the MDR strain. In 2005, the WHO approved the Stop TB strategy to supplement DOTS with new objectives of universal access to treatment and protection of individuals from HIV/AIDS and MDR tuberculosis, and an increased emphasis on research for tuberculosis control.

While the MDGs did specifically name reduction in tuberculosis as a goal, it clearly fit in with one of the MDGs to halt and reverse the incidence of malaria and "other major diseases." The WHO found this goal, as related to tuberculosis, to be achieved by 2015 as the global incidence of the disease declined by 18 percent since 2000 (World Health Organization 2015a). As with HIV/AIDS and malaria, the SDGs called for a more ambitious goal of ending the epidemic of tuberculosis by 2030. To coincide with this SDG target, the WHO decided in 2014 to move from Stop TB to an End TB strategy for 2016–2035. The targets to achieve by 2035 for this strategy include a 95 percent reduction in tuberculosis deaths and a 90 percent reduction in the global incidence rate from 2015 levels. To accomplish this task, the End TB strategy emphasizes patient-centered care and prevention (including early diagnosis and treatment), a political commitment to funding as well as universal health coverage and poverty alleviation, and more intensive research and innovation (World Health Organization 2017d).

An effective tuberculosis eradication program, just as with malaria, will ultimately be dependent on political will and the availability of funding. Funding rose in recent years from US$3.3 billion in 2006 to US$6.9 billion in 2017 (World Health Organization 2017d). Although funding has been increasing, the WHO estimates the funding for 2017 was still US$2.3 billion short of what would be needed to meet the demands of the End TB strategy. International funding in 2017 for tuberculosis, 80 percent of which was provided by GFATM, was just over US$1 billion, far behind that of HIV/AIDS, which was well over US$6 billion (World Health Organization 2017d). Tuberculosis presents a complex problem for global health. A vaccine and effective treatment for most cases have been around for several decades, yet it remains one of the major threats to human health. Its association with HIV/AIDS suggests that successful control of one disease is important for successfully controlling the other. The SDGs and the End TB strategy represent a good opportunity to move toward elimination of this disease as a global health burden. Historically, tuberculosis has also been related to a number of social causes, ranging from poverty and poor sanitation to poor diets, tobacco use, and excessive alcohol consumption. Global health governance has focused its attention on drugs, health care services, and intergovernmental cooperation to combat the disease. Progress has been made, but as indicated by the success of developed countries in combating tuberculosis, economic development may be a large part of the puzzle and the most significant obstacle to overcome.

HIV/AIDS

HIV/AIDS is perhaps the most visible issue in global health. As previously mentioned, it is the only health issue to have received attention by the UN Security Council and was the first disease specifically mentioned by the MDGs. It was also one of the three diseases (along with malaria and tuberculosis) that the SDGs targeted to end as an epidemic by 2030. HIV/AIDS has consistently ranked as one of leading causes of death in the world, although it was not in the top ten in 2015 (WHO 2017b). In 2016, over 36 million people globally have been infected by this disease along with 1 million deaths as a result. As with malaria, HIV/AIDS disproportionately affects Africa, which is home to over 25 million of the world's infected population (UNAIDS 2017). On the positive side, HIV has been on the decline in the twenty-first century. The number of people that acquired the virus in 2016 was 16 percent fewer than in 2010. AIDS-related deaths are lower as well, with a decline from 1.9 million in 2005 to 1 million in 2016 (UNAIDS 2017).

Unlike malaria and tuberculosis, HIV/AIDS is a relatively new health threat to humans. The discovery of the virus began in the late 1970s and early 1980s as increased incidences of unusually rare diseases of pneumonia caused by *Pneumocystis carinii* and a cancer called Kaposi's sarcoma were identified in the United States. These diseases appeared most frequently in New York and San Francisco and occurred primarily among homosexual males. The growing incidence of these diseases was associated with a weakened immune system common to these individuals. It was initially referred to as *Gay-related Immune Deficiency Syndrome* (GRID). This condition, however, was soon called *Acquired Immunodeficiency Syndrome* (AIDS) as it was also discovered in non-homosexual drug users and people who became infected by the disease through blood transfusions (Barnett and Whiteside 2006). By 1981, the disease developed a global scope as cases of AIDS were found in Africa, Europe, and Latin America.

The virus that causes AIDS, the Human Immunodeficiency Virus (HIV), was identified in 1983. As further research demonstrated, HIV was not as easy of a virus to acquire as many other infectious diseases. Transmission could only be through bodily fluids. Most cases of spreading the infection have been through sexual intercourse, although infections from mothers to unborn children, blood transfusions, and intravenous drug use have also led to acquisition of the virus. A distinguishing feature of AIDS, compared to other infectious diseases, is that the infection takes a much longer time to develop into an illness (Barnett and Whiteside 2006). This feature makes it a very difficult disease to detect, and the fact that AIDS does not currently have a cure, makes it an extremely challenging disease for health authorities to control.

In addition to the difficulty in treating the disease, HIV/AIDS created much more of a political and social problem than other infectious diseases in the 1980s. It was perceived as a "gay cancer" and a disease that was acquired due to personal irresponsibility rather than misfortune. Individuals, who contracted the disease, especially during its first decade, faced a social stigma. In the United States, for example, "Ronald Reagan, the U.S. president under whose watch the epidemic first exploded, failed to utter the word AIDS for the first six years of his two terms in office" (Shepard 2007: 174).

HIV/AIDS began to emerge as an international issue in the mid-1980s. As it became a growing epidemic in sub-Saharan Africa, greater realization began to develop that the disease had a much wider scope of transmission than just homosexual behavior (O'Manique 2004). The predominant mode of transmission in Africa was through heterosexual contact and prenatal transfers. A global governance response to HIV/AIDS began when the WHO initiated the Global Programme on AIDS (GPA) in 1986. The next step was a WHA resolution in 1987, which endorsed a global strategy for the prevention and control of AIDS. Until this time, the WHO primarily had only been engaged in collecting and disseminating information about the disease. The uncertainty surrounding its nature and scope, as well as the WHO's emphasis on promoting primary health care as the main part of its agenda, contributed to the organization's hesitancy to assume a leadership role on AIDS (Mann and Kay 1991). The global strategy was aimed at persuading states to develop strong national programs to prevent the spread of AIDS; cooperate fully with one another and with the WHO to share information, technology, and financial assistance to combat the disease; and to establish the WHO as the coordinating agent in global governance. This role for the WHO was confirmed by the UN General Assembly by a resolution it adopted in October 1987. The GPA was the focal point for the WHO. A main point of early emphasis for the program was to provide support for national governments to develop their own domestic AIDS programs. Due to the demand by states for this assistance, the GPA emerged as the WHO's largest program by 1988 (Mann and Kay 1991).

A number of problems had clearly developed for the GPA by the early 1990s. Infection rates of HIV continued to increase, especially in sub-Saharan Africa. States, especially major donors, became discontented with its performance. A particular point of criticism was that the GPA did not work well with other UN agencies in coordinating cooperative arrangements (Poku 2002). As Patterson (2007) suggests, a major reason for this outcome was due to philosophical differences on the best approach to the epidemic. The GPA supported a view that AIDS was related to socioeconomic factors, such as poverty, education, and human rights. In this view, these social factors needed to be effectively addressed for a global campaign against AIDS to be successful. Key WHO officials, including the Director-General, and major donor states, in particular the United States, wanted to focus resources on a technical, scientific approach to develop a cure.

The dissatisfaction with the GPA led to the formation of another international organization to replace it and take the lead in the form of UNAIDS in 1996. UNAIDS was designed to improve cooperation among the various UN actors that addressed AIDS-related issues. It is sponsored by ten UN-affiliated organizations including the WHO, World Bank, the International Labor Organization, and UNICEF. At the time that it was formed, UNAIDS was a unique arrangement by bringing together these different organizations to coordinate a unified policy. Its goals were similar to those of the GPA: to provide international leadership on HIV/AIDS, assist national governments in developing AIDS programs, promote cooperation, and raise awareness and financial contributions. In addition to its position outside of the WHO's formal structure, another major difference that UNAIDS had with the GPA was that its objective was to coordinate funding among its co-sponsors rather than directly provide funds for HIV/AIDS programs. In the short-term, this created a problem for some national programs that were dependent on GPA funds for support (Das and Samarasekera 2008). Another major challenge for the launch of UNAIDS was the decline in funding. Although UNAIDS represented a significant change in global governance from GPA's leadership, donor states had become disenchanted with the system. UNAIDS staff was over 50 percent below that of the GPA with a budget that was 15 percent less than that of the GPA (Poku 2002).

Despite its slow start, much progress was made in the global campaign against HIV/AIDS in the 2000s. The UN Security Council's resolution on HIV/AIDS adopted in July 2000 was followed a couple months later by the Millennium Declaration and the corresponding MDGs, which prominently included the halting of the spread of HIV/AIDS as a global objective. The next year, a UN General Assembly Special Session on the issue produced a Declaration of Commitment on HIV/AIDS. This agreement, while not creating a legal obligation, provided an acknowledgment by the international community that the disease was connected to poverty and economic development. It also recognized that individuals infected with HIV/AIDS should be protected against discrimination as a human right.

As was the case with malaria and tuberculosis, funding for HIV/AIDS received a boost with the creation of GFATM in 2002. The Bill and Melinda Gates Foundation also emerged as a major actor in global health during this time, and HIV/AIDS was one of its priorities for funding. To supplement these financial resources, in 2003 U.S. president George W. Bush announced the President's Emergency Plan for AIDS Relief (PEPFAR). This initiative was a commitment by the United States to provide US$15 billion to fifteen African and Caribbean states to assist them in the prevention, treatment, and care of AIDS. PEPFAR was later extended under the Obama and Trump administrations. Since the program began, the United States has provided over US$57 billion for bilateral HIV/AIDS programs and over US$13 billion to GFATM from 2004 to 2017 (President's Emergency Plan for AIDS Relief 2017). The World Bank also devoted much more of its efforts to stop epidemics in the 2000s as well as increasing its funding from US$500 million in 1998 to US$4 billion by 2008 (Merson et al. 2008). The WHO continued to be a major actor in the campaign, announcing a "3 by 5" initiative in conjunction with UNAIDS to provide antiretroviral (ARV) therapy to 3 million people with HIV living in developing countries by 2005. UNAIDS benefited from the increased political visibility of HIV/AIDS as well, as it experienced significant growth in its budget and staff members over the decade.

What contributed to the enhanced response of global governance to the epidemic compared to the relatively lackluster reply in the 1990s? Patterson (2007) credits the increased interest of developed states, especially the United States in combating the disease, as well as the effective work of nongovernmental organizations (NGOs) and civil society in raising its political profile. The establishment of PEPFAR provides a good example of these features. The United States had both security and economic concerns about the HIV/AIDS epidemic in Africa. The devastating effect of this disease on these countries contributes to poverty and political instability, which could in turn contribute to terrorism (Stolberg 2008). The connection between HIV/AIDS and poverty also contributed to fears of a growing presence of the disease and potentially destabilizing effect of it on countries such as China, India, and Russia (Merson et al. 2008). The United States also had a public relations incentive to support this program. The 2003 war in Iraq was globally unpopular, especially in developing countries. The announcement of PEPFAR during the same year was viewed as a means to improve American relations with some of these countries. Although the U.S. trades and investments very little in Africa compared to the other regions of the world, PEPFAR could also be viewed as a way to heighten U.S. presence in the region, especially in light of China's growing influence.

In regard to the activity of NGOs, faith-based organizations (FBOs) played a key role in the development of PEPFAR. The program had 248 FBOs as partners when it began, and 25 percent of its funds went through these organizations (Bartsch and Kohlmorgen 2007). In addition to security and economic interests, the significant involvement of FBOs in supporting and implementing the program indicates a strong moral incentive as well. Another actor that has received praise for the improvements of the global campaign against HIV/AIDS in 2000s has been UNAIDS and its director at the time, Peter Pirot. In particular, UNAIDS was considered to be instrumental in including NGOs as an important part of the campaign and a strong and effective advocate that was successfully able to make the case for AIDS expectionalism, which refers to the idea of HIV/AIDS control as a primary objective of global health governance.

Although significant progress was achieved in the global campaign against HIV/AIDS in the 2000s, in terms of international cooperation, funding, decreases in new infections, and deaths some obstacles continued to be present. In 2006, the UN General Assembly convened another special session on HIV/AIDS to reaffirm its commitment to combating the disease. The negotiations at this session were much more contentious than those in 2001. A new declaration was produced, but it omitted language specifically referring to high-risk groups such as homosexual men, prostitutes, and drug users. It also did not include financial targets. The interests of the United States, in particular, were associated with this outcome. The United States, along with some Islamic states, did not want to name the high-risk groups for moral reasons. The United States also did not want to include financial targets because, as the world's largest contributor to GFATM and with PEPFAR, it did not want to appear accountable if the funding targets were not reached (Patterson 2007). The UN General Assembly, however, did reconvene with another special session in 2011 to adopt another declaration on HIV/AIDS. The 2011 declaration was a more comprehensive document that did specifically mention the high risk groups, who were omitted from the 2006 declaration. It also included expanded provisions on the prevention of HIV/AIDS and human rights.

Political issues also emerged with respect to funding. While the Bill and Melinda Gates Foundation has served as one of the world's largest contributors to the global campaign against HIV/AIDS, some concerns exist over its role in global health. The Gates Foundation is an active donor with members that are associated with several other global health partnerships. It has been influential not just in providing funds but also in global health policy and research agendas. The fact that a private actor that does not have political accountability to a constituency wields so much power in defining the policy agenda for global health has raised some criticism of the foundation (McNeil 2008). Its policies have tended to support specific disease programs and technological solutions rather than general health care and social causes of disease. Also, the fact that the Gates Foundation gives a large of amount of funding to U.S. organizations, especially compared to health organizations in developing countries, has also raised questions(McCoy et al. 2009b).

Despite this issue, funding from PEPFAR has been even more controversial. Although it has been a substantial source of global funding for HIV/AIDS, it has had some conditions attached. In 2004, the legislation allocating the dispersal of PEPFAR funds called upon a third of the funds for prevention and education to be spent on abstinence promotion programs, and none of the funds could be spent on syringes or needles for drug users. Recipients of the funds were also called on to rebuke prostitution (Garrett 2005). The fact that a significant portion of the funds are channeled through faith-based organizations, including those that have not had much experience with global health has led to the critique that religious groups have used PEPFAR to promote conservative religious beliefs. The ideological underpinnings of PEPFAR have also been indicated in its fifteen focus countries. Although these states represent the majority of HIV-infected persons in the world, much of the funding has also been distributed to states such as Kenya, Ethiopia, South Africa, and Uganda who have been supportive of U.S. anti-terrorism policies (Ingram 2009). The abstinence funding requirement was dropped in 2008; however, the policy is still encouraging promotion and funding for abstinence programs. The emphasis on abstinence, along with the anti-prostitution clause for foreign NGOs continues to be PEPFAR's policy.

Because HIV is a lifelong condition that currently has no cure, treatment for the disease has been based on ARV. This form of treatment involves the use of combinations of drugs to manage the virus. ARV treatment of HIV infection has proven to be fairly successful. It is considered to be one of the most powerful treatments devised by medical science for a deadly disease. An infected individual with access to ARV treatment can slow down the progression of AIDS considerably, and with consistent treatment, can possibly extend life expectancy by decades. One study suggests that an individual with HIV in Europe or North America who begins ARV treatment at age twenty in 2008–2010 could expect to live to ages sixty-three to sixty-seven on average depending on other health and lifestyle factors. If the individual had a low viral load and over a year of treatment, then that person could expect to live to age seventy-eight (The Antiretroviral Therapy Cohort Collaboration 2017).

Due to the progress of ARV treatment in the 2000s, contraction of the HIV/AIDS virus is no longer considered to be a "death sentence" to the extent that it was in the 1980s and early 1990s, especially for individuals in developed countries. Despite the scientific breakthroughs in addressing HIV/AIDS, ARV treatment does have some negatives. Because these drugs manage and do not cure the virus, they must be taken over a lifetime. They may also lead to side effects, and even though ARV treatment may prolong life, they do not tend to extend life beyond that of a person who does not have the virus, because treated individuals may be more vulnerable to chronic diseases as they age due to their weakened immune system (Volberding and Deeks 2010). Nevertheless, thanks to the improvement in drugs, HIV-positive individuals in developed countries who have access to ARV treatments can still expect to live a fairly long and healthy life.

The most significant aspect of ARV treatment, however, is access to the necessary drugs. The issue has two important dimensions: (1) the availability of funding so that the poor, especially in developing countries can receive this medication and (2) the business practices of pharmaceutical companies and the protection of their patents under international law that produces a high cost for these drugs. Progress has been made in both these areas over the past decade. Politically, universal access to ARVs has been endorsed by the

MDGs, the SDGs, and UN General Assembly declarations on HIV/AIDS. In terms of distribution, the number of people with HIV globally receiving ARV treatment was 46 percent by 2016. In eastern and southern Africa, the region with the highest infection rate in the world, the number of individuals with HIV that are covered by ARV treatment increased from 24 percent in 2010 to 54 percent by 2016 (UNAIDS 2016). The growth of international funding for HIV/AIDS was a critical factor in this increase.

As discussed in chapter 2, a leading authority of intellectual property law is the WTO's Agreement on Trade-Related Aspects of Intellectual Property Rights (TRIPS). This agreement provides international legal protection for pharmaceuticals. In 2001, the WTO adopted the Declaration on the TRIPS Agreement in public health, also known as the Doha Declaration. This declaration by the WTO permitted the use of compulsory licenses by member states so that they could produce drugs that were to be used for an urgent health need, including HIV/AIDS, malaria, and tuberculosis, without the permission of the patent holder. In implementing the agreement, the TRIPS council of the WTO also permitted states that did not have the capability to sufficiently produce the drug to import generic drugs produced under a compulsory license by other states. This decision led to a considerable decrease in the cost of ARVs for HIV treatment. In 2006, ARV combination therapy could cost an individual in a developed state about US$10,000 per year. When generic ARVs were introduced into the international market, the cost of treatment could be less than US$200 a year, making treatment much more affordable (Wise 2006).

Although the international community's objectives for HIV/AIDS control have not been reached by some countries, much progress has been made in the campaign since 2000. HIV/AIDS has emerged into a priority health issue for global health governance, and it still receives more international funding than other communicable diseases. A future objective will need to include more emphasis on prevention. Although 2 million more people were receiving ARV treatment in 2016 compared to 2015, this number was somewhat offset by the 2 million new HIV infections in 2015 (UNAIDS 2016). HIV/AIDS is a significant target for the SDGs to ensure healthy lives. As with malaria and tuberculosis, the SDGs call for an end to the AIDS epidemic by 2030. Additionally, the SDGs call for affordable access to medicines in accordance with the Doha Declaration. To follow the SDGs, the UN General Assembly held a high-level meeting in June 2016 on ending AIDS. The meeting produced a political declaration, which reaffirmed the commitment by UN member states to end the AIDS epidemic by 2030, and intensify efforts at prevention, treatment, and care of the disease. The fact that this meeting and its declaration addressed only the end of the AIDS epidemic indicates how this disease continues to be a high priority and has a special place in the agenda of global health governance.

BOX 4.1 NEGLECTED TROPICAL DISEASES: AN EMERGING AREA FOR GLOBAL HEALTH GOVERNANCE

Neglected tropical diseases (NTD) refer to infectious diseases that are "considered 'neglected' when there is a lack of effective, affordable, or easy to use drug treatments" (Yamey 2002). These particular diseases are also labeled as "tropical" because they are predominantly associated with warm climates in equatorial regions of the world. The tropical designation also implies that these are diseases largely endemic to relatively poor countries. The WHO has identified seventeen infectious diseases that it classifies as NTDs (WHO 2012). These diseases include dengue, onchocerciasis, blinding trachoma, and Chagas disease, among others. The WHO estimates that more than one billion people may be affected by these diseases or what Hotez et al. (2009) refer to as the "bottom billion."

As with other infectious diseases, notable progress addressing these diseases has been made since 2000. Between 2000 and 2007, drug and vaccine development partnerships for six diseases were developed despite a lack of commercial demand (Yamey and Hotez 2007). The WHO began to introduce the strategic interventions of preventive chemotherapy and intensified disease management in 2003 to target these diseases, and in 2010, Director-General Margaret Chan issued the WHO's first report on neglected tropical diseases to substantiate the WHO's progress in addressing these diseases (World Health Organization 2012a). Additionally, the World Health Assembly passed a comprehensive resolution on NTDs in 2013. The most significant achievement for NTDs in global health governance, however, was the inclusion of these diseases in the SDGs as target to end as an epidemic by 2030. As the case with the "big three" diseases, sufficient funding and the political will by national governments, intergovernmental organizations, and private actors will be necessary to achieve this goal.

ASSESSING GLOBAL HEALTH GOVERNANCE'S RESPONSIVENESS TO INFECTIOUS DISEASES

The "big three" diseases of malaria, tuberculosis, and HIV/AIDS are among the highest priorities for global health governance. The importance of these diseases to the international community is indicated by their inclusion as an

MDG and how the SDGs have targeted the end of the epidemics of these diseases by 2030. These diseases are also primary funding areas for GFATM and the Bill and Melinda Gates Foundation. In addition to being the three deadliest infectious diseases, the cases and fatalities associated with these diseases are most prevalent in impoverished areas of the world, sub-Saharan Africa in particular. On the positive side, the incidence of these diseases has been significantly reduced in the twenty-first century. Of the "big three," HIV/AIDS does stand out. Unlike malaria and tuberculosis, which have been around for centuries, AIDS was completely unknown forty years ago. Its political profile is far beyond any other disease due to international recognition of its relationship to human rights and even state security. Although HIV/AIDS receives much more funding than malaria and tuberculosis, it is also more expensive and difficult to treat.

As previously noted, realists view infectious disease as the most important area in global health due to its potential impact on state security. The ability for these diseases to spread great distances and cross borders has been a concern for global governance since the nineteenth century. Infectious diseases are also more likely to impact younger people, who are productive members of society, than chronic diseases do, which are associated more with aging. As international funding and attention by the UN Security Council indicates, HIV/AIDS is especially significant as a security issue. Infectious disease control is related to the national interest for all states, however, as explained in chapter 1, a realist analysis of global governance is based on the assumption that it is structured by the interests of great powers. In examining the cases of malaria, tuberculosis, and HIV/AIDS, it is apparent that the great powers, in particular, the United States, have had mixed motives in regard to the global control of these diseases. On the one hand, as a security priority, great powers do have to be concerned that the diseases may spread into their territory and harm its citizens. On the other hand, great powers also need to be concerned about how a pandemic may affect other states. Such a pandemic could weaken those states significantly and contribute to instability and conflict, as well as prove damaging to economic interests. With twenty-first century globalization, great powers increasingly have an interest in other regions of the world due to potential benefits they may receive from their markets and resources.

The burden of a pandemic in another state could potentially harm the economy of a great power, or draw it into a military conflict if the pandemic leads to the collapse of a state's infrastructure and political instability. Also, as the PEPFAR example may indicate, great powers can use their support of infectious disease control as a means to improve relationships with and even gain leverage over states that are greatly affected by these diseases. For instance, the "big three" diseases are predominately diseases of the developing world. Tuberculosis and especially malaria are unusual diseases for developed states. In addition, these states also have fairly easy access to effective treatments. HIV/AIDS has more of an impact on developed states, but with access to ARV treatments, it has become a manageable disease for states with sufficient financial resources. It is apparent that great powers have an interest in global infectious disease control, but it is not a major priority for them.

Because realists assume that global governance is dominated by great powers, the WHO, World Bank, UNAIDS, and other non-state actors are considered to play a limited role. For international infectious disease control to be effective, according to realists, it will ultimately depend on the actions by powerful states. Tremendous strides were made against malaria when the United States determined that the disease was hindering its war effort. Global mortality from tuberculosis and HIV/AIDS has declined since 2000 as the United States has increased its international funding for addressing those diseases. The history of malaria and tuberculosis, however, also indicate that when great powers no longer believe that they are directly threatened by the disease, they lose some political will to combat it.

Neoliberal institutionalists, in contrast, would provide greater credit to the evolution of non-state actors and especially international law and international regime development as to the improvement in infectious disease control. The WHO has provided a significant leadership role in the cases of malaria and tuberculosis. The Roll Back Malaria Initiative and the DOTS program have been effective in reducing the burden of these diseases. UNAIDS played a critical role in raising AIDS awareness to such an extent that it became the first health issue to be addressed by the UN Security Council. The World Bank, GFATM, and the Bill and Melinda Gates Foundation have assisted significantly in raising funding. Despite these achievements, however, neoliberal institutionalists would also find that global governance is still relatively weak when it comes to infectious diseases. The IHR is the only international law covering this area, and although it has become a stronger agreement, its lack of mechanisms to promote compliance makes it difficult to ensure that states will follow its obligations. The WHO has no direct power over states. WHA and UN General Assembly resolutions, such as those related to the MDGs and SDGs, are not legally binding. States are under no legal obligation to provide funding for infectious disease control, which indicates the continuing problem of free-riding in this area. Although international cooperation has improved in the twenty-first century and the SDGs demonstrate a clear international consensus to eliminate the "big three" diseases, the overall lack of institutionalization or rules-based solution in this area reflects that infectious disease control remains a challenging collective action problem, especially if eradication is the goal.

A constructivist analysis of global health governance and infectious diseases suggests that the system is driven by norms and identities rather than state interests or institutional rules. The norm for global infectious disease control has fluctuated over time. In the cases of malaria and tuberculosis, the scientific discoveries of effective means to combat these diseases increased the expectation and will of powerful states and the WHO to effectively reduce the global burden of these diseases in the late 1940s and 1950s. After these diseases became effectively contained in developed states, the norm began to weaken. It was not until the 1990s when the WHO, World Bank, and civil society organizations were able to successfully convince states that these diseases were a significant global problem. Their influence was effective in strengthening the norm, leading to the MDGs and GFATM in the 2000s and the call for elimination by the SDGs in the 2010s.

The norm for HIV/AIDS control is certainly newer and has not exhibited the same kind of fluctuation. When it was discovered during the early 1980s, it did not elicit much of response in global politics largely due to its perception as a "gay cancer." The growth of HIV cases in Africa during the 1980s and the efforts of the WHO and civil society organizations in the 1980s and 1990s and UNAIDS in the 1990s heightened AIDS awareness to such as an extent that it emerged as the priority issue in global health. According to constructivists, states are more compelled to reduce the global burden of infectious diseases today than they were thirty years ago. The norm for infectious disease control, however, is still evolving. It is not yet quite strong enough to reach the international community's goals for funding and the elimination of these diseases as a burden on global health.

In terms of identity, the identity of global infectious disease control has shifted between eradication and control. Eradication, of course, is the more attractive option. The experiences of malaria and tuberculosis, however, reveal that even with effective treatment and preventive measures, achieving eradication is difficult because once significant progress is made; the actors of global health governance have tended to lose some interest and focus on other issues. The SDGs represent a current identification of global governance for the "big three" diseases to either be eradicated or at least be close to eradication by 2030. Whether or not this framing of the global response to these infectious diseases will hold remains to be seen.

Marxist-based approaches would point to a strong relationship between infectious diseases and economic inequality. The fact that the "big three" diseases predominately impact the world's poorest countries demonstrates this claim. Globalization is a driving factor in the impact of infectious diseases. Developed states have become enriched by international capitalism to the detriment of developing states. The economic development of these states is hindered by their dependence on rich states for economic capital. Because poor states are at a disadvantage in international economic transactions and many are subject to significant foreign debt obligations, they lack the resources to provide sufficient means of prevention and treatment of these diseases. Marxists are particularly critical of multinational corporations and how their incentives for profit have hindered access to essential medicines to the world's poor. Even as international organizations such as the UN and WHO have called for universal access to treatment, MNCs have continued to shield their profits through the WTO and political support by developed states. From a Marxist perspective, for global health governance to effectively manage the infectious disease burden, it must not only act to compel states and MNCs to provide greater support for prevention and treatment of these diseases, but it must also convince these actors to provide a greater effort in addressing the deeper issues of poverty and economic development that are linked to them. The SDGs represent a trend in this direction by their holistic approach to health, but as the case with neoliberal institutionalists, the lack of a robust rules-based approach to this problem will likely lead Marxist-based approaches to be skeptical regarding the prospects for eliminating these diseases.

These different views suggest some important considerations for global health governance. As noted, international infectious disease control fits well with the concept of a collective good. Because these diseases can move from person to person and country to country, all will benefit from effective control of these diseases. Realism, neoliberal institutionalism, constructivism, and Marxism, however, offer some significant challenges for this good to be provided to all. The interest of great powers is certainly related to all of these perspectives. Realists consider this factor to be especially critical because without political and economic support from powerful states, effective infectious disease control on a global level will not be adequately provided. Neoliberal institutionalists have more faith in international institutions to enhance cooperation in this area; however, they also acknowledge that without the support of great powers in developing strong institutions, these institutions will be relatively ineffective in facilitating the provision of this good. Constructivists would highlight that humanitarian and moral considerations are also very relevant factors, in addition to material interests, to understand the motivations of great powers in supporting effective disease control. To assess their level of commitment, it will be necessary to account for the strength of infectious disease control as an international norm and the degree to which great powers have been socialized by it. If either of these are lacking, then the commitment of great powers to infectious disease control will be limited, and then it can be expected that the good will be undersupplied. Marxist-based approaches, of course, view great powers as promoters of globalization and international capitalism. Due to their vested interest in maintaining the capitalist system, their support for international infectious disease control will be dependent on how it impacts their economic growth and the profits of their business interests. Unless these areas are adversely affected, then committing to an effective system of controlling these diseases will not be a significant interest for these states, and collective action will be ineffective.

The fundamental question regarding the establishment of an effective system for international infectious disease control is what is to be done to improve the current system? One approach that would correspond in particular to neoliberal institutionalist views but also to constructivists would be through enhanced international legalization. Fidler (1999) has proposed a framework convention on infectious disease prevention and control that would complement the revised IHR. The key components of this treaty are (1) legal principles for states to follow in the areas of surveillance, trade-restricting health measures, human rights, and environmental protection; (2) specific commitments that states would be required to take to achieve effective prevention and control of these diseases; (3) a financial mechanism supported by developed states, which can be used to assist developing states in managing the burden of infectious diseases; (4) potential for protocols to address specific diseases and other health issues; and (5) mechanisms for monitoring compliance.

Although the revised IHR and GFATM have moved the infectious disease control regime more in the direction of this framework since 2000, the fundamental objective of Fidler's (1999) proposal is to solidify an "international legal code" for infectious disease. Such a code would provide both guidance and obligations for states to contribute to an improved regime. Neoliberal institutionalists would support the view that this proposed agreement would strengthen the regime and would be more effective at providing control. If such an agreement were to be adopted, constructivists would regard it as a manifestation of the development of a stronger norm. It would represent a greater interest by states to provide the global good of infectious disease control. Realists, in contrast, would be pessimistic at both the prospects and effectiveness of such a treaty. They would suggest that powerful states are not yet sufficiently threatened by infectious diseases to make such a legal commitment to this issue. Even if such an agreement were to be accepted, realists would maintain that compliance with its provisions would be subject to the national interests of the most powerful states. Marxists would also be wary about the prospects of such an agreement. While Marxists would consider enhanced regulation as an important component in reigning in capitalism and compelling developed states to assist developing states with infectious diseases, they would be skeptical as to whether such rules could effectively regulate the policies of rich states and the activities of MNCs in their overriding desire for economic gain.

CONCLUSION

Historically, infectious disease control has been the most prominent health issue in international politics. Major advances in this area have taken place in global health governance over the past twenty years as exhibited by greater attention to this issue by the United Nations, World Bank, the creation of GFATM, and significant increases in funding. The prevalence and fatalities from three of the world's major infectious diseases, malaria, tuberculosis, and HIV/AIDS, have declined as a result, and the MDG targets for addressing these diseases have been considered successful. Nevertheless, more progress needs to be made to satisfy the SDG expectations of the international community for 2030. Prevention of infectious diseases and access to medicine, in particular, remain elusive goals. Different theories of international relations provide some useful guidance for why infectious disease control continues to be a challenging issue for global health governance despite costing millions of lives on an annual basis. Realism emphasizes the role of great powers and their interests. While infectious disease control is related to security, the relatively small impact that these diseases have on these states limits their support. Neoliberal institutionalists focus on the lack of international law in this area as a factor, while constructivists believe that effective control on a global level is still an evolving norm in international politics. Marxist-based approaches tend to find that infectious diseases are related to economic inequality. As long as globalization continues to increase the gap between developed and developing states, the poor will continue to suffer a vast amount of the burden brought by infectious diseases. Even as science and technology improve, rich states will be reluctant to share these innovations with poor states unless the poor states are willing to pay a substantial cost for them. The SDGs represent an opportunity to end the global epidemic of the "big three." However, for global governance to continue to make progress in this area, state and non-state actors must devise effective means to overcome these obstacles.

DISCUSSION QUESTIONS

1. What is a collective good, and how may infectious disease control be considered a collective action problem in international politics?
2. The World Health Assembly called for eradication of malaria in 1955, and sixty years later, the United Nations' Sustainable Development Goals have targeted an end of the malaria epidemic by 2030. With this long-standing political support in global governance, why has it been so difficult to put an end to this disease?

3. What have been the advances and the challenges for global governance in addressing tuberculosis?
4. Why is HIV/AIDS considered to be an exceptional disease in global health? How do theories of international relations explain why HIV/AIDS is a promising area for international health cooperation?

SUGGESTED READINGS

Barnett, Tony, and Alan Whiteside. 2006. *AIDS in the Twenty-First Century: Disease and Globalization*. Second Edition. New York: Palgrave Macmillan.

Provides a thorough analysis of the origins and global impact of HIV/AIDS.

Fidler, David P. 1999. *International Law and Infectious Disease*. Oxford: Clarendon Press.

Offers a comprehensive analysis of the relationship between international law and infectious disease.

Harman, Sophie. 2012. *Global Health Governance*. New York: Routledge.

A good overview of malaria, HIV/AIDS, tuberculosis, and neglected diseases.

Smith, Richard, Robert Beaglehole, David Woodward, and Nick Drager. 2003. *Global Public Goods for Health: Health Economics and Public Health Perspectives*. Oxford: Oxford University Press.

Edited volume that includes a number of health-related case studies to analyze health through an economic analysis of a global public good.

Chapter 5

Securitizing Global Health

This chapter examines the security aspects of global health. Security is a key component of the study of international politics, but it is also an elusive concept. As Wolfers (1952) noted over sixty years ago, national security is "an ambiguous symbol" in that it is based on the subjective determination of what a particular state values. Although frequently used as an explanatory variable in theory and policy analysis, this ambiguity remains an issue today. In fact, Baldwin (1997: 26) argued that "no social science concept has been more abused or misused than national security." Realists have long assumed that security is associated with military force by national governments. Constructivists emerged as the chief opponents of this view as they consider security to be a much more fluid concept resulting from social interactions. Buzan et al. (1998), for instance, propose that any public issue can be placed on a spectrum that can range from "non-politicized" (where it is not addressed by the state) to "politicized" (where the state will be required to make decisions to address it) to "securitized" (where the state takes extraordinary measure to protect it from outside threats). Whether a policy issue is "securitized" depends on if an actor (i.e., the state, political leader) can convince the audience (i.e., the state, citizens, or even all of humankind) to accept the idea that the issue represents such a significant threat that it is above "normal politics" and should be treated as a top priority and addressed by exceptional means.

According to Rothschild (1995), liberal thought during the eighteenth century understood security to be both an individual and collective good. Individual security was associated with political rights and economic freedom, in which the state provided an apparatus that would both be a source of security and insecurity for individuals. In contrast, realist thinking about international relations heavily associated security with military protection by the state against external threats. This idea was shaped by the experience of the French

Revolution and the Napoleonic Wars during the late eighteenth and early nineteenth century, respectively, and was reinforced by the devastation of the two world wars in the first half of the twentieth century. Survival of the state was viewed as paramount to the national interest of the state. The Cold War continued the perception that security was related to military force based on the rivalry between the United States and the Soviet Union and the threat of nuclear war (McInnes and Lee 2012). The post–Cold War world, which has seen a significant decline in interstate war, however, provides an opportunity to expand the concept of security beyond national security to individual and global dimensions (Rothschild 1995).

From a rationalist perspective, framing health as a security issue fits best with liberal perspectives of international relations. Concern over the welfare of the individual has been a focus of classic liberal thought. Liberals are also more flexible than realists in their understanding of the national interest of the state. Although realists may focus their conceptualization of security on military force and consider health to be more in the realm of "low politics," they may still be amenable to considering health as a security issue. This consideration, however, would most likely require a potentially significant health impact on a state's military strength or political stability.

Due to the emphasis by constructivists on framing issues based on social interaction and the adoption of norms through socialization, health could become established as a fairly extensive international security issue as long as it becomes accepted as such by foreign policy elites. Marxists approaches tend to consider security as involving more of the protection of the capitalist economic system and capitalist ideas. If on one hand, a health issue were to threaten international travel, tourism, or commerce, Marxists would expect a robust response from the actors from global governance, especially if wealthy states and interests of multinational corporations were affected. On the other hand, interest in securing health will be constrained by whether or not such measures would infringe on profit-maximizing economic activities.

This chapter will explore the issue of global health security by first examining the evolution of health as an issue for global security. Second, it will examine two health issues that have strong connections to security: the spread of infectious diseases, especially newly emerging infectious diseases, and biosecurity. McInnes and Lee (2006) have identified these areas as the dominant health issues in international security policy. Third, it will consider the utility of global health governance in providing health security and the prospects for a more robust response to protecting health at the global level. The key questions that may be considered in this chapter include the following: Is global health, in fact, a security issue, and if so, what is the nature of the connection between health and security? Has global governance effectively addressed problems emanating from emerging infectious diseases? What is the nature of the threat from biological weapons and bioterrorism, and is the current system of global health governance equipped to sufficiently respond to this threat?

EMERGENCE OF HEALTH AS A GLOBAL SECURITY ISSUE

Although health did not become effectively addressed as an international security issue until the post–Cold War era, it has long been featured as a security concern for states. As noted by Brundtland (2003: 417), "disease was often seen as an impediment to exploration and a challenge to winning a war." As discussed in more detail in chapter 2 on intergovernmental organizations (IGOs), the origins of global health governance were based on security as European states established the standard practice of quarantines to prevent the spread of infectious diseases from entering their country. Hoffman (2010) identifies four different time periods of global health security governance: (1) unilateral quarantine regulations (1377–1851), (2) multiple sanitary conferences (1851–1892), (3) international sanitary conventions and international organizations (1892–1946), and (4) the hegemonic leadership of the WHO (1946–present). The international sanitary conventions of the nineteenth and twentieth centuries were devised as a solution to assist states to move beyond unilateral measures and begin to coordinate their quarantine efforts with other states, as well as to mitigate their impact on international commerce. Historically, states have tended to address infectious disease as an internal security matter. This characterization was the case even with the international sanitary conventions. Under these conventions, states had a duty to notify other states regarding outbreaks of limited set of diseases. This obligation, along with a standardization of measures to be taken for quarantines, was the maximum extent of international cooperation institutionalized by these agreements. They were mostly designed to assist the state in protecting itself from outside diseases than promoting a collective good.

The World Health Organization (WHO) became the lead institution for global health following its establishment in 1948. Three years later, the WHO's World Health Assembly (WHA) adopted the International Sanitary Regulations to replace the existing conventions. Although these regulations covered only the diseases of smallpox, cholera, yellow fever, typhus, relapsing fever, and the plague, they did require that states notify the WHO of the occurrence of these diseases in their territory. The International Sanitary Regulations were revised in 1969 to be renamed as the International Health Regulations (IHR). Other than the removal of typhus and relapsing fever, there was little difference between the IHR and the International Sanitary Regulations.

The limited rules and obligations of the conventions, the International Sanitary Regulations, and the IHR, however, conveyed little sense that health was a matter of international security. As discussed in chapter 2, the WHO focused its efforts during the Cold War at first on the control of certain infectious diseases, such as the eradication of malaria, followed by the promotion of primary health care and the "health for all" objective during the 1970s. Outside of disease surveillance, the WHO did not promote a security connotation with the global health agenda.

The Concept of Emerging Infectious Diseases

The emergence of the concept of global health security began in the mid-1990s. Weir (2015) credits a report by the U.S. Institute of Medicine on the threat of emerging infectious diseases to the United States as the impetus for the formation of global health security. This report established the concept of emerging infectious diseases and discussed how they could threaten the United States and how the United States would require international cooperation to detect and respond to such diseases that originated beyond its borders. The United States used its diplomatic influence to convince other states to support this action. In 1995, the WHA passed a resolution, which both endorsed the emerging infectious disease concept and supported an improvement in the WHO's capacity for surveillance and response to these diseases.

The acceptance of the emerging infectious disease concept in global health governance, along with outbreaks of cholera in Peru, plague in India, and the global HIV/AIDS epidemic, contributed to sufficient political support to commence negotiations to revise the IHR during this time. The limited applicability of the IHR's disease coverage and a general lack of compliance with its provisions convinced member states that the IHR (1969) was an outdated and ineffective instrument. These events involving the increased recognition of emerging infectious diseases and the negotiations over the IHR coincided with the rise of the concept of human security in global governance. This concept was first elaborated in a 1994 United Nations Development Programme (UNDP) report, which suggested that security should be reinterpreted to focus on the protection of human beings, rather than the traditional perspective of security as defense of territory. It argued that most people's lives were threatened by everyday dangers rather than external military force. Health certainly fit into this conceptualization, which contributed to the growing momentum of the idea that health, in fact, had an international security dimension.

To implement the WHA's resolution on emerging infectious diseases, the WHO created a new division covering these diseases separate from the preexisting division on communicable diseases. This new division began development on the Global Outbreak Alert and Response Network (GOARN), which started in 1997 and was formalized in 2000. GOARN was a mechanism outside of the IHR that would allow the WHO to use all possible sources of information to surveil outbreaks of infectious diseases around the world independent of official government notification. As noted by Fidler (2005), GOARN provided a means to empower the WHO while negotiations over the IHR remained unsettled. Without the adoption of an additional formal legal framework, GOARN allowed the WHO to monitor diseases outside the scope of the IHR, permitted the WHO to significantly expand its data on infectious diseases by incorporating information gathered from the Internet and reports from non-state actors, and assisted the WHO in investigating several outbreaks of infectious diseases that were not required to be reported under the IHR (Fidler 2005).

Another breakthrough for global health security was the resolution passed by the United Nations Security Council in 2000 to acknowledge that the HIV/AIDS epidemic could pose a risk to state security. This occasion was the first time that the Security Council adopted a resolution regarding a health threat. It also served to legitimize the disease as a security issue (McInnes 2006). Such recognition by the highest security institution in global governance provided an indication that health specifically, and human security more generally, would become part of the international security agenda in the twenty-first century.

While HIV/AIDS moved to the center of global health security with the UN Security Council resolution, the WHA continued to push the inclusion of emerging infectious diseases, as well as WHO influence, as part of this agenda. In 2001, the WHA passed a resolution that equated global health security with epidemic alert and response. It urged member states to participate in surveillance and information sharing about health emergencies with the WHO and other relevant actors such as other intergovernmental and non-governmental organizations, while IHR negotiations were still ongoing. The following year, the WHA passed another resolution that addressed the intentional use of biological, chemical, or radioactive agents as a threat to global health. What is most notable about this resolution is that it expanded the WHO's scope of activity to cover bioterrorism, an area that was associated with traditional international security institutions and was not covered by the WHO constitution or the IHR (Weir 2015).

International Health Regulations (2005)

Agreement on the revised IHR was finally reached in 2005, after the international outbreak of SARS in 2003. This IHR's (also discussed in chapters 2 and 4) purpose is to provide surveillance and response to diseases that could spread across borders and coordinate the detection and control of these threats. Unlike the WHA resolutions, the IHR is a legally binding instrument on all member states. Its coverage of diseases is much broader than IHR (1969), but also less specific. With the exception of a few diseases that always require notification (i.e., smallpox, new subtype influenza, and SARS), any disease events considered to be of significant international concern are required to be reported to the WHO by national governments. States are also obligated to establish national focal points to serve as a contact for communication with the WHO and develop national emergency plans and a public health preparedness infrastructure to respond to health risks.

Gostin (2014) describes the IHR (2005) as a balance among international trade, human rights, and public health interests. In regard to trade, the IHR requires that health measures cannot be more restrictive on trade than necessary to reduce the risk to health. Human rights protections include a commitment that health response measures were to be applied in a non-discriminatory manner and that international human rights law must be taken into account by national governments in their treatment of persons when attempting to reduce health risks. The public health component was based upon scientific methodologies. Both the determination of whether an event qualifies as an international health emergency and the implementation of health measures in response are required to be based on scientific evidence.

The IHR (2005) also formalized the legal basis for the WHO's steps taken since 2000 in expanding its influence into international security. Although a proposal to include a requirement that member states notify the WHO and give it all relevant data if chemical, biological, radioactive, or nuclear weapons were used in a country was rejected, the WHO still gained some authority in this area through IHR (2005). Both the "all risks" approach taken for IHR notification and the IHR's mention of intentional or unintentional release of toxic and hazardous materials as an example of an event with a high public health impact indicates that the WHO has been granted an international security mandate through this instrument (Weir 2015).

The Road to the Global Health Security Agenda

The securitization of health reached another milestone with the WHO's world health report in 2007, which was based on the theme of public health security. This report emphasized the collective threat that infectious diseases posed to all states in the era of globalization. The WHO advocated a collective response in terms of reporting and surveillance of these diseases. It also relied, however, on each state to effectively contribute to the response, due to its lack of authority to enforce compliance. The report pointed out that even though SARS did not evolve into a global pandemic and was limited to just over 8,000 infections, the economic cost to the Asian countries that were affected amounted to over US$2 million per infected person (World Health Organization 2007: 39). The fear of contracting the disease reflected by decline in tourism and consumer spending, rather than treating the disease itself, provided most of the economic cost. A global pandemic would prove to have far more of an impact both upon human life and economic costs.

Despite the SARS outbreak, the swine flu (H1N1) pandemic in 2009, and the WHO report, the conceptualization of health as a security issue lost some momentum in the late 2000s. One reason has to do with the problem of defining health security (Aldis 2008). Developed states tend to view health security as defense of their populations from bioterrorism or infectious diseases that are outside of their country. Developing countries consider health security as based on the provision of adequate health care for all individuals, a much broader perspective. The WHO report did not promote either perspective, as it focused on health security as compliance with the IHR. The lack of consensus on the meaning of health security has curtailed its impact.

The second reason has to do with the evolution of HIV/AIDS as a security issue since 2000. The Security Council did not address the issue again until passing a resolution in 2011. McInnes and Rushton (2010) suggest that this delay was due to the fact that the consensus on 2000 resolution was not particularly strong, due to the rise of terrorism as a security concern since 2001 and the lack of empirical evidence linking HIV/AIDS with state stability. Because HIV/AIDS had been the only health issue to reach the "high politics" realm of the Security Council, its fall from the agenda indicated less visibility of health as an international security issue than was the case in the late 1990s and early 2000s.

Nevertheless, the rising political profile and economic costs of emerging infectious diseases in the 2000s was significant enough to lead to some diplomatic progress on global health cooperation. In February 2014, the U.S. announced a global health security agenda in partnership with the WHO, the Food and Agriculture Organization (FAO), the World Organization for Animal Health, and over 40 countries (The White House 2016). The goal of the Global Health Security Agenda (GHSA) is to:

> to strengthen both the global capacity and nations' capacity to prevent, detect, and respond to infectious diseases threats whether naturally occurring, deliberate, or accidental—capacity that once established would mitigate the devastating effects of Ebola, MERS, other highly pathogenic infectious diseases, and bioterrorism events. (Global Health Security Agenda 2016)

Its purpose is not to compete or duplicate the IHR but rather facilitate and accelerate its implementation (Frieden et al. 2014). The GHSA provides a mechanism to assist states that lack the core capacity to put their responsibilities under the IHR into practice. It seeks to bring health security above the ministerial level to that of national leaders. During its first meeting in Helsinki, Finland, in May 2014, an "Action Package" concept was established to promote GHSA objectives. The packages are directed at eleven areas such as antimicrobial resistance, zoonotic disease, biosafety and biosecurity, immunization, as well as measures for detection (i.e., nationwide laboratory network) and response (i.e., emergency operations center) to infectious diseases. They include "the relevant five-year target, an indicator by which to measure progress, desired impact, current country commitments, five-year action items, and lists of baseline assessment, planning, monitoring, and evaluation activities necessary to implement the action items" (Centers for Disease Control and Prevention 2016). If effective prevention, detection, and response programs are established, countries may protect both their nationals and vulnerable populations around the world from the threat of infectious disease (Frieden et al. 2014).

At this point, the GHSA is in its early stages of implementation, and it was launched at the beginning of the Ebola outbreak, so its impact in addressing the international spread of infectious disease is yet to be determined. On one hand, it could be viewed as a means to strengthen the IHR. Gostin and Katz (2017), for instance, suggest that the GHSA should be harmonized with the IHR, as the IHR provides the primary international legal criteria for global health security, but the GHSA action packages may provide a significant source of funding in support. Alternatively, however, the GHSA could be perceived through a realist lens as a response to the inadequacy of an IGO to address a major international threat, and the need for the U.S. government to step in and address a gap in global governance (Lancet 2014). Regardless of which path will be taken by the GHSA, it represents how the link between health and security has continued to grow in the early twenty-first century, and how states are becoming more willing to accept that infectious disease is a collective threat that requires international cooperation to help resolve.

PANDEMIC THREATS AND EMERGING INFECTIOUS DISEASES

HIV/AIDS

Notwithstanding the rise of the concept of emerging infectious diseases in the mid-1990s, the first health issue to cross over into international security was HIV/AIDS. In early 2000, following a Central Intelligence Agency (CIA) report that suggested the spread of HIV/AIDS in Africa could create problems for international and U.S. security, U.S. president Bill Clinton declared the disease to be a threat to national security (Flint 2011). This development spurred the UN Security Council to consider whether it should endorse this position in regard to international security. As discussed in July 2000, the Security Council passed resolution 1308, marking the first time that it identified a health issue as a threat to international peace and security.

How did HIV/AIDS evolve from a domestic social problem to an international security threat? Elbe (2010) identifies three areas where this disease was considered to threaten security. The first area was a presumed connection between HIV/AIDS and the military. In particular, some evidence indicated that military personnel were much more likely to acquire the HIV virus than civilians. This finding was especially the case in sub-Saharan Africa. Second was a presumption, also aimed at sub-Saharan Africa, that HIV/AIDS could threaten political and social stability of states with high prevalence of infections. The fear, in this case, was that such instability would exacerbate violent conflict, which may result in outside military intervention. The third area was the relationship between the spread of HIV/AIDS and international peacekeeping. As more peacekeeping operations included soldiers from countries with a high prevalence of HIV/AIDS, the concern was that these individuals could spread the disease in the country of their deployment as an unintended consequence of their mission.

Resolution 1308 was a significant milestone in securitizing health in global governance. Rushton (2010), however, argued that despite passing the resolution, members of the UN Security Council in 2000 still did not consider HIV/AIDS to be a genuine threat to international peace and security. One factor involved in the successful passage of this resolution was the effective politicking by the United States and the Clinton administration. The United States put the issue on the Security Council's agenda. Some states had major reservations on supporting this issue (China, France, and Russia). While they were eventually persuaded by the United States to pass the resolution, such support may have been due more to American diplomatic pressure and possible reputational costs in opposing a human rights issue than a genuine belief that HIV/AIDS was, in fact, a threat to security. To support this contention, Rushton (2010) points out that during the UN General Assembly's special session on HIV/AIDS, which was held less than a year after the passage of resolution 1308, only 33 percent of the speeches given during this meeting even mentioned HIV/AIDS as a security issue. Resolution 1308 was rarely mentioned at the event. Far more references were made to HIV/AIDS as a development or human rights issue. Another factor that Rushton (2010) contributes to the successful passage of resolution 1308 was that the relationship between HIV/AIDS and security was couched in soft language in the operative clause of the resolution with much of its focus on peacekeeping rather than state stability. Even the resolution's non-binding preamble stated that HIV/AIDS "may" pose a risk to stability and security.

As discussed in chapter 4, the Security Council resolution was part of a significant international policy effort in the early 2000s to address HIV/AIDS. Between 2001 and 2003, the UN General Assembly approved the Declaration of Commitment on HIV/AIDS, and the Global Fund to Fight AIDS, Tuberculosis, and Malaria (GFATM), as well as the President's Emergency Plan for AIDS Relief (PEPFAR), were created. After 2005, however, the securitization of HIV/AIDS began to lose momentum. A continuing examination of empirical evidence on the areas that tied the disease to security suggested that the concern over these issues may have been overstated. Research indicated the lack of a direct relationship between HIV/AIDS and state stability. Additional studies also did not find a strong connection between the spread of the disease and the military and whether it was in conflict zones or during peacekeeping operations (McInnes and Rushton 2010). The UN Security Council did pass another resolution addressing HIV/AIDS in 2011; however, the meeting in 2011 was not a high-profile event as the 2000 session (McInnes and Rushton 2013: 130). Although the empirical link between HIV/AIDS and security may be tenuous, the disease did serve to place health on the security agenda, and it continues to have a security connotation in the discourse of global health governance.

SARS

HIV/AIDS is not the only new infectious disease that has developed over the past forty years. According to the WHO (2007), over forty of these new diseases have been identified since the 1970s. The severe acute respiratory syndrome (SARS) was the first new disease to become a global pandemic in the twenty-first century. The SARS virus originated in Guangdong, China, a province on the coast of the South China Sea. It is not entirely known how the disease originated, but the most common belief is that it originated in animals and was later transmitted to humans.

This region of China was known for the slaughter and consumption of certain wild animals as delicacies, and it is widely believed that this practice was responsible for the transfer of the virus. The first case of a SARS infection in a human was indicated at a local hospital in the province in January 2003. It was diagnosed as an unusual form of pneumonia, but it was not reported to the WHO. As the disease began to spread in the region, the WHO slowly became aware of the scope of the epidemic through e-mail and Internet reports as information was difficult to obtain from the Chinese government. Once the WHO approached the government about the disease, they acknowledged the outbreak of this unknown disease, but they also indicated that the spread of the disease had peaked and was now effectively under control (Fidler 2004). In February 2003, a doctor who had been treating SARS patients in Guangdong went to a hotel in Hong Kong and infected sixteen others (Fidler 2004).

One of the infected individuals, an American businessman, traveled to Hanoi, Vietnam, and checked into a hospital. The disease was soon spread to hospital staff, and by March 15, 2003, forty-three cases of individuals with SARS had been reported in Vietnam (WHO 2003a).

Around this time, the WHO issued a global alert about this mysterious disease, which identified the location of the outbreak (Guangdong, Hong Kong, and Hanoi), the relevant symptoms, and recommended the isolation of individuals exhibiting the signs of the disease. The WHO also requested that any cases of the disease should be reported to the national government and issued an international travel advisory. The issuance of this alert was also the first instance of the disease given the name of SARS by the WHO (Fidler 2004). The WHO worked quickly to establish a global network of doctors to share and disseminate information about this new disease.

The cross-border transfer of SARS occurred rapidly. In addition to the spread of the disease from Hong Kong to Hanoi, two other guests infected at the Hong Kong hotel had soon after traveled to Singapore and Canada, spreading the disease to those countries in the process. By April 2003, the WHO (2003b) had found over 1,800 cases of SARS in fifteen countries. Due to the rapid spread of the disease, the WHO decided to take a much more aggressive response than was customary. Its actions included the issuance of a travel advisory for SARS "hot zones," which was criticized by the Canadian government because Toronto was included as one of these areas. The WHO was also publicly critical of the Chinese government and accused it of greatly underreporting of the number of SARS cases in the country (Fidler 2004). The Chinese government became more cooperative following the confrontation with the WHO. At this point, according to Heymann et al. (2013: 780):

> Official reporting and effective national outbreak control followed, and, in what became perhaps the greatest legacy of SARS, disease reporting changed almost overnight from being approached with hesitancy and preoccupation with concern about the economic fallout from such transparency, to something that was simply expected and respected.

The global spread of the disease peaked by the end of April, and the disease was effectively under control by July as the WHO declared the transmission chain among humans to have ended (WHO 2003c). By this time, 8,456 cases of SARS had occurred in thirty states, and resulted in 809 deaths. Almost half of the cases were in China (Fleck 2003). The SARS epidemic of 2003 was truly a reflection of twenty-first century globalization. Its spread around the world in only a few months from southern China was a result of international air travel. The response, however, was largely based on monitoring of the disease from e-mail and Internet reports by non-state actors, which was an unprecedented measure in controlling an infectious disease. Despite the fear generated by the rapid speed and distance covered by SARS, the cost of life was relatively low compared to past pandemics, as well as the annual impact of malaria, tuberculosis, and HIV/AIDS on global health. The fact that a new disease was discovered and effectively halted in only a matter of months was an impressive accomplishment for global health governance. David Fidler (2004: 105) considered that the global response to SARS "will undoubtedly rank as one of the great success stories in the history of global public health efforts on infectious diseases, and the greatest achievement in this realm since the eradication of smallpox in the late 1970s." The experience of the SARS epidemic motivated the WHA to substantially revise the IHR. The new version was accepted in 2005 and went into force in 2007.

H1N1 (Swine Flu)

The first challenge for the revised IHR was the introduction of another new virus, H1N1, discovered in the United States in April 2009. It was later determined that the virus had previously been contracted in Mexico. It was a virus that had not been identified before in humans or animals (Centers for Disease Control and Prevention 2010). Because the virus was similar to influenza viruses originating in pigs, it became referred to the "swine flu," even though it was transmitted by human contact. Soon after its identification, the WHO declared the virus as a "public health emergency of international concern" (PHEIC) under the rules of IHR, and advised states to monitor unusual cases of influenza. By June, WHO Director-General Margaret Chan announced that the global alert for H1N1 was raised to level 6 on the influenza pandemic scale, its highest level designating a global pandemic.

Although the H1N1 virus was globally widespread, some governments and experts disagreed with the WHO that the severity of the disease was significant enough to warrant the "pandemic" designation, making the decision somewhat controversial (Fidler 2009). The WHO's pandemic alert lasted until August 2010 when the outbreak of H1N1 was considered to be in a post-pandemic phase. A study on the first year of the pandemic estimated that approximately 284,000 people worldwide died due to the H1N1 virus. A great majority (80%) of these deaths were to individuals under age sixty-five, and 51 percent of the deaths related to the virus were in the developing regions of southeast Asia and Africa (Dawood et al. 2012). Although the number of deaths due to the H1N1 influenza was high, it was not too dissimilar from that of normal, seasonal influenza, which continues to make the WHO's pandemic designation for this outbreak to be questionable (Doshi 2013).

BOX 5.1 IS AVIAN INFLUENZA THE NEXT GLOBAL PANDEMIC?

A great fear for health professionals is the potential spread of avian influenza (H5N1). This virus was first discovered as an infection in chickens in 1878. Outbreaks of this disease among wild birds have occurred several times in a variety of countries over the past forty years (Horimoto and Kawaoka 2001). It was not considered to pose a danger to humans until 1997 when it was transmitted in Hong Kong poultry markets from selling live birds to eighteen people, six of whom died from exposure. Because the virus had never before appeared in humans, no treatment or cure was available.

Avian influenza did not appear again until 2003 when two people in Hong Kong became infected. This time, however, the disease spread beyond China as it emerged over the next three years with human infections in Vietnam, Korea, Thailand, Cambodia, Indonesia, Turkey, and Iraq. Despite this spread, acquiring avian influenza is rare for humans. Since the 2003 outbreak, the countries that have reported the greatest number of cases have been Egypt (359), Indonesia (200), Vietnam (127), and Cambodia (56) (World Health Organization 2018a). Even though avian influenza has had only a relatively small impact on human populations, the major concern for the disease is its potential to become the next great global pandemic. Cases of the disease have occurred primarily in transmissions from poultry to humans. The fear, however, is that the virus could mutate to become a contagion spread by human to human contact. Given that the H5N1 virus has killed almost half of those infected, along with the lack of any natural immunity to the virus for humans, greatly influences the fear of this possibility. Although an avian influenza global pandemic may never occur, it is a genuine fear in global health governance.

Ebola

The SARS and H1N1 pandemics contributed to concerns that other new diseases emerging from animal to human transmissions could lead to future, and even more deadly, pandemics. The 2014 outbreak of the Ebola haemorrhagic fever (or Ebola virus) demonstrated this fear. Depending on the particular strain of the Ebola virus, the risk of death caused by infections from the Ebola virus can range between 25 percent and 90 percent (Feldmann and

Geisbert 2011). This virus was first discovered in Zaire (now the Democratic Republic of the Congo) and Sudan in 1976. It is not known how the virus originated, but its presence in humans has been attributed to contact with infected animals. Apes and fruit bats have been found to be a common carrier of the virus. Additionally, it can also be transmitted by infected humans. Five different subtypes of the Ebola virus have been discovered. Prior to 2014, the largest outbreak occurred in Uganda in 2000 with 425 cases, with 53 percent resulting in death (WHO 2012b). Although the Ebola virus has proven to be extremely deadly, it is a rare disease that has previously largely been restricted to central Africa. Contemporary globalization, however, has made the global spread of this disease possible. The virus, in fact, was first found in the United States in 1989. Shipments of monkeys sent from the Philippines were found to be infected at a facility in Reston, Virginia. Although no humans were infected, the presence of an extremely fatal disease in the United States, which until that point had only been found in central Africa, was alarming at the time.

The 2014 Ebola outbreak, however, dwarfed all of the combined previous outbreaks of the virus both in the number of cases and its global spread. Fauci (2017: 21) described the outbreak as a "perfect storm" in that it was associated with "poor countries with histories of conflict, political unrest, and resultant mistrust of government; densely populated cities; severely limited healthcare infrastructure; and long-standing cultural practices that enhance the potential for contact with infectious bodily fluids." By April 2016, more than 28,000 cases of Ebola infections were reported with over 11,000 deaths (WHO Ebola Response Team 2016).

This epidemic originated in a village in the West African country of Guinea in December 2013. It soon spread beyond this village to other parts of Guinea as well as its neighboring states of Liberia and Sierra Leone. The fact that the epidemic began in West Africa, by itself, was unusual. Prior to 2014, only one case of Ebola had been diagnosed in West Africa. That infection, which proved to be non-fatal, took place in Cote d'Ivoire rain forest in 1994 (Feldmann and Geisbert 2011). The transmission of the virus in Guinea was not diagnosed until March 2014, several weeks after the wave of deadly illnesses had begun.

The WHO proved to be slow in responding to the growing number of Ebola cases in West Africa. Only thirty-eight personnel were placed in Guinea by March of 2014, and it was not until August 8, 2014 after 1,000 deaths from the disease did the WHO declare the Ebola outbreak to be a PHEIC under the revised IHR (Sack et al. 2014). At this point two American aid workers had been affected, and an infected individual had entered into Nigeria. The American aid workers were sent to the United States for treatment, the first time a patient with the virus had been treated at an American hospital. The

WHO did not recommend a travel ban to the affected West African states, but it did say that these states should declare a national emergency, activate emergency management measures, and engage the community in education about the disease, as well as early identification and treatment (World Health Organization 2014a).In September 2014, the UN Security Council further demonstrated global governance's concern about the outbreak by unanimously passing a resolution declaring it to be a "threat to international peace and security." The UN General Assembly also supported the effort by authorizing the UN's first public health mission, the United Nations Mission for Ebola Emergency Response.

The virus began to spread outside of Africa in October 2014. The first case was when a nurse in Spain, who treated two victims of the virus in Madrid, became infected with Ebola. It also soon spread to the United States when a Liberian national, Thomas Eric Duncan, became infected with the Ebola virus and then traveled to Dallas, Texas. He died soon after his arrival in the United States from the disease. During the process of his treatment, however, two health care workers also became infected. Although these health care workers were successfully treated, the fact that Ebola had spread to the United States created a national panic. The situation exacerbated as later that month an American doctor, who had been treating Ebola patients in Guinea, became infected with the virus and returned to New York City before becoming aware that he had contracted the disease. In response, New York and New Jersey decided to quarantine many travelers from the affected West African countries. Australia, despite not having any reported cases of Ebola, went even further by closing its border to all citizens from the affected countries (Flanagin 2014).

Unlike the successful response to SARS in 2003, for the most part, the WHO's response to the 2014 Ebola outbreak has been considered to be inadequate (Farrar and Piot 2014; Gostin and Friedman 2014). One of the main points of criticism has been that the WHO deferred too much to the interests of member states rather than take a leadership role on its own. Director-General Chan's response to these contentions has been that it was the policy of the WHO to delegate authority to its office in Africa in the early stages of the epidemic and that the WHO's purpose was to assist the national governments in addressing the disease rather than replacing them as health care providers (Sengupta 2015). The WHO also faced criticism for not challenging the official reports from Guinea, Liberia, and Sierra Leone, which understated the severity of the epidemic in these countries. According to Kamradt-Scott (2016), this passive response was surprising given the reputation that these countries had for weak health care and a lack of a comprehensive disease surveillance system. The criticism that the WHO received from being overly aggressive with its response to H1N1 may have contributed to the organization's slow response (Kamradt-Scott 2016). Regardless of whether it was bureaucratic inefficiency or passive leadership, the credibility of the WHO in effectively addressing future pandemics has become questionable after the review of its performance in addressing the outbreak.

Zika Virus

The most recent declaration by the WHO of a public health emergency of international concern (PHEIC) was with the outbreak of the Zika virus in 2016. This virus is primarily spread to humans through mosquito bites. The first reported case of Zika was found in Uganda in 1947. During the next decade it spread through Africa and India. From the 1960s through the 1990s, the virus was found across equatorial Africa and spread into India, Pakistan, Indonesia, and Malaysia. For the most part, however, the disease was rarely found in humans, and when someone became infected, any symptoms tended to be moderate (Kindhauser et al. 2016).

The first outbreak of the Zika virus did not occur until 2007 in the island of Yap in the Federated States of Micronesia. Prior to this outbreak only sixteen cases infected with Zika had ever been reported. In this case, over 70 percent of the population on this small island was infected with the virus, although there were no reports of any serious illness (Kindhauser et al. 2016). In addition to the surprising fact that such a rare disease was so prevalent in a particular population was the tremendous distance that the virus had traveled from Africa and Asia where the earlier infections of the diseases had been discovered. Another outbreak of the virus in French Polynesia in 2013 revealed that Zika may not have been as mild of a disease as had been believed when it became associated with a simultaneous rise in Guillain-Barré syndrome. While most Zika infections were mild and might result in a fever, skin rash, muscle discomfort, or headache, Guillain-Barré syndrome was a neurological condition, which could lead to loss of sensation in a person's limbs and possibly paralysis (World Health Organization 2016b). In 2015, Zika virus infections were detected in Brazil, the first case in the Americas. The infections of pregnant women in Brazil revealed a link between the virus and microcephaly, which is a birth defect that leaves a baby with an abnormally small head and an underdeveloped brain at birth. The outbreak in Brazil also revealed that not only could Zika be transmitted via mosquitoes and prenatally, but by sexual intercourse as well. Over the next year over 500,000 people in the Americas became infected with Zika in over forty countries and territories (Ali et al. 2017).

The WHO had a difficult time addressing the Zika epidemic as the effects and transmission of the disease were not well known, especially in the Americas where the population may not have immunity (World Health Organization 2016). In February 2016, WHO Director-General Chan declared the Zika epidemic as a PHEIC, the first such declaration since the Ebola outbreak in 2014. Despite the PHEIC declaration, the global governance response to the epidemic could still be viewed as inadequate. The WHO calculated that it would need US$112 million to effectively implement its strategic response plan to Zika. By the end of 2016, however, it received only US$24.9 million in direct contributions (World Health Organization 2017e). Additionally, the WHO terminated the PHEIC declaration by November 2016. In doing so, the WHO decided to consider Zika as a seasonal mosquito-borne disease that was still a serious threat to health but as with malaria or other tropical diseases, would no longer be regarded as a global health emergency. Critics of the WHO's decision claimed that it was premature, would reduce funding for Zika control efforts, and make the disease less visible as a threat to health and as a global and a domestic health issue (McNeil 2016). The WHO, however, continues to assist countries in controlling the Zika virus through its strategic response plan.

BIOSECURITY: BIOLOGICAL WEAPONS AND BIOTERRORISM

Although biological weapons are labeled as "weapons of mass destruction" along with chemical and nuclear weapons, they operate quite a bit differently. While all three types of weapons have the potential to indiscriminately kill a massive numbers of people, biological weapons are the only type of weapons, however, that continue to be a threat after release by spreading from person to person as an infectious disease (Elbe 2010). In this sense, these weapons have much relevancy to global health governance. These weapons demonstrate that diseases not only spread naturally but also by intentional actions of human beings. Unlike chemical weapons, biological weapons are naturally occurring agents. This characteristic may change in the future as genetic engineering could lead to the weaponization of man-made viruses, but at this point in time only natural agents have been used in biological warfare (Carus 2015).

The use of biological weapons in war is not new. In fact, their use can be traced back to ancient Greece and Rome as dead animals were used to contaminate the drinking water of enemies (Elbe 2010). The use of such weapons over the past century, however, has been rare. The earliest instance of converting biological agents into instruments of modern warfare can be traced to Germany during World War I. These measures, however, were directed more at the horses and mules that provided transport for the supplies of their enemies rather than human beings. France was the only other state to engage in similar activities but apparently to a much lesser degree (Carus 2015).

After the war, the use of biological weapons was addressed by the Geneva Protocol in 1925. This agreement provided only a blanket statement banning the use of biological weapons in warfare. It was silent regarding other issues such as possession, stockpiling, or the development of a biological weapons program. The protocol was ratified by all major powers with the exception of Japan and the United States. France, nevertheless, proceeded with its biological weapons program after the protocol went into force. Its commitment to the protocol, however, and the German occupation in the 1940s both served to constrain the program's development (Guillemin 2005).

The most extensive case of a state using biological weapons as part of their military operation was by Japan in the 1930s and early 1940s (Carus 2015). The impetus for Japan's tactic was its 1931 invasion of Manchuria in northern China. The invasion was highly successful for the Japanese military and led to the conversion of Manchuria into the Japanese puppet state of Manchukuo. A Japanese military doctor, Shiro Ishii, attempted to persuade the military that with Western states committed to the Geneva Protocol, Japan could gain a military advantage by developing a biological weapons program on its own (Guillemin 2005). The occupation of Manchuria provided such an opportunity. After years of experiments on human test subjects, the Japanese military began to use biological weapons to launch several attacks on Chinese cities. Tactics included the use of fleas to start outbreaks of the plague and infection of water supplies with typhoid and cholera (Guillemin 2005). Despite its early experimentation and research with biological agents and warfare, Germany did not use biological weapons in its military operations during World War II. Evidence suggests that Japan was the only country that used these types of weapons in military operations during the war. Although some assessments indicate that resistance movements associated with the Soviet Union and Poland used biological attacks against German soldiers (Carus 2015).

The United Kingdom and the United States examined the potential for military applications for biological organisms during the 1940s. Unlike the United Kingdom, however, the United States did not ratify the Geneva Protocol, so it was not legally bound to ban the use of biological weapons in warfare. Nevertheless, the United States elected to not use such weapons during the Cold War even as it had significantly invested in research, development, and testing of such weapons after World War II. According to Guillemin (2005), the Korean and Vietnam wars posed ample opportunities for the United States to deploy biological weapons in combat. Although the United States faced allegations from North Korea and China that it used biological weapons during the Korean war, its leadership role in a UN-approved coalition and lack of effective biological bombs would seem to be significant reasons in preventing it from doing so. In the Vietnam case, political controversy over the American use of chemical agents such as riot control gases and herbicides seemed to deter the United States from deploying biological weapons during the conflict (Guillemin 2005: 94).

By the 1960s, interest in biological weapons was declining in both the United Kingdom and France due to their Geneva Protocol commitments, as well as their development of atomic weapons. The United States, under the pressure of international criticism for the use of chemical agents in Vietnam, began to reassess the utility of its biological weapons program. In 1969, American president Richard Nixon, announced that the United States would remove the potential use of biological weapons in combat from its military doctrine. Nixon's decision was not based on a compulsion to adhere to the principles of the Geneva Protocol as was the case with the Western European countries but rather realist logic in determining that it was not a cost-effective military program (Fidler and Gostin 2008). The U.S. decision and the growing international norm against the use of chemical and biological agents in combat during the Vietnam conflict contributed to an impetus to move beyond the Geneva Protocol to establish a more comprehensive international agreement addressing the use of biological weapons.

While the United States became more willing to accept the ban of biological weapons, its preference was to separate legal commitments for biological weapons from those it may accept for chemical weapons. The use of chemical agents by the United States in Vietnam made it more politically problematic for the United States to agree on a chemical weapons ban as that conflict was ongoing. The Soviet Union initially opposed the separation between these types of weapons but ultimately accepted this separation in return for a treaty commitment by all parties to continue to negotiate an agreement to ban chemical weapons in the future. In 1972, the Convention on the Prohibition of the Development, Production, and Stockpiling of Bacteriological (Biological) and Toxin Weapons and on their Destruction (BWC) was open for signature. It received a sufficient number of ratifications to enter into force in 1975. Currently, 175 states are parties to the BWC. Only some small states in Africa and the Pacific Ocean, along with Israel, have not accepted the agreement, making it almost universal in scope.

The BWC imposes much more significant obligations than the Geneva Protocol. Instead of merely banning the use of biological weapons in warfare, the BWC prohibits states from developing, producing, stockpiling, acquiring, or retaining biological agents that are not intended to be used for peaceful purposes or any biological weapons. States were also obligated to destroy such agents and weapons already in their possession and to not assist other states or international organizations from acquiring them. To put it another way, the purpose of the BWC was to make biological weapons a taboo subject.

Despite this fairly comprehensive scope of commitments, Fidler and Gostin (2008) noted some deficiencies in the rules of the BWC. First, the prohibition on biological weapons was based on intent, meaning that as long as biological agents and toxins were used for peaceful purposes, development and production were permitted. The treaty did not address how such intent was to be discerned. Second, although the BWC required states to execute its provisions into domestic law, it did not specify exactly what measures were to be taken or include a mechanism to ensure compliance. Although the BWC demonstrated the strength of an international norm prohibiting biological weapons, it also "created a regime that allowed cheaters maximum technological flexibility and political deniability" (Fidler and Gostin 2008: 48).

These weaknesses became apparent during the Cold War, as Salerno et al. (2004) identified three confirmed cases where states violated the provisions of the BWC. The first was the Soviet Union. In the 1970s and 1980s, the Soviet Union undertook a significant biological weapons program, which included research, testing, production, and deployment of offensive and strategic weapons. Although it is not entirely clear why the Soviet Union elected to build up their biological weapons program after signing the BWC, Guillemin (2005) speculates that it was due to either a Soviet belief that cheating on the agreement would give it a military advantage or that it believed that the United States was also secretly continuing its own program. After the Soviet Union dissolved in 1991, Russian president Boris Yeltsin declared an end to the biological weapons program (Salerno et al. 2004).

Another case was Iraq, which had signed but not ratified the BWC. Iraq had been considering the development of a biological weapons program since the mid-1970s. By the late 1980s, Iraq was preparing for the production of viruses including anthrax and botulinum toxin to be weaponized in the form of missiles and bombs. Iraq, however, did not use these biological weapons against U.S. forces during the 1991 Gulf War. After the war, the UN Security Council passed a resolution requiring Iraq to ratify the BWC and destroy all chemical and biological weapons under the supervision of a special UN commission. After the commission uncovered evidence of a biological weapons program during its investigation, Iraq confessed to an offensive program in 1995 (Kellman 2001). Iraq claimed that it had destroyed its biological weapons program in 1991 in light of the UN inspections. Despite Iraqi subterfuge, the 2003 invasion of Iraq by the United States seemed to confirm that Iraq had discontinued the program after its alleged 1991 termination date (Salerno 2004). South Africa also developed a modest biological weapons program in the 1980s to potentially counter the activities of anti-apartheid groups, This South African program researched and produced some biological agents such as anthrax, cholera, and the plague before the program's termination in 1993 (Salerno 2004).

The Soviet Union and Iraq cases, in particular, revealed the difficulty in detecting violations of the BWC. Both programs were undetected for years until the extraordinary events of a collapse of a state (Soviet Union) and war (Iraq) led to an end to these programs. In 1993, a Chemical Weapons Convention (CWC) was finally signed. The CWC included stronger provisions than the BWC, such as an international organization (OPCW) to implement the CWC's terms by inspecting former chemical weapons facilities and assisting with the destruction of these weapons. These events and the end of the Cold War provided an incentive to strengthen the BWC in the 1990s. During the third review conference of the BWC in 1991, parties agreed to establish a group of experts, who would meet at a special conference to develop enhanced verification procedures for the treaty.

After years of negotiation, the group's working paper for a BWC Protocol was rejected by the United States in 2001. The George W. Bush administration took this position despite the fact that the United States experienced an anthrax attack through the mail just weeks before the fifth review conference of the BWC. In fact, not only did the United States reject the draft protocol, but it also called for a dissolution of the group of experts who had been negotiating the terms of the document. Due to this action, the parties to be BWC reconvened the conference for 2002. Although the group of experts was not abolished, the draft protocol had been effectively terminated (Sims 2011). A number of factors can be attributed to the difficulties in strengthening the BWC. In rejecting the draft protocol, the Bush administration cited military secrecy and burdens that the agreement would place on the pharmaceutical industry as its justification (Guillemin 2005). Additionally, the concern that an enhanced BWC would not address the growing fear of bioterrorism was another consideration in the failure of the process (Fidler and Gostin 2008).

As an alternative, the United States was the most ardent supporter of addressing the issue of biological weapons through the UN Security Council rather than another multilateral treaty (Parker and Pate 2005). The UN Security Council decided to undertake a measure to strengthen not only the BWC but also the CWC and the nuclear non-proliferation treaty (NPT) by passing a resolution addressing these agreements in 2004. This resolution complemented the BWC, but it also expanded its reach somewhat in that it was binding on all members of the UN, not just those states that ratified the BWC. Under the resolution's terms, states were to refrain from providing support to any non-state actors in developing, manufacturing, or acquiring chemical, biological, or nuclear weapons. States were also required to take effective law enforcement measures to prevent non-state actors from gaining any access to these weapons. This resolution served as a response to the fact that not only the BWC did not address non-state actors, but also several states did not have criminal laws in place to prohibit the possession or use of biological agents that could be weaponized (Parker and Pate 2005). This resolution supported American interests in a couple of ways. First, it served as a diplomatic consolation to the international community following its rejection of the BWC protocol process. Second, it directed the attention of the possession of biological agents toward prospective terrorists and away from commercial industry.

American policy on the issue of a BWC Protocol did not change with the transition to Barak Obama's administration in 2009. Obama, however, did develop a different strategy for biological weapons. While the Bush administration focused on *biodefense*, which refers to an emphasis on preventing the intentional use of a biological agent as a weapon against the United States, Obama administration invoked a broader strategy based on *biosecurity*, which would address both the potential intentional and natural threats posed by biological agents. It is also a strategy that is more globally oriented as Obama has supported the BWC as the international center for biosecurity issues and the expansion of the WHO's surveillance and response capability with the revised IHR to assist with detection of potential biological threats worldwide (Koblentz 2012). The announcement by the United States for the GHSA in 2014 was another step toward developing a stronger international regime for detection, prevention, and cooperation in regard to all biological threats.

Bioterrorism

Bioterrorism has emerged as perhaps the most significant security issue for the potential use of biological weapons in the post-9/11 environment. Historically, however, not only have biological attacks by non-state actors been very rare, but also terrorist organizations have shown little interest in using such weapons as part of their tactics (Carus 2015). According to a report by the National Consortium for the Study of Terrorism and the Responses to Terrorism, only seventeen attacks involving a biological agent were used by terrorists from 1990 to 2011 (Pinson et al. 2013). In evaluating the impact of these attacks, however, not only have most of these attacks been unsuccessful, but they have also tended to be criminal actions aimed at selected targets for personal grievances or monetary gains rather than political, religious, or ideological motivations (Jansen et al. 2014).

The most active organization in biological attacks has been the Aum Shinrikyo cult, which carried out seven biological attacks in Japan during the 1990s (Pinson et al. 2013). This doomsday cult's most notable attack involved chemical weapons as the group launched a sarin gas attack on the Tokyo subway system in 1995 that killed twelve people and injured thousands more. Aum Shinrikyo, however, had developed an extensive biological weapons program as well. Before the sarin gas attack, the cult had built a laboratory in Japan to search for a usable biological agent to effectively weaponize. Their first attempt was with botulinum toxin, a substance that can be lethal in only small doses. To deliver this agent, members of Aum Shinrikyo used a vehicle to spray an area near the Japanese parliament as well as near a U.S. naval base and an international airport. All of these attacks proved to be unsuccessful. The cult also experimented with a bacterium that causes anthrax, but its efforts to spread this toxin also failed to contribute to any injuries or deaths. These fruitless attempts, however, motivated Aum Shinrikyo's decision to abandon bioweapons and turn to sarin gas for its fatal 1995 attack (Rosenau 2001).

The Aum Shinrikyo attack and the 1998 bombing of American embassies in Tanzania and Kenya spurred the United States into attempting to enhance its defense from a biological attack. Protective measures included US$10 billion for annual funding of the weapons of mass destruction domestic preparedness program. Additionally, President Clinton included a civilian component to biodefense by integrating public health measures, especially disease surveillance into the program (Guillemin 2005). Nevertheless, the United States soon faced its most significant biological attack with the anthrax letters of September and October 2001. A week after the September 11 terrorist attack, letters containing anthrax spores were mailed to a variety of mass media offices. These letters were unopened, however, a photo editor for a tabloid became infected with anthrax at his office and later died. A couple of weeks later, a second set of letters was mailed including letters to Democratic Senators Thomas Daschle and Patrick Leahy. The Daschle letter was opened, resulting in contamination and closure of the Hart Senate Building near the U.S. Capitol.

The scope of the attack contributed to twenty-two infections, five of which resulted in death (Warrick 2010). Further investigation revealed a connection of the anthrax spores to an Army laboratory at Fort Dietrick, Maryland. After an eight-year inquiry, the Federal Bureau of Investigation (FBI) concluded that an Army microbiologist who worked at the biodefense lab in Fort Dietrick was responsible for the attacks (Warrick 2010). This scientist had demonstrated indications of mental instability and committed suicide two years before the FBI had concluded its investigation.

Aum Shinrikyo's biological weapons program and the 2001 anthrax attack reveal some important lessons for understanding the current state of bioterrorism. In Rosenau's (2001) analysis of why Aum Shinrikyo's program failed, he suggests that three factors, in particular, contributed to its failure. First, was the difficulty in developing a lethal strain of bacteria. Lethal strains of botulinum toxin are extremely difficult to cultivate from the soil and purify in large quantities, which Aum Shinrikyo attempted to do. While the bacteria that causes anthrax is naturally occurring, it requires significant scientific training and experience to develop the bacteria into a toxic form. Dissemination of the biological agent was also an obstacle. For an agent such as anthrax to cause a mass killing, an aerosol cloud must be created, which requires very large and expensive research facilities. Besides the scientific and technical challenges facing Aum Shinrikyo, Rosenau (2001) also finds that irrational leadership, poor judgment, and dysfunctional decision-making hampered the group's efforts.

The fact that the 2001 anthrax attack was attributed to a scientist with significant training and experience with biological agents further supports the idea that it is very difficult for non-state actors to acquire the scientific expertise necessary to develop a viable biological weapon. The crude delivery of anthrax in 2001 also indicates that in addition to scientific knowledge, the technical requirements for significant dissemination of a biological agent will not only be scientifically burdensome but also expensive to acquire. Nevertheless, the potential for mass destruction provided by biological weapons should continue to be an attractive prospect for a terrorist organization with some form of a genocidal or apocalyptic agenda.

GLOBAL GOVERNANCE AND THE SECURITIZATION OF HEALTH

Framing health as a security issue would, perhaps, give increased relevance to global health as a part of states' national interest, according to a neorealist view of international politics. Neorealists, in particular, emphasize that states are driven by security maximization. As Mearsheimer (2001: 31) notes, "specifically, states seek to maintain their territorial integrity and the autonomy of their domestic political order." Historically, this view of security associated the threat to the state to be the military power of other states. Health, even with its security dimension, does not fit neatly into this neorealist conception of security. The threat posed by biological weapons would be more applicable to the neorealist view than naturally occurring infectious diseases. As indicated by Peterson (2002/2003), however, the spread of infectious disease could be relevant to conflict in a number of ways. Beside the intentional use of biological agents, infectious diseases could also erode a state's capacity to defend itself in a conflict, contribute to foreign policy disputes between states over responses to a disease outbreak, and create general domestic instability that could lead to civil war or contentious relations with other states.

Price-Smith (2009) has supported a variation of realism that can better account for the role of health, especially the threat of infectious diseases, outside of its potential impact on military conflict. This republican version of realist theory would concur with neorealism and its assumptions that the international system is based on anarchy and interstate competition and the view of the state as the principal actor in international relations. Where this republican version of realism differs from neorealism, however, is that it does not assume that states base their decisions on rational choices, nor that domestic politics is a separate sphere of activity from international politics. These differences mean that in the republican version, decision-making comes from powerful elites who may be influenced by a psychological bias and that domestic political problems may impact a state's foreign relations with other states.

According to this view, emerging infectious diseases pose a security threat that can impact the economic, political, and social cohesion within states. They may weaken worker productivity, challenge the capacity of national governments to provide basic services including public safety, and exacerbate differences among the social classes and their access to a potentially overburdened health care system. These problems cannot be contained internally. As Price-Smith (2009) argues, the impact of infectious disease may destabilize trade and commercial relations, and serve to amplify cooperation deficiencies among national governments inter se or with IGOs. The cases involving the international spread of emerging infectious diseases demonstrate these negative externalities. Price-Smith (2009) found that the SARS outbreak had a substantial adverse effect on the Chinese economy in 2003, especially its service sector, due to fear of disease, which impacted tourism. He notes that if SARS had continued to spread, China could have experienced further economic harm from the possibility of a quarantine of Chinese manufactured goods by other states and a loss of foreign investment due to a decline in economic productivity. During the H1N1 influenza pandemic in 2009, it was estimated that Mexico lost US$ 8.2 billion billion due to its effect on tourism, as well as experiencing a US$ 27 million million deficit in the trade of pork (Rassy and Smith 2013). In addition to the massive loss of life from the 2014 Ebola outbreak, the three afflicted West African countries faced a combined economic impact estimated to be US$2.8 billion (World Bank 2016a). International political cooperation also proved to be suboptimal in these cases. Both the spread of SARS (China) and Ebola (Guinea, Liberia, and Sierra Leone) exhibited instances of national governments underreporting the severity of these diseases to the international community.

A realist assumption that may be very relevant to understanding the implementation of global health security policies through global governance is that a determinant of international politics is based largely upon the power of the states. In the current international system, which realists assume is more or less structured around the unipolar power of the United States, realists would consider much of global health security policy to be based on U.S. interests and states that are aligned with it. The cases on emerging infectious diseases and biosecurity provide support for this view. The United States initially identified the threat of emerging infectious diseases and used its influence in the

WHO to promote the adoption of the concept in the international community. When the Clinton administration declared HIV/AIDS to be a threat to global security, the United States pushed for a UN Security Council resolution to concur with this position only a few months later. Additionally, realists would view the establishment of the GHSA as not merely a means to improve international security against threats of infectious disease but as a mechanism for the United States to promote its interests in health as an international concern. In terms of biosecurity, both the creation of the BWC and the failure to revise the agreement through a subsequent binding protocol were consistent with the U.S. position on biological weapons.

Neoliberal institutionalists believe that international institutions may play key roles in developing and improving global health security. The central institutions for global health security are the WHO and the IHR. Even with the establishment of the GHSA, Katz et al. (2014) finds a substantial overlap between the targets and objectives of the IHR and GHSA. The biological weapons regime is currently governed by the Geneva Protocol and the BWC. Although the revised IHR (2005) provides a more comprehensive response to global health security threats, it still exhibits some significant flaws. One problem is non-compliance. In Katz and Fischer's (2010) study on the H1N1 influenza pandemic, they point out how some national governments acted without WHO guidance, including bans on imports of pork from North America and Mexico and quarantines by China and Singapore on some travelers from these countries. Another weakness of the IHR is the lack of enforcement mechanisms, such as a sanction for not notifying the WHO of an international public health emergency. The efficacy of the IHR is also dependent on the surveillance capacity of states and their willingness to share relevant information with the WHO and other national governments (Katz and Fischer 2010). As demonstrated in the 2014 Ebola outbreak, the lack of resources and weak public health infrastructure in some developing states, as well as the incentive for some states to not be completely transparent about a possible public emergency for fear of economic repercussions may contribute to a suboptimal global policy response to infectious disease, even with a stronger security regime.

While surveillance has emerged as a relative strength in global security against emerging infectious diseases, it is a major weakness against the threat of biological weapons. The Geneva Protocol and the BWC provide clear prohibitions on the use and stockpiling of biological weapons, however, the absence of verification or inspection mechanisms is problematic for global governance's provision of effective security. Diplomatic efforts at adding more international agreements such as a BWC Protocol with a formal verification system have not been successful. The international biological weapons regime remains very much dependent on the voluntary compliance by national governments. As Fidler and Gostin (2008: 231) state, "of the new treaties recently adopted, only the IHR 2005 creates new authority for an intergovernmental organization that impinges on the exercise of state sovereignty." To that effect, institutions may be useful guides to formulate an effective response to the threat of biological weapons by global governance, but their impact is certainly constrained.

Neoliberal institutionalists, nevertheless, may attribute the relative non-use of biological weapons to the role and influence of the Geneva Protocol and the BWC. Constructivists, however, would attach greater weight to the development of an international norm against their use due to the weaknesses of these agreements. In addition to the influence of norms, constructivists also find the framing and identification of concepts and social relationships to be significant factors for understanding global health security. As previously noted, Buzan et al. (1998) explained how any public issue could be securitized if an actor can convince a target audience that the issue is an extraordinary threat. In regard to the securitization of health, Fidler (2007: 42) has suggested that "the use of security as a trope has become ubiquitous in how experts frame public health governance." This process of securitizing health was evident in the revised IHR. A growing collective security interest in health provided the motivation for the member states of the WHO to expand the scope of the IHR and empower the WHO to play a greater role in detecting and responding to emerging infectious diseases on a global scale.

The GHSA can also be viewed as a further extension of the framing of health as a security issue. One implication from this growing trend is that if it continues, health could begin to become more associated with the realm of "high politics" on states' foreign policy agendas. Based on the Ebola experience, however, Fidler (2017) found the political commitment to global health security to be greatly lacking. In terms of a shift from framing health as a human rights issue to a security issue, he notes, "the exposure of this shift as more rhetorical than transformational leaves global health vulnerable to the marginalization that characterized this policy before it became associated with national and global security" (Fidler 2017: 143). If framing health as a global security issue is indeed superficial, then global health will unlikely develop into a significant interest for powerful states.

A different perspective on the framing of global health has been suggested by Elbe (2010). He criticizes the securitization framework for understanding global health because "this security logic remains fairly unchanged and indeed dominates in terms of producing a range of (often undesirable) political effects" (Elbe 2010: 15). As a result, securitization theory does not directly address how the practice of security may change if health is considered to be linked to the concept. As an alternative, he suggests that the process is guided by a medicalization of security. This framework involves defining social issues as medical problems. In doing so, medical professionals and institutions become more powerful actors in social life and policy. Through this view, Elbe (2010) suggests that insecurity becomes associated as a medical problem. The fear of disease motivates the actors of global health governance to respond via some form of a security instrument or institution. The UN Security Council's resolution on HIV/AIDS, the expansion of the IHR, the greater prominence of the threat of biological weapons following the 9/11 attacks and the Bush administration's War on Terror, and the formation of the GHSA are illustrative of this point. Whether health is becoming more securitized or security is becoming more medicalized, both of these perspectives suggest a growing dimension of security in global health governance.

Neo-Marxist approaches highlight the division of interests between rich and poor countries in global health security. While poor countries face a much greater health burden than developed states, the identification of global health risks is dominated by its relationship to global capitalism. In regard to the relative lack of attention to diseases in global governance that are more endemic to poor countries, Labonté (2008: 468) states, "Rather, and in ethically troubling ways, the securitisation of health privileges those diseases most likely to inconvenience global trade and finance or to travel to high-income nations." The cases of emerging infectious diseases and biological weapons could be consistent with this view. The three infectious disease outbreaks that placed and expanded the issue of health on the global security agenda (HIV/AIDS, SARS, Ebola) were diseases that had a deleterious impact on the world's largest economies (North America, China, and Europe). Other infectious diseases that pose an even greater health burden on developing countries, such as neglected tropical diseases, have not fit the global health security agenda. Other maladies that have more of an impact on developing countries such as tobacco-related chronic diseases have also not been securitized. From a neo-Marxist perspective, the relative robustness of the biological weapons regime can be associated with the fact that biological weapons programs are expensive and require significant scientific and research expertise to implement. These programs are much more likely to be produced by and target richer countries.

In assessing the utility of global health security, it appears that security has now become a more accepted dimension of global health. The revised IHR, in particular, also demonstrates a commitment to stronger institutionalization for health security at the international level. These different perspectives of international relations, however, all reveal some significant flaws in the system. Realists and neo-Marxists can both demonstrate how the global health security agenda is biased toward the interests of powerful states, or alternatively, global capitalism. Neoliberal institutionalists can point to weaknesses in the design of the global health security agenda, such as the lack of sanctions or enforcement mechanisms to ensure compliance. Constructivists may look on the emergence of an international security norm more optimistically, but at the same time, this could be viewed as fairly novel and limited in scope. For global health governance to develop more efficient responses to health-related security problems, stronger and broader international institutions and norms will most likely be necessary to mitigate the challenges posed by realists and neo-Marxists.

CONCLUSION

Potential external threats to public health have long been a security concern of national governments. With the exception of the biological weapons regimes, health did not become firmly established as an international security issue until after the end of the Cold War. Over the past two decades, global health security has been addressed in UN Security Council resolutions and has contributed to an enhanced International Health Regulations and an empowered World Health Organization. Nevertheless, the scope of global health security has been fairly limited in its focus on the potential threats of emerging infectious diseases and biological weapons. For policies of global governance to be more effective, stronger and broader international institutions, as well as greater recognition and acceptance of an international norm of human security, rather than national security, may be necessary.

DISCUSSION QUESTIONS

1. What is the role of the World Health Organization (WHO) and the International Health Regulations (IHR) in global health security?
2. How did HIV/AIDS transition from a humanitarian issue to a security issue in global governance?
3. Why was the response of global governance to the SARS outbreak in 2003 considered to be fairly successful while the response to the 2014 Ebola outbreak has been widely criticized?
4. Has global governance adequately addressed the issue of biological weapons? Why or why not?
5. To elevate health on the agenda of global governance, would it be better to frame it as a human rights or humanitarian issue or as a security issue and why?

SUGGESTED READINGS

Elbe, Stefan. 2010. *Security and Global Health*. Cambridge, UK: Polity.

An innovative examination of the relationship between security and health.

Fidler, David P. 2004. *SARS, Governance and the Globalization of Disease*. New York: Palgrave Macmillan.

Detailed account of the role of international politics and law during the 2003 SARS outbreak.

Guillemin, Jeanne. 2005. *Biological Weapons: From the Invention of State-Sponsored Programs to Contemporary Bioterrorism*. New York: Columbia University Press.

Provides a thorough account of the history of biological weapons.

Kamradt-Scott, Adam. 2016. "WHO's to blame? The World Health Organization and the 2014 Ebola outbreak in West Africa." *Third World Quarterly* 37(3): 401–418.

An excellent analysis of the World Health Organization's role during the 2014 Ebola outbreak in West Africa.

Price-Smith, Andrew T. 2009. *Contagion and Chaos: Disease, Ecology, and National Security in the Era of Globalization*. Cambridge, MA: MIT Press.

Comprehensive and insightful perspective on the nature of disease as a security issue.

Chapter 6

The Global Politics of Chronic Diseases

Infectious diseases were severely curtailed in most regions of the world by the late 1960s, which produced a major change in the pattern of diseases. Chronic or non-communicable diseases, such as heart disease, cancer, and diabetes, which by definition are long-term and incurable, replaced infectious diseases as the major threat to health worldwide. As mortality rates from infectious diseases declined, people began living longer on average to the point that chronic diseases became more prevalent and emerged as the leading cause of death. According to the World Health Organization (WHO), chronic diseases were responsible for 68 percent of the world's deaths in 2012 (World Health Organization 2014b). A significant number of these deaths (40%) were premature, which the WHO identified as death for individuals under seventy years old.

While all states face significant health threats from chronic diseases, developing states, in particular, confront a daunting challenge. For instance, the WHO (2014b) found that almost 75 percent of total deaths from chronic diseases and 82 percent of those deaths that were considered to be premature occurred in middle- and low-income countries. The WHO (2008a) forecasts that by 2030, deaths due to infectious diseases, especially HIV/AIDS and tuberculosis will decline in both middle- and low-income states. Deaths from chronic diseases, however, will increase rapidly in these states. Although the longer life span and aging among world populations will be a major cause in the future growth of chronic disease as a cause of death, smoking will also continue to grow as a hazard to human health. By 2030, almost 10 percent of all deaths globally will be related to tobacco use according to the WHO's (2008a: 23) forecast. Tobacco use also has significantly negative economic effects. It is estimated to be responsible for almost 6 percent of all global spending on health, and the economic cost of smoking is equivalent to almost 2 percent of the world's gross domestic product (GDP) (Goodchild et al. 2017). The prevalence of tobacco-related chronic diseases is especially adverse for developing states. For instance, the highest proportion of smokers in the world (68%) is men living in middle-income countries (World Health Organization 2017f). Overall, 80 percent of the world's smokers live in middle- and low-income countries with China, India, Indonesia, and Russia ranking as the world's top four countries for the highest number of smokers (Jha 2009). Middle- and low-income countries are also expected to bear the burden of 40 percent of the world's economic costs for smoking (Marquez and Moreno-Dodson 2017).

Another problem will be the increasing prevalence of cardiovascular disease. Mortality rates for cardiovascular disease have been declining in the United States, United Kingdom, and other advanced industrialized states due to improvements in diet, exercise, medical care, and a reduction in smoking. This trend, however, is not evident in developing states where cardiovascular disease tends to affect the younger population. For states like China, Russia, India, Brazil, and South Africa, cardiovascular disease will increasing kill or disable workers of a productive working age (thirty-five to sixty-four) in the forthcoming decades. China, for example, is expected to have 9 million deaths by cardiovascular disease in 2030, over half of which will be by individuals in the thirty-five to sixty-four age group (Leeder et al. 2004: 23). Diabetes is on the rise as well in developing countries. In 1980, for example, there were 108 million cases of diabetes worldwide compared to 422 million in 2014 (World Health Organization 2016c). Again, China is the world leader with some 92 million cases, followed by India with 73 million and the United States with 30.7 million. Some 80 percent of all deaths from diabetes occur in middle- and low-income countries (World Health Organization 2016c).

Evidence indicates that chronic diseases have a significant impact on economic development. Chronic diseases have also been found to have a significant impact on economic development. The annual direct cost of diabetes alone was estimated to be US$827 billion in 2013 (World Health Organization 2016c). Combine diabetes costs with heart disease, cancer, and other chronic diseases, and the cost can be as high US$1.7 trillion annually. Chronic diseases place a substantial economic burden not only on individuals but also on households, employers, and national economies. Improved health care, especially to those individuals that are in the productive working age range, will be an important factor for successful development in middle- and low-income states. The dilemma for developing states is that while the future increase in chronic diseases will be a threat to their economic productivity, mitigating the impact of these diseases will require considerable costs to improve health care, especially for costs aimed at treatment.

Chronic diseases are placing and are expected to continue to place a greater burden on global health than infectious diseases. Horton (2005) has characterized these diseases as a "neglected epidemic." He notes that despite the fact that cardiovascular disease, cancer, respiratory diseases, and diabetes accounted for a little over half of all projected deaths globally in 2005, reduction of chronic diseases was not included as one of the UN's Millennium Development Goals (MDGs). The issue of this neglect of chronic diseases has also been addressed by Stuckler, Hawkes, and Yach (2009). They explain why this particular aspect of global health has not received greater attention. They note that historically, health care systems have been primarily directed toward infectious, or communicable, diseases. Despite the statistical evidence indicating the growing danger of chronic diseases, these systems are still oriented toward infectious diseases. Other factors have to do with the association between chronic diseases and a natural part of aging, as well as their association with being "diseases of the wealthy." Individual choice is also associated with chronic disease risk. The historical tendency in global health is to view individuals with infectious diseases as victims, while those suffering from a chronic disease contributed to their conditions by choosing to smoke tobacco, drink alcohol, and maintain an unhealthy diet. These perceptions, however, according to Stuckler, Hawkes, and Yach (2009), do not hold in comparison with the current data on global health. They point out how these diseases are afflicting younger and poorer populations to a greater degree. Even individual choice, they argue, is mitigated by the lack of constraints on trade and foreign investment and extensive marketing campaigns by multinational corporations (MNCs) distributing unhealthy products worldwide. Enhanced global governance is needed for prevention and control of these diseases because of their global scope.

Despite the fact that chronic diseases have lagged behind infectious diseases in terms of attention and funding, the 2010s have signaled an unprecedented focus on chronic diseases in global governance. In 2010, the United Nations (UN) General Assembly passed two resolutions on the prevention and control of non-communicable diseases. These resolutions led to a high-level meeting in 2011 on the issue, marking the first time that the General Assembly met for a health issue other than HIV/AIDS. The General Assembly held another high-level meeting on non-communicable diseases in 2014 and called upon states to increase their efforts in controlling these diseases and set national targets to reduce risk factors associated with these diseases by 2025.

The omission of chronic diseases in MDGs was remedied by the adoption of the UN's Sustainable Development Goals (SDGs) in 2015. In a much more comprehensive targeting of global health issues, the SDGs called for a one-third reduction of premature deaths from these diseases by 2030. Additionally, the SDGs included targets related to chronic disease such as the prevention and treatment of substance abuse (specifically mentioning narcotic drugs and alcohol) and substantially reducing deaths and illnesses from pollution.

Global health governance is a complex process involving many different actors, institutions, and interests. To assess its utility in addressing chronic diseases, case studies of the role global governance plays in the area of chronic disease will be analyzed, and the different theoretical approaches will be applied to provide insight into the process. Cardiovascular disease, cancer, and diabetes are some of the significant chronic diseases that may be somewhat preventable through effective intervention. These case studies are based on international efforts to regulate three major risk factors that have demonstrated links to these diseases: tobacco, unhealthy diets, and alcohol. The primary instruments that have been developed to address these risk factors are listed in table 6.1. Some important questions to consider in this chapter include the following: Have the institutions of global governance been effective in addressing the global burden of chronic diseases? Are the efforts aimed at tobacco control applicable to the risk factors of diet and alcohol?

TOBACCO CONTROL

Despite the scientific findings demonstrating the hazards of tobacco, its use continues to be extensive worldwide. According to the WHO (2015b), 21 percent of adults globally are smokers. One factor in explaining its prevalence is that tobacco is an addictive product due to its nicotine content, and its use creates a difficult habit to break. Another major factor is the long and successful advocacy efforts by the tobacco industry. The tobacco industry has historically been able to limit the U.S. government's regulation of the product. In fact, between 1950 and 1982, the federal government did not increase taxes on cigarettes (Studlar 2008). The Food and Drug Administration (FDA), which was officially created in 1930, has continually confronted some major political obstacles in its efforts to regulate tobacco. Several decades after FDA's creation, the U.S. Supreme Court even ruled that the FDA lacked jurisdiction over tobacco in the 2000 case of *FDA vs. Brown and Williamson Tobacco Corporation*. The FDA was finally given the authority to regulate

Table 6.1. Major Chronic Disease Risk Factors and Primary Instruments to Address Them in Global Politics

Risk Factor	*Instrument*
Tobacco	Framework Convention on Tobacco Control (2003)
Unhealthy diet	The Global Strategy on Diet, Physical Activity and Health (2004)
Alcohol	Global Strategy to Reduce Harmful Use of Alcohol (2010)

tobacco products in 2009 when President Barack Obama signed the Family Smoking Prevention and Tobacco Control Act.

Even though the United States has made some greater efforts in recent years to regulate tobacco, the tobacco industry has a global reach, penetrating many markets around the world. The end of the Cold War and the acceleration of globalization enhanced the distribution of tobacco as tobacco facilities have moved away from their traditional base in the United States and Western Europe. One explanation for this movement has been traced to the neoliberal economic policies promoted by the International Monetary Fund (IMF) and World Bank, which encouraged developing states to embrace foreign investment and privatization (Hammond 1998). Another factor had to do with the desire of former communist states such as Russia and China to transition to a market-based economy. For instance, two large foreign investors in Russia are tobacco companies, Philip Morris and British American Tobacco. The lack of regulations in the transition from the Soviet system proved to be very attractive to the tobacco industry (Gilmore and McKee 2004). The tobacco companies have also gained a major foothold in China. British American Tobacco was a heavy lobbyist in support of China's entry in the World Trade Organization (WTO), so it could export tobacco products into its market more easily (Zhong and Yano 2007). Nevertheless, the China National Tobacco Corporation and the State Tobacco Monopoly Administration serve as the dominant actors in China's cigarette market. The tobacco industry in China employs millions of people and provides a significant source of revenue for the government (He et al. 2012). In addition, Chinese tobacco companies are major actors in the international market. They account for 40 percent of cigarette sales globally and do not face as restrictive domestic regulations as Western or Japanese tobacco companies because of their close connection to the national government (Yach 2014).

Trade liberalization has also facilitated the global distribution of tobacco products. In addition to the establishment of the WTO, the 1990s saw a number of regional free trade agreements including the North American Free Trade Agreement (NAFTA) and the ASEAN Free Trade Area (AFTA). Tobacco consumption increased as a result of this trend during the 1990s (Taylor et al. 2000). This pattern was particularly the case in developing countries. Although evidence indicates that openness to free trade is related to tobacco consumption, national governments still have the capacity to regulate it, even under WTO rules. States are permitted to impose measures regulating tobacco imports as long as these measures are applied to all states and do not discriminate against any particular tobacco-producing state. In 1990, Thailand's decision to ban imports and cigarettes resulted in a trade dispute with the United States, which was addressed by the dispute settlement procedure of the WTO's predecessor, the General Agreement on Tariffs and Trade

(GATT). In this case, the GATT panel decided that smoking was a risk to human health, but any restrictions on importing tobacco had to be limited in order to be consistent with GATT. An import ban was viewed as being inconsistent with the agreement but labeling of hazards associated with tobacco was not. The panel ruled that while Thailand could not ban tobacco imports, they could place labeling and advertising restrictions on tobacco as long as they were applied in a non-discriminatory manner (Emslie 2005).

Tobacco regulation has traditionally been within the purview of national governments, and this system continues to be largely in place. The WHA passed a resolution on smoking, and a WHO committee issued a report on hazards associated with smoking in the 1970s, but the WHO did not attempt to pursue a treaty-based strategy to address this issue even though it had the power to do so under its constitution. Over the past twenty years, however, more of an effort to manage tobacco distribution and consumption has been made in global governance. The first step involved a collaborative effort between two American scholars, Ruth Roemer and Allyn Taylor. They believed that the WHO could become a much more powerful actor in global health if it were to utilize its authority to adopt treaties under Article 19 of its Constitution. Although the WHO had never used this power in its history, Roemer and Taylor concluded that a treaty addressing tobacco control might have a chance to be approved due to growing scientific evidence demonstrating the harm posed by tobacco, as well as the fact that the World Health Assembly (WHA) has passed a series of anti-smoking resolutions since the 1970 (Roemer et al. 2005). They were successful in advocating for such an international agreement and the WHA's resolution 48.11 in 1995 that requested the WHO Director-General to make a report regarding the possibility of a potential treaty for tobacco control. Following a favorable report, the WHA passed another resolution in 1996, which called on the Director-General to pursue the process of developing such a treaty.

A combination of various circumstances between 1998 and 2000 led to a tobacco control treaty to become a reality. The selection of Gro Harlem Brundtland as the WHO's Director-General was a significant factor. Brundtland made tobacco control a priority of her agenda and was supportive of a treaty-based approach to the problem. She began the WHO's Tobacco Free Initiative (TFI) in 1998. The purpose of this program was to increase knowledge and awareness of the hazards of tobacco use. One important aspect of TFI was for WHO to develop partnerships with other IGOs to help curb tobacco use. The World Bank was a natural partner in this effort due to the Bank's growing influence in health-related matters. This collaboration resulted in a World Bank report in 1999, which suggested how national governments could try to control tobacco consumption in their states and how doing so could contribute to economic productivity (World Bank 1999). This report was instrumental in providing information to developing states that indicated effective regulation of tobacco was economically beneficial, even though tobacco companies could provide a source of foreign investment (Collin 2004). Its detailed analysis on the economics of tobacco control developed more of an awareness of the costs associated with the consumption of tobacco and how income acquired from the sale of tobacco may not be as valuable to a state's economy as previously thought. Strong scientific research on the detrimental effects of tobacco consumption played a pivotal role on promoting demand for an international agreement (Warner 2005).

Another significant development was a 1998 settlement in the United States between four major tobacco companies (Brown & Williamson, Lorillard, Philip Morris, and R. J. Reynolds) and forty-six attorney generals from American states. As part of the settlement, these tobacco companies agreed to release confidential industry documents. The WHO used these documents to produce a report in 2000, which comprehensively detailed how the tobacco industry had exerted its influence to purposely undermine the WHO in many of its tobacco control efforts (Zeltner et al. 2000). In addition, these documents revealed that tobacco companies had known for decades about the addictive and harmful effects of consuming tobacco products (Glantz et al.1995).

Maintaining transparency and including civil society in the negotiating process were part of the WHO's strategy in gaining acceptance of its first international treaty. The WHO conducted its first public hearing on this issue in 2000, giving the opportunity for both non-governmental organizations (NGOs) and the tobacco industry a chance to participate in discussions on the proposed agreement. Treaty negotiations on the development of the Framework Convention on Tobacco Control (FCTC) lasted until 2003. Four coalitions emerged during FCTC negotiations, each expressing a different interest. A group of NGOs known as the Framework Convention Alliance (FCA) wanted a strong agreement that would pose significant requirements on member states to regulate tobacco consumption. Another coalition composed of developed states such as the European Union, Canada, and Australia also supported an agreement with substantial obligations but with less precise regulations than desired by the FCA. The United States, Japan, and Germany did not support an agreement with significant regulations, and so they advocated for flexibility in its obligations. These states continued to resist control measures that have proved to be effective, such as advertising restrictions, but would be detrimental to the economic interests of the multinational tobacco corporations (Warner 2005). The tobacco industry, of course, directed its efforts at promoting an agreement with weak international obligations, although they were willing to accept some degree of tobacco control (Collin 2004).

Despite their relative weakness as political actors, NGOs played an important role in the FCTC negotiation process. Lencucha et al.'s (2011) study of

Canadian NGOs during the negotiation found that these organizations were involved in monitoring, lobbying, offering technical expertise, brokering information, and promoting inclusion. These NGOs reviewed various drafts of the agreement. They also provided knowledge to the participants not just based on the scientific evidence regarding tobacco, but they also acted to help educate some of the national delegates of the business practices of the industry. In terms of inclusion, the Canadian NGOs examined in this study also helped to fund NGOs from developing countries so that they could participate in efforts for tobacco control. They were particularly influential in persuading low-income states that an international agreement on tobacco control would be in their best interest. While the expertise of NGOs was influential, the final product of negotiations rested with the states. NGOs were granted only limited access to the negotiations and were largely removed from the final phase of deliberations (Collin 2004).

The WHA officially adopted the FCTC in May 2003, which was the first time that a treaty had been adopted by the WHO in its history. The treaty went into effect in 2005, after it had received forty ratifications of national governments. Currently, 181 states have ratified the FCTC. The United States did sign the FCTC in 2004 but has yet to ratify the agreement. Germany and Japan decided to ratify despite their supportive position toward the tobacco industry.

A number of obligations regarding tobacco control were placed on the states that ratified the agreement. These included a comprehensive ban on advertising and a regulation of contents of tobacco products. States also pledged to implement various domestic control measures such as the promotion of public awareness regarding the hazards of tobacco use and raise taxes on tobacco products. Key provisions of the FCTC are listed in table 6.2.

Table 6.2. Key Provisions of the Framework Convention on Tobacco Control (2003)

Price and tax measures to reduce the demand for tobacco (Article 6)
Protection from exposure to tobacco smoke (Article 8)
Regulation of the contents of tobacco products (Article 9)
Regulation of tobacco product disclosures (Article 10)
Packaging and labeling of tobacco products (Article 11)
Education, communication, training and public awareness (Article 12)
Tobacco advertising, promotion and sponsorship (Article 13)
Demand reduction measures concerning tobacco dependence and cessation (Article 14)
Illicit trade in tobacco products (Article 15)
Sales to and by minors (Article 16)
Liability (Article 19)
Research, surveillance and exchange of information (Article 20)
Reporting and exchange of information (Article 21)
Cooperation in the scientific, technical, and legal fields and provision of related expertise (Article 22)

As with domestic policy on tobacco control, the tobacco industry has constrained international management as well. Despite the FCTC and the movement to ban tobacco advertising, tobacco companies have been increasing spending on marketing campaigns (Yach et al. 2007). The power of the tobacco industry poses a substantial regulatory challenge for developing states. According to the WHO (2017f) only 25 percent of states have a national agency for tobacco control with more than five staff members. A great majority of the states that do not have a national agency are middle- and low-income countries (World Health Organization 2017f). In addition, of the revenue from excise taxes on tobacco collected globally, 95 percent of this revenue spent on tobacco control efforts is from high-income states (World Health Organization 2017f: 104). This lack of staffing and funding for tobacco control in developing states could make them more vulnerable to political lobbying and marketing efforts by the tobacco industry.

Even developed states are not insulated from this influence. Cooper and Kurzer's (2003) study on Germany's reluctance to support the FCTC found that German political parties received financial contributions from the tobacco industry, and correspondingly, these parties did not support strict tobacco regulation. The tobacco industry's success carried over into international negotiations as another study by Grüning et al. (2011) argued that Germany played a significant role in influencing other states, such as European Union and Central American governments, to accept a relatively weak agreement. A similar explanation can be made for the recalcitrance of the United States regarding the FCTC. In Luke and Krauss's (2004) study on the U.S. Congress from 1997 to 2000, they discovered that tobacco industry contributions influenced the voting behavior of Congress. Republicans, in particular, were susceptible to the tobacco lobby as they voted pro-tobacco three times as often as Democrats. This voting pattern was significant in that the Republican Party had a majority in both houses during this time.

Although the FCTC represents an effective instance of international cooperation in global health, its major omission was that it did not address trade. This issue was a very contentious one during FCTC negotiations. The debate focused on concerns of tobacco control becoming another form of trade protectionism. The political compromise in the negotiations was to leave out any trade provisions in the agreement, which would continue to leave this issue in the hands of the WTO and other free trade agreements (Mamudu et al. 2011). As Collin (2010) points out, the final version of FCTC indicates the superior interest in international trade over global health and a partial victory for multinational tobacco corporations. As a result, the final agreement reflected an approach designed to reduce that demand for tobacco, while not attempting to reduce the supply of the product.

Research has indicated that the FCTC, even before it came into effect, has influenced national tobacco control policies. In their study of tobacco control policy adoption among 193 WHO member states between 1996 and 2005, Wipfli and Huang (2011) found that over time, national governments became more willing to adopt stronger measures for tobacco control that fit with the WHO's recommendations. Interestingly, they did not believe that pattern of adoption was based upon a thorough legislative review by each national government. Alternatively, they argue that this global proliferation of tobacco control reform was based on a process of diffusion where national governments were motivated to adopt this legislation because other states were making similar policies.

Since the FCTC went into force in 2005, the trend for WHO member states has been to adopt domestic legislation consistent with the agreement. To provide an assessment of the implementation of tobacco control policies, the WHO established MPOWER, which refers to several tobacco control policies including (1) raising taxes on tobacco, (2) banning advertising, (3) providing second-hand smoke protection, (4) raising public awareness about the hazards of tobacco, and (5) monitoring the use of tobacco. When the WHO introduced MPOWER in 2008, it found that only 5 percent of the world's population was covered by smoke-free laws, and of those states that had such laws, most of them did not have strong enforcement. In terms of tobacco taxes, a measure that the WHO considers to be the most effective measure for decreasing tobacco consumption, only four states had taxes over 75 percent of the product's price (World Health Organization 2008b).

The World Bank has also continued to be a strong supporter for tobacco control since its 1999 report. A major point of emphasis for the World Bank has been on raising taxes on tobacco. In 2017, the World Bank issued a report on tobacco control that was designed to use economistic terminology to demonstrate the economic benefits of tobacco taxes to policy-makers. The report claimed that tobacco excise taxes would effectively reduce consumption of tobacco, which in turn could reduce mortality and poverty and provide the state with more resources for economic development (Marquez and Moreno-Dodson 2017). Specifically, the report cites examples of states such as the Philippines, Ukraine, and Botswana, which experienced significant benefits from increasing taxes on tobacco.

For the most part, consistent progress seems to have been made. In its 2017 tobacco report, the WHO noted that 121 states, which together composed two-thirds of the world's population, were covered by at least one of the MPOWER strategies. This represented a significant increase from only forty-two states covering 15 percent of the world's population in 2007 (World Health Organization 2017f). Some gaps in global tobacco control, however, continue to remain. The WHO's report found that in 2016 only 10 percent of the world's population lived in countries with an adequate tax on tobacco products, and only ten additional states had taxes more than 75 percent of the product's price since the MPOWER strategies were established. Most of these states were also high-income countries (World Health Organization 2017f). Success in reducing the prevalence in smoking seems to be related to the implementation of the FCTC by national governments (Gravely et al. 2017). Despite some deficiencies, tobacco control is an area where global governance has demonstrated some significant measurable success within the past twenty years.

BOX 6.1 ARE E-CIGARETTES A HEALTHIER ALTERNATIVE FOR SMOKING?

Electronic cigarettes (e-cigarettes) are products that create an aerosol (vapor) by heating a liquid that usually includes nicotine, a drug associated with the addictive quality of tobacco products. This product was developed in 2003 by a Chinese pharmacist, Hon Lik, as a substitute for cigarette smoking and as an aid to help people to quit smoking (Boseley 2015). Of course, the main issue regarding e-cigarettes is whether they are in fact safe to consume. This question is difficult to answer because the health effects of e-cigarette smoking are still being studied. The Center for Disease Control (2017), however, notes while e-cigarette vapor contains harmful substances, it does tend to have fewer toxic substances than smoke from tobacco-based cigarettes.

On the positive side of e-cigarettes, Wagner et al. (2012) have emphasized that smokers tend to use them as a step toward quitting smoking altogether. They also tend to provide less of a craving than regular cigarettes, and they are a less toxic source of secondhand smoke. On the negative side, Grana et al. (2014) argue that the use of e-cigarettes could also contribute to dual use of both cigarettes rather than encouraging users to quit smoking. In addition, they express concerns regarding the potential health harm posed by nicotine, especially for young people, and how these vapors can still be a source of indoor air pollution. In terms of global governance, the FCTC does not address e-cigarettes, so regulations are largely left to national governments. Although the health impact of this product may be debatable, there may be some genuine uneasiness in the future of tobacco control as to whether the sale of e-cigarettes may empower tobacco companies and whether they may be used to circumvent smoking laws and weaken anti-smoking norms.

MANAGEMENT OF DIET AND OBESITY

Chronic diseases such as heart disease, cancer, and diabetes have been linked to poor diet and obesity. These diseases have traditionally been viewed as a health problem for richer, developed states. Certainly, poor diet is a major health problem for these states. More than one-third of American adults and 17 percent of youth could be considered obese (National Center for Health Statistics 2015). Obesity is also a growing health concern in Europe, where the rates of obesity have doubled since the 1980s (James et al. 2004). Obesity is not just a problem for affluent nations but is now increasing in middle- and low-income countries, particularly in urban areas because of increased intake of energy-dense foods high in fat and sugar, along with a decrease in physical inactivity due to the sedentary character of many types of work and changing forms of transportation (World Health Organization 2018b). In this respect, obesity has been emerging as a global phenomenon. As poverty is reduced, nutrition deficiencies decline globally. Rising incomes, however, tend to lead to increasing obesity rates (Htenas et al. 2017). As middle- and low-income states begin to rival developed states in terms of obesity rates, Popkin (2011) has noted that developing states are facing great challenges in addressing significant malnutrition and poverty issues along with growing obesity rates simultaneously.

Why does this rise in obesity create such a worry for national governments? Elbe (2010) identifies two reasons for concern. The first has to do with the link between obesity and disability or premature death from a chronic disease (i.e., heart disease and cancer). As mentioned, these diseases could negatively impact the productivity of a state's workforce. The other reason is based on the burden that an epidemic of these diseases could have on a state's health care system. An obesity epidemic may constrain the possibility for a state's economic growth or economic development. It is estimated that obesity costs almost US$2 trillion per year globally, which puts obesity only behind smoking and armed violence in terms of human-caused social burdens (McKinsey Global Institute 2014).

The global changes in diet and the rise in obesity are related to the process of globalization and economic development. These changes are referred to as a *nutrition transition*. Demographic changes in population, urbanization, and dietary trends have contributed to a global diet and lifestyle that increases risks of obesity and chronic disease on a global scale (West et al. 2006). The major demographic change in population is the aging of the global population coupled with a decline in population growth. Global life expectancy increased from 46.5 years in the 1950s to 65 years in the 1990s. The fertility trend indicates a declining growth rate. At the world level, fertility of women declined from 5 children per woman in 1950 to about 2.5 children per woman today (Roser 2017). Among countries that are European Union members, the fertility rate is much lower with 1.58 live births per woman in 2015, which is below the replacement rate of 2.1 (European Commission 2018). This trend indicates an older population, especially in the developed states that have lower fertility rates, which will be more susceptible to the burden of chronic disease risk factors in their society.

In addition to older populations, urbanization, and growing income levels, the two traits associated with globalization, have contributed to the nutrition transition. The growing population shift from rural to urban areas over the past few decades has had a major negative effect on diet (Popkin 1998). Urban populations in low- and middle-income countries tend to be more obese than rural populations. Reasons for this difference include less physical activity and greater access to food in urban areas (Ford et al. 2017). In terms of income, the increasing economic growth of developing states has led their populations to move away from traditional diets rich in fiber and grains to more "Western-oriented" diets with increased fat and sugar. In the case of China, income increases are in proportion to the increased consumption of animal fat (Popkin 2006). More and more poor states have access to high-fat diets, which has made the traditional distinction between diets in high-income and low-income states less relevant (Drewnoski and Popkin 1997). Monteiro et al. (2013) find in their study of the distribution of ultra-processed foods, which are foods that are ready to consume and are mostly made from industrial ingredients and additives (i.e., pizza, pasta, and chicken nuggets), that these foods are dominant in the food supplies of high-income countries, and are increasingly growing in middle-income countries such as Brazil.

Increased global trade liberalization through GATT and the WTO has impacted diet and this rising consumption of high-processed foods globally. In particular, the decision during the Uruguay Round of trade negotiations to include agricultural products within the GATT framework was significant. Among developing states, food imports doubled as a percentage of GDP from 1974 to 2004, with most of the increase share being in processed foods (Hawkes 2006). Trade in products with vegetable oils serve as an example of a link between trade and diet. Vegetable oil has been regarded as a major source of calories available globally. From 1990 to 2004 oil crop production increased by 60 percent, while consumption of vegetable oil increased by 25 percent in the United States and Western Europe, 50 percent in India, and doubled in China (Hawkes 2006). Trade liberalization has also served to affect domestic food chains. As markets have become more open to foreign imports of food, local food supplies face more competition, and in some markets processed foods may replace locally produced goods as part of a state or a community's food chain (Rayner et al. 2006).

Foreign direct investment (FDI) also plays a role in the nutrition transition. FDI from the United States in food processing rose from US$9 billion in 1982 to US$36 billion by 2000 (Hawkes 2005). Much of this FDI has to do with the spread of supermarkets and the fast-food industry. Supermarkets provide an ample supply of processed foods with high fat and sugar content. More and more consumers around the world are receiving their food from supermarkets more now than ever before. In the United States, 80 percent of retail sales of food come from supermarkets, while in Latin America it is 60 percent (Popkin 2006). The fast-food industry has rapidly spread around the world. By the end of 2010, the Subway restaurant chain surpassed McDonald's with 33,749 restaurants worldwide, while McDonald's operates 32,737 stores globally (Jargon 2011). Other American fast-food chains, such as Burger King, Kentucky Fried Chicken, and Pizza Hut have locations in many countries outside the United States. This diffusion of fast-food has also contributed to the proliferation of local chains in some countries to compete with the American franchises (Watson 2006).

Global governance did little to address the issue of obesity until the tobacco initiative provided some momentum in the WHO to improve international cooperation in reducing other risk factors associated with chronic diseases. In fact, James (2008) has argued that the WHO largely ignored the obesity issue until the 1990s because it was deemed to be a fairly manageable condition that could be addressed by simply decreasing the consumption of food. Obesity began to slowly receive more attention as more evidence indicated a connection between obesity and cardiovascular disease. The issue grew in importance on the WHO's agenda with its plan to deepen its analysis on understanding the risk factors for premature death and disability (James 2008). A significant step had taken place in 1998, when the WHA passed resolution 51.18, which requested the WHO Director-General to develop a plan to more effectively address non-communicable diseases. This resolution was followed by a report by the WHO and the Food Aid Organization (FAO) in 2002 that recommended a significant reduction in the consumption of fat, salt, and sugar (World Health Organization and Food and Agriculture Organization 2003).

While the process regarding diet control had some similarities with tobacco, such as an increasing interest in the WHO to develop some degree of international regulatory standards and increasing scientific evidence that reduced consumption of these products would improve health, some major differences between the two made international cooperation much more difficult in this area. The most significant issue is that while the scientific evidence regarding the harm caused by tobacco is quite strong relative to studies on food, the complexity of the relationship between diet and health provides more difficulty in developing a policy response to the issue (Lee 2006).

Another issue has to do with the connection between diet and lifestyle. While tobacco is inherently harmful, eating foods that are high in fat and sugar may not necessarily pose a health risk to an individual as long as intake of these foods is moderate, the diet is also balanced with fruits and vegetables, and the individual also engages in regular physical activity.

Additionally, unlike the situation with tobacco, the food and sugar industries did not suffer the same loss of credibility that the tobacco industry did with its litigation settlements in the late 1990s. The tobacco industry did support some control initiatives in order to try to appear as a more responsible actor, but the food and sugar industries took a more aggressive approach against the possibility of a treaty-based approach in the area of nutrition. The U.S. sugar industry challenged the scientific evidence in the WHO/FAO report and encouraged the United States to withhold funding to the WHO if it was to continue to promote flawed research (Norum 2005).

The WHO has even treated the food and sugar industries differently than tobacco industries despite their forceful response. A more cooperative approach was taken despite the food industry acting strategically similar to tobacco industry by paying scientists to promote research favorable to the industry, and also act as advisors and consultants to promote its image as socially responsible (Brownell and Warner 2009). The WHO expressed openness to work with the food industry as partners to effectively develop a strategy to improve the global diet. Such a possibility was not open to the tobacco industry (Barraclough 2009). A combination of the exposure of tobacco industry's efforts to undermine the WHO, along with the much stronger scientific evidence as to harm directly caused by its product, indicate that the WHO was more inclined to take a softer approach in regard to diet despite the similarities in the political practices of both industries.

In 2004, the WHA approved a resolution to adopt the Global Strategy on Diet, Physical Activity, and Health (DPAH). This strategy is composed of the following goals: (1) to reduce risk factors for non-communicable diseases that stem from unhealthy diet and physical inactivity; (2) increase awareness and understanding of the impact of diet and physical activity on health; (3) encourage the development and implementation of global, regional, national, and local policies to improve diet and increase physical activity; and (4) monitor scientific data on diet and physical activity. DPAH is a comprehensive plan that involves a number of actors at different levels of global governance. Due to the contentious nature of the WHO/FAO report, negotiation led to the report not to be included or referenced in DPAH (Norum 2005).

The policy response to diet is quite different than tobacco control. While the FCTC represents a "hard law" response with a multilateral treaty that has been ratified by a vast majority of the world's states, the DPAH is a "soft law" approach, which is based on non-binding declarations and recommendations.

In this sense, it is a much weaker policy response. Even with the "soft" policy approach to diet, the DPAH still faced political and economic obstacles. During the negotiations of the DPAH, the United States indicated that it had some philosophical reservations regarding the regulation of food based on the WHO's guidelines. The United States based its reservations publicly on scientific evidence and sovereignty concerns. Cannon (2004), however, argues the U.S. position was primarily motivated by its view that it would represent a costly constraint on U.S. economic power. The conflict between the WHO and the United States was such that a senior scientist of the WHO's obesity campaign charged the U.S. government of making health a "hostage of fortune" due to its support of the sugar industry and soft drink manufacturers (Dyer 2004: 45). Sugar-exporting states were also reluctant to endorse the strategy due to a potential loss in income. Due to these conflicts of interest the final version of the strategy had to be softer than what the WHO had envisioned (Zarcostas 2004).

The WHA followed DPAH with resolution 63.14 in 2010 regarding marketing of food and alcoholic beverages to children. This resolution called on WHO member states to take steps to reduce the impact that these products may have on children. This measure was designed to give even greater attention to the negative health effects of diet on a vulnerable population. Nevertheless, the fact that it was a WHA resolution and also did not contain much in the way of obligatory or precise language further indicated the lack of a political commitment to regulate diet at the global level.

On the heels of the UN General Assembly's high-level meeting on non-communicable diseases, obesity was addressed again by the WHO in 2013 with its Global Action Plan for the Prevention and Control of NCDs 2013–2020. This plan included nine global targets for member states to meet by 2020. One of the targets was to halt the rise in diabetes and obesity. The indicators included with these targets are adoption of national policies to reduce salt consumption and saturated fats, implementation of WHO policies on marketing of food and non-alcoholic beverages to children, and implementation of the International Code of Marketing of Breast-milk Substitutes (World Health Organization 2017g).

Because of the close connection between diet and chronic diseases, obesity is a relevant concern to the UN's SDGs for 2030 as one of its targets for its health goal called for a reduction in premature deaths resulting from non-communicable diseases. Although this target provides some indirect recognition for diet and physical inactivity as global sustainable development issues, as pointed out by Hawkes and Popkin (2015), the SDGs do not provide much of a focus on building healthier food systems. The global food system is of particular concern as states may be able to implement some national regulations to promote healthy eating, but the globalization of the food chain may mitigate the impact of these efforts.

CONSUMPTION OF ALCOHOL

In addition to tobacco and diet, the consumption of alcohol has also been regarded by health experts as a major risk factor for chronic diseases. As mentioned in chapter 2, one measure used for assessing the impact of disease is disability-adjusted life years (DALYs). This measure demonstrates the number of years lost due to poor health. In its comprehensive report on the risks to global health, the WHO (2009) considered alcohol consumption to be one of the five leading risk factors (along with childhood malnourishment, unsafe sex, unsafe water, and high blood pressure) responsible for 25 percent of the world's deaths and 20 percent of the world's DALYs. Alcohol use was regarded to be responsible for 3.3 million deaths, almost 6 percent of global total, and 139 million DALYs worldwide in 2012. (World Health Organization 2014c).

Alcohol is similar to tobacco and unhealthy food in that heavy consumption can be linked to an increased risk of a chronic disease. In fact, alcohol has been linked to several diseases, including various gastrointestinal diseases, cancer, and cardiovascular disease. A major difference, however, between alcohol and these other products is that heavy consumption can also contribute to a greater propensity for motor accidents, intentional violent actions, and social harm to others. Men are particularly susceptible to the harmful use of alcohol, as it contributed to over 7 percent of deaths of men globally compared to 4 percent of women (World Health Organization 2014c). On a positive note for alcohol, however, is that unlike tobacco, consumption of alcohol may still have some health benefits. There is research indicating that drinking alcohol in moderation could be associated with reduced rates of cardiovascular disease and diabetes (Carroll 2015). Nevertheless, heavy consumption is a health hazard.

As with tobacco and unhealthy food, heavy alcohol use also has a great economic cost for states. A study by Rehm et al. (2009) found that these costs were over 1 percent of the GDP for high- and middle-income states. For high-income states, the U.S. loss was 2.7 percent of its GDP, while South Korea had the highest rate for a middle-income state at 3.3 percent. According to the WHO's findings, high-income states have more alcohol consumption than low-income states. Developing states, however, face a greater burden from alcohol-related diseases than richer states (World Health Organization 2014c).

The issue of alcohol and global governance can be traced back to the League of Nations in the 1920s. The topic, however, left the League's agenda by the early 1930s after the end of prohibition in the United States (Room 1984). The WHO did not address alcohol per se when it was founded in 1948, but it chose to deal with the condition of alcohol addiction. Despite its place as an early agenda item for the WHO, the issue of alcoholism did not receive much attention from the organization from the late 1950s until the late 1960s (Room 1984). It was not until 1979 when the WHA passed resolution WHA

32.40 that called for member states to develop "appropriate legislation and other measures enabling effective action to be taken" to reduce the harmful effects of alcohol (World Health Assembly 1979). The WHA followed this resolution with another one in 1983, which went a step further and asked states to form a comprehensive national alcohol policy. After this resolution, alcohol began to fade from the WHO's agenda. The WHA would not pass another resolution regarding alcohol for over twenty years.

As with diet and obesity, the FCTC motivated the WHO and several national governments to pursue a more comprehensive policy on alcohol at the global level. The momentum led to the adoption of resolution WHA 58.26 in 2005. In addition to continuing to encourage states to continue developing and implementing national programs to reduce the harmful effects of alcohol, it also asked the Director-General to work with the states, IGOs, and relevant non-state actors to promote effective policies and programs (World Health Assembly 2005). Given the nature of the product, the more comprehensive data and greater scientific evidence linking alcohol to disease since the 1980s and the success of the tobacco control movement, an expectation developed that alcohol would also be politically suitable for a treaty-based response. At least in the short term, this outcome has not been the case. The negotiations during the WHO's Executive Board in January 2005 revealed a lack of consensus on alcohol control. Pakistan and Thailand, along with some support from Russia, advocated for a Framework convention on alcohol. France objected to this proposal, and the United States was "strongly opposed to it—in the delegate's view, food and alcohol differed from tobacco" (Room 2005: 1396). The United States was also a strong proponent of including the alcohol industry as collaborators in any global alcohol control efforts (Room 2005).

Resolution WHA 58.26 was the negotiated outcome. As noted, it encouraged the development of global strategy for reducing the harmful effects of alcohol, but it did not place any obligations on the member states. The WHA reviewed a subsequent proposed resolution in 2007, but it failed to pass despite the support of forty states (Casswell and Thamarangsi 2009). The following year, the WHA did pass a resolution requesting the Director-General to work with member states and other relevant actors to draft a global strategy for alcohol. After two years of deliberations, the global strategy to reduce the harmful use of alcohol was endorsed by the WHA in 2010.

Similar to DPAH, the global strategy for alcohol functions as a series of non-binding recommendations. The strategy lists five objectives: increased global awareness of harm caused by alcohol; increased knowledge both for science and policy initiatives; increased technical support to states to develop effective alcohol control policies; enhanced cooperation among all stakeholders (states, IGOs, and non-state actors); and improved monitoring, information gathering, and policy development (World Health Organization 2010). Suggested policy areas of coverage include age limits for purchasing alcohol and legal penalties for drunk driving. As the title of the strategy indicates, the use of alcohol is not viewed as an inherent health hazard as the case with tobacco. The word "harmful" was used to describe the type of alcohol use that was targeted. Another similarity with DPAH and its lack of a standard for excessive food consumption is the lack of a scientific measure for the level of consumption of alcohol to be considered "harmful." The global strategy for alcohol does mention the number of deaths that can be attributed to alcohol but does not contain any other numerical data.

As with the tobacco and food industries, the alcohol industry is rich, powerful, and has a global reach. It also has a very concentrated market as the ten largest manufacturers of alcoholic beverages produced 48 percent of the sales of global brands in 2005. The largest corporations such as Anheuser-Busch, headquartered in the United States, rank among the world's top corporations for revenue production and global advertising (Jerrnigan 2009). In addition to its market power, the alcohol industry has proactively established social organizations to influence alcohol policy at the global and national levels. These organizations have advocated policies based on the health and social benefits of alcohol. They have encouraged governments, through various means, to promote responsible drinking rather than curb overall alcohol consumption (Anderson 2004).

Strategically, the alcohol industry has acted in the same manner as the tobacco and food industries to counter control policies by appearing to be socially responsible and offering biased evidence to support their position. Alcohol companies have funded campaigns addressing the prevention of drinking and driving as well as the sale of alcohol to underage drinkers. They have also influenced research and have questioned research findings that have supported the harmful effects of alcohol (Casswell and Thamarangsi 2009). As noted earlier, the alcohol industry was supported by the United States in the global policy deliberations. This inclusion was designated in the WHA's 2008 resolution, which included the term "economic operators" as one of the actors that the WHO Director-General is requested to consult (World Health Assembly 2008).

Compared to the tobacco control movement in civil society, NGOs advocating for similar policies were not nearly as powerful. Casswell and Thamarangsi (2009) noted that a major reason behind their weakness has to do with a lack of funding. They have not received the same kind of financial support from cancer organizations as the anti-tobacco groups. Global networks of NGOs for alcohol control, however, are relatively new. The Global Alcohol Policy Alliance began only in 2000 but has established affiliates in Europe, the United States, South America, India, and Southeast Asia. It is still an emerging movement within global health governance. Zeigler (2013) has suggested that these NGOs should establish networks with groups affected by alcohol use but not part of the policy movement, such as groups that support the protection of young people and groups involved with victims of sexual violence, to strengthen their base of support. Even with this strategy, however, he also argues that increased funding for these NGOs will be critical for global alcohol policy to go beyond the WHO's 2010 global strategy.

In addition to political support by the WHO, the global movement for alcohol control has also received increased backing by the World Bank. While the World Bank had historically supported the alcohol industry for its investment in economic development, the World Bank's view on the industry has changed, especially in light of its 2007 report on the negative economic impact of chronic diseases. It has now encouraged national governments to improve their alcohol regulations, including raising taxes and restrictions on advertising (Casswell and Thamarangsi 2009).

Despite the increased awareness of the harm related to alcohol use and the emergence of the global movement to regulate alcohol, as with tobacco, international trade law remains as a significant obstacle to reduce consumption. A key principle of the WTO is trade liberalization. Any restrictions on alcohol could be interpreted as a violation of free trade by limiting foreign access to domestic markets. Two of the major treaties under the purview of the WTO are the General Agreement on Tariffs and Trade (GATT) and the General Agreement on Trade in Services (GATS). Both of these agreements allow for states to take measures to protect human health, as long as such measures are necessary and did not discriminate against foreign goods. In a trade dispute before a WTO panel, this standard of necessity will be strictly construed to avoid the potential of permitting a protectionist trade practice if it is mixed with a public health justification. Baumberg and Anderson (2008) argue that despite this interpretation, an alcohol control policy that had a minimal, non-discriminatory effect on trade based on a "pure health" ground could be approved by the WTO. Even with this possibility, it would seem that alcohol control would be more likely to be successfully defended by the WTO if it had a stronger basis in international law. As previously noted, the FCTC did not address international trade, with the exception of illegal smuggling. In comparison with tobacco, it would seem that political will would even be weaker to support carving out a health exception in international trade agreements for alcohol control.

GLOBAL HEALTH GOVERNANCE AND THE BURDEN OF CHRONIC DISEASE

The cases of tobacco, diet, and alcohol have a number of similarities, but they exhibit some key differences as well. In terms of similarities, all involve products that if consumed can increase the risk of contracting a chronic disease for the user. The potential harm of these products has also been backed by more scientific evidence. Another similarity has been the stronger advocacy by the WHO and health-related NGOs since the late 1990s in calling for an enhanced role for government in regulation of both products. Additionally, in all cases, powerful industries with widespread reach in the global market have contested this regulatory movement. National governments, particularly governments of richer, developed states, which are home to most of these industries, have also demonstrated reluctance in supporting international regulations of these products. In all three cases, while global health governance has supported a greater awareness of these issues, they both have not been successfully managed at either the international or the national level to prevent them from becoming greater health risks to human populations, especially in the developing world.

The issue of tobacco has some distinctive differences. First, while the scientific evidence on the harm posed by tobacco is fairly strong, food, even that which is high in fat, sugar, and salt content, is not hazardous per se. The chronic diseases risks linked to the consumption of "bad" food can be mitigated by moderate consumption and regular physical activity. The evidence against alcohol is more compelling, but low consumption of alcohol has been linked to a reduced risk of cardiovascular disease. Second, the advocacy efforts by the WHO and NGOs have been much more successful in the realm of tobacco than in diet and alcohol control. These efforts are reflected in the "hard law" response in regard to tobacco as demonstrated by the FCTC compared to the "soft law" consensus reflected in the DPAH and the global strategy to reduce the harmful use of alcohol. Even though the FCTC has some inherent weaknesses with some of its language, coverage, and with its implementation problems, it still represents the most significant example of an international political commitment to a health issue. The creation of the FCTC, however, brings up a number of different questions regarding the prospects for international cooperation and health, such as (1) is the treaty approach applicable to other chronic disease health risks? (2) what is the likelihood that the FCTC could be revised to become a more restrictive agreement? and (3) will a treaty-based approach be an effective way for global governance to regulate, or at least manage, other health risks for chronic diseases?

The hypotheses regarding global health governance that have been previously posed in chapter 1 provide some insights into analyzing these questions. The realist view is that because cooperation in health does not bear a strong relationship to the state security, cooperation in this area may be only likely, as long as it serves the mutual interests of states. This cooperation, however, will be structured around the interests of the most powerful states with international institutions and non-state actors playing a limited role in the process.

This proposition does seem to fit the nature of global governance and chronic disease. In all these cases, the United States, the most powerful actor in health, indicated its reluctance to establish a strong international regulatory regime in the areas of tobacco, diet, and alcohol. The primary reason for its position has to with economic expansion and American power. The tobacco, food, and alcohol industries have a substantial presence in the U.S. economy. Unduly restrictions on the international sale of tobacco, processed foods, and alcohol would negatively affect the economy, which could constrain the power of the United States. In the area of tobacco, other powerful states with large economies, Germany and Japan, were also advocates of a softer tobacco agreement, although both states did ratify the agreement, unlike the United States. The most ardent supporters of the FCTC represent a diverse group of states around the world, such as mid-level powers including Australia, Norway, and South Africa, as well as less powerful states such as Ghana. In the realist view, the global governance response to tobacco, diet, and alcohol has revolved around American interests in soft management of the products, rather than a more restrictive approach, which is backed by an international consensus of weaker states.

While the realist view provides a persuasive explanation as to the outcome of global governance's response to chronic disease, it overlooks some elements of the process, particularly the role of the WHO in sponsoring initiatives to address both tobacco and diet, as well as the strong response of the international community to confront these issues, which until recently, have been considered as issues for domestic policy. The view from neoliberal institutionalism would look at international cooperation in health as a collective goods problem. In order to provide a reduced risk of chronic disease to the global community, global governance must develop a strong institutional framework to facilitate national political commitments to health and reduce the incentive for states to free-ride on these commitments. In this view the WHO has played a key role in sponsoring initiatives leading to the FCTC, DPAH, and the global strategy for alcohol. These initiatives provide a framework for managing tobacco, diet, and alcohol for global governance. The weaknesses of these agreements, however, limit their utility in addressing collective action problems, particularly on a global scale.

In addition to the lack of restrictions placed on these products, another problem is the dearth of funding available for states to implement the provisions of these agreements, which makes it difficult to manage these risk factors. In 2016, the Bill and Melinda Gates Foundation funded US$1, 197,000 for global health, of which HIV/AIDS received 18 percent and malaria received 17 percent. In comparison, tobacco control received 6 percent of the US$513,000 funded to global policy and advocacy (Bill and Melinda Gates Foundation 2018). The World Bank's Strategy for Health, Nutrition, and Population Results recognizes the problems that chronic diseases place on national economies and the importance of prevention and control of these diseases. Problems of weak domestic institutions, corruption, and economic incentives from multinational corporations engaged in tobacco, sugar, fast-food, and alcohol industries increase the difficulty of implementing the global health frameworks in developing countries. Although the development of such frameworks directed at a global response to chronic disease is a significant achievement, the weakness of institutionalization makes compliance and an effective response to the problem inadequate under the current system of global governance.

While the neoliberal institutionalist assessment differs from that of realists in that it views the undersupplied nature of protection from chronic disease as primarily resulting from a lack of institutionalization and an overall weak regime in global public health, it does share a state-centric explanation for this phenomenon. The lack of institutionalization in this area is due to an aggregation of the preferences of national governments. It is in the interests of states to provide greater health regulations to both improve the quality of life for their citizens and to promote economic development by maintaining a healthy and vibrant workforce. At the same time, the industries that produce unhealthy products serve as a significant source of revenue for both their home states and their host states as a resource for foreign investment. The WTO's rules and its fundamental principles of trade liberalization and non-discrimination enhance the difficulty for global governance to effectively manage distribution and consumption of these products.

Constructivism provides a different perspective in understanding the problem in managing chronic disease at a global level of analysis. This approach moves away from the central role of states and national interests to a process based upon international norms and shared ideas that are reflected in state action but are also associated with NGOs and civil society. The progression in international negotiations that has led to the FCTC, DPAH, and the global strategy for alcohol represents a strengthening norm in international relations that tobacco, unhealthy foods, and alcohol are global "bads" and the powerful actors of global governance are pressured to address these issues. This norm, however, is competing against another strong norm in global politics, and that is neoliberal economics. Neoliberalism has become a staple of both international and domestic politics since the end of the Cold War. It is reflected in the policies of the World Bank, WTO, and the United States. It has even influenced the policy at the WHO, the world's leading health institution. States clearly recognize, to a greater extent than ever before, that tobacco, and to a lesser extent high-fat and high-sugar foods and alcohol, pose a threat to human health. At the same time, their political commitment to health is also shaped by neoliberal economic policy. The convergence of these norms relates to the outcomes in the form of the FCTC, DPAH, and the global strategy for alcohol. The greater legalization of tobacco control is due to the much stronger norm of the threat of tobacco to health compared to the less pervasive beliefs regarding the health threats of diet and alcohol.

A Marxist analysis of chronic disease focuses on how the problem has been exasperated by the global capitalist mode of production. Powerful MNCs make a tremendous amount of income from the global sale of tobacco, unhealthy food, and alcohol. Global demand for these products is very high, despite their role in increasing the risk of chronic disease. Even though tobacco control has received greater attention with the FCTC, Marxists would point to how these MNCs are now increasingly directing their marketing and supply efforts at poorer states that are not able to regulate tobacco as effectively as rich states. Not surprisingly, these states are experiencing a greater share of the burden of chronic diseases. The MNCs that are selling these products are also headquartered in core capitalist economies that are protective of them in international negotiations. The United States, in particular, has tended to be opposed to international regulations for these products. Neo-Gramscians would also emphasize the strength of the free market ideology that is supported by the IMF, World Bank, and the WTO in addition to the world's rich countries. Their pressure to develop support for neoliberal economic policies and their socialization of other actors to accept it, have influenced poor states to maintain open markets in regard to tobacco, unhealthy foods, and alcohol. Worldwide increases in diseases associated with these goods are a by-product of globalization.

Although greater scientific evidence and stronger advocacy by the WHO and NGOs managed to enhance the issue of chronic disease on the global health agenda in the 2000s, its conflict with market interests have limited its impact. Moodie et al. (2013) make the case that including industry self-regulation and public-private partnerships in the policy process will not lead to effective policies for addressing chronic disease risk factors at the national or global level of politics. Because the fundamental goal of these actors is to maximize profits, they have incentives to undermine or weaken these policies in negotiations. As a result, they suggest that significant government regulation with support of civil society will be needed to constrain the influence of these private actors and more effectively address public health concerns. In general, Marxist-based approaches would tend to argue that global governance and its actors and institutions would need to act to limit or deemphasize capitalist political and economic practices for the burden of chronic disease to be effectively curtailed at the global level.

What does this analysis suggest about the prospects for global health governance and international cooperation in health? The first question is whether the treaty approach taken with tobacco is applicable to other chronic diseases? Yach et al. (2003) examined the potential relevancy of the FCTC to diet and physical activity. They found a number of its provisions such as pricing and taxes, labeling, education campaigns, and advertising restrictions could be similarly applied to food. A treaty-based approach does have some potential given the similar obstacles that exist for diet that the FCTC was able to overcome, such as opposition by the United States and multinational corporations. The main problem, however, as identified by constructivists has to do with global norms rather than material interests. Until a stronger global norm emerges that identifies unhealthy food, alcohol, or any products that create increased risks to health as global "bads" to the same extent as tobacco then political support within the structure of global health governance will not be sufficient to legalize these other areas to the same degree. Even though powerful states, such as the United States, have tried to limit international regulation in this area, the tobacco norm grew to be strong enough to compel these states to ultimately support the agreement, and even the United States signed the treaty in 2004. The nutrition norm is at a much earlier stage of development, and it will undoubtedly need to become stronger for a treaty-based approach to become a feasible option for cooperation in this area.

Alcohol control is also a norm that is early in development. Taylor and Dhillon (2013) have analyzed the feasibility for a Framework Convention on Alcohol Control. They conclude that a treaty-based response, similar to the FCTC, is not the best option at the present time. Alternatively, they argue that pursuing non-binding international legal agreements would be a more optimal short-term strategy for global alcohol control. A couple of problems exist for a legalized solution to alcohol. First, Taylor and Dhillon (2013) suggest that political will and the current state of scientific evidence have been too weak to develop a global consensus that alcohol use needs to be regulated by an international treaty. Second, they point out that if the legal strategy happens to fail, then the entire global movement for alcohol control could be set back by a number of years. The norm for alcohol control must be first strengthened. Before the FCTC, the WHA passed seventeen tobacco control regulations in twenty years (Taylor and Dhillon 2013: 455). Comparatively, alcohol has had only four WHA resolutions between 1983 and 2010.

The second question is what is the likelihood that the FCTC will become a more restrictive agreement? The answer to this question can be found under realist, neoliberal institutionalist, constructivist, and Marxist analyses. All of these views would suggest that renegotiation for a stronger agreement is unlikely. Global tobacco politics features a number of significant conflicts of interests among powerful actors. The FCTC represents a satisficing solution, which was the most feasible outcome of negotiations given the nature of the political conflict. The most powerful actor in global health governance, the United States, has still not ratified the agreement. Given these circumstances, it does not appear to be in the interests of the key actors in global governance to strengthen the current agreement. For many states, implementation of the FCTC is more of a challenge than making a political commitment to it. A more restrictive agreement would require an even stronger anti-tobacco norm, especially to overcome the prevailing sentiment that tobacco control should not be unduly burdensome on international trade. At this point it seems that tobacco control is making some progress, but the lack of states placing high taxes on tobacco products also does not indicate much political support for a stronger treaty.

The third question is will a treaty-based approach be an effective way for global governance to regulate, or at least manage, health risks related to chronic disease? Abbott and Snidal (2000) and Taylor and Dhillon (2012) suggest that informal arrangements have advantages in that these arrangements pose less of an infringement on sovereignty and can promote compromises among different actors. Even though informal approaches are often favored solutions by actors in resolving cooperation problems, the global epidemic of chronic disease requires a greater degree of regulation to constrain powerful market forces that are promoting unhealthy products. A treaty-based approach is important to serve this end due to the failure of markets to address chronic disease prevention. The major obstacles to this approach will be the number of obstacles presented in the case studies: political commitment, political will, international and domestic institutional capacity, and embedment of an effective health regulation regime in a global structure based on capitalism and market-based economic policies.

CONCLUSION

Chronic disease has been traditionally associated as a health problem of affluent countries but has become a growing threat to populations in the developing world since the end of the Cold War. While global governance is now directing more attention to problems of global health than ever before, most of its focus has been on the dangers of infectious diseases. Global governance involves a complex process of many actors, interests, and institutions. Realism, neoliberal institutionalism, constructivism, and Marxism provide different explanations and insights for understanding why prevention of chronic diseases has been undersupplied at the global level. Realism views the deficiency based upon the lack of interest by powerful states in addressing this problem through global governance. Neoliberal institutionalism finds that the limited response to chronic diseases is based on a weak institutional structure. The lack of firm agreements in the health area and the mix of cooperation and competition among international organizations in the development of global health policy make it difficult for global governance to develop effective management. Constructivism views the undersupply of global heath as due to the lack of a strong international norm in this area. Even though recognition of the problem is much stronger, as a regulatory norm it is still fairly weak, especially in areas other than tobacco control. Marxism views the burden of chronic disease as linked to the power of MNCs and the pervasiveness of neoliberal ideology on a global scale. Global health governance will continue to be deficient as long as capitalist economic interests are prioritized by the world's most influential actors. Taken together, these approaches suggest that global health governance is shaped by a variety of underlying interests and values. Conflicting views and a lack of a consensus as to the nature and the extent of the threat posed by chronic diseases significantly constrain effective management of this growing problem.

DISCUSSION QUESTIONS

1. Why have chronic (or non-communicable) diseases received less attention than infectious (or communicable diseases) in global health governance?
2. How was the World Health Organization (WHO) able to successfully promote an international treaty for tobacco control, the first global health treaty under its authority?
3. Why does trade liberalization, or neoliberal economic policies in general, provide a significant obstacle for tobacco control, even with the Framework Convention on Tobacco Control (FCTC)?
4. Why has the international legal response to unhealthy food and beverages, as well as alcohol, been much weaker in comparison to tobacco? How may theories of international relations explain this difference?

SUGGESTED READINGS

Barraclough, Simon. 2009. "Chronic Diseases and Global Health Governance: The Contrasting Cases of Food and Tobacco." In Adrian Kay and Owain Williams (eds.) *Global Health Governance: Crisis, Institutions, and Political Economy*. New York: Palgrave Macmillan. 102–128.

A book chapter that provides a good assessment of the potential for global health governance to address the global obesity epidemic based on its experience with tobacco control.

McGrady, Benn. *Trade and Public Health: The WTO, Tobacco, Alcohol, and Diet*. Cambridge, UK: Cambridge University Press.

Provides a comprehensive analysis of international trade law and its relationship to tobacco, alcohol, and food.

Norum, Kaare R. 2005. "World Health Organization's Global Strategy on Diet, Physical Activity and Health: The process behind the scenes" *Scandinavian Journal of Nutrition* 49: 83–88.

Provides a short but detailed account on the negotiations for the Global Strategy on Diet, Physical Activity, and Health.

Roemer, Ruth, Allyn L. Taylor, and Jean Lariviere. 2005. "Origins of the WHO Framework Convention on Tobacco Control." *American Journal of Public Health* 95: 936–938.

Description of the genesis of the Framework Convention on Tobacco Control by two scholars (Roemer and Taylor) closely involved with its origins.

Chapter 7

Health as an International Human Right

Do human beings have a right to good health? While an affirmative answer to this question has been gaining greater acceptance at both the international and national levels, it has taken a long time to develop as a principle of global governance, let alone as an enforceable right. In fact, the areas of health and human rights did not significantly begin to connect until the 1980s campaign against HIV/AIDS (Gruskin et al. 2007). Despite the fact that both health and human rights are necessary conditions for the well-being of individuals, two factors, in particular, can account for this delay. The first had to do with the evolution of human rights as an issue in international relations. Before World War II, a government's treatment of its own people was considered part of its sovereignty. States did, however, have a duty as an international custom to provide respectful treatment to nationals from other states. This responsibility was driven by an incentive to maintain cordial relationships with other states as opposed to a recognition that all people were entitled to an inherent set of rights (Henkin 1990). While international concerns for the treatment of non-nationals began to emerge over time in regard to slavery and the treatment of persons living under colonial rule, it was not until the humanitarian disaster and atrocities of World War II that human rights became incorporated into global governance and the practice of international politics.

The second factor had to do with a disconnect between the concepts of health and human rights. With the exception that they both shared one objective in protecting individuals from violent actions, they were essentially viewed as different concepts without a natural link. Much of the reason for this disparity had to do with different philosophical, cultural, and methodological interpretations of what constituted health and human rights (Mann et al. 1994). It was not until the end of the twentieth century when these two concepts began to develop a more generally accepted connection. Despite the progress that health has made as a principle of human rights, however, it remains uncertain as to exactly what kind of "health" are individuals entitled to as an international human right.

The purpose of this chapter is to consider the place of global health within a human rights framework by examining the development of international human rights law after World War II and the connection between the concepts of health and human rights. This analysis will include case studies of HIV/AIDS and chronic diseases in a human rights context. Prospects for the effective implementation and enforcement of an international right to health will also be examined. Important questions to be considered in this chapter include the following: What is the nature of the relationship between health and human rights in international law and politics? Can a human-rights-based approach be useful in promoting a standard of good health for all in global governance?

THE DEVELOPMENT OF INTERNATIONAL HUMAN RIGHTS LAW AFTER WORLD WAR II

The base for modern international human rights comes from the Charter of the United Nations (UN). The Charter was signed by fifty states on June 26, 1945, and entered into force on October 24 of that year. With the exception of some amendments addressing the enlargement of the UN Security Council and Economic and Social Council (ECOSOC) and some procedural matters, the UN Charter retains the same text and obligations as it did at its inception. Although the preamble to the Charter is not legally binding on member states, it states at its outset that the purpose of the organization is "to reaffirm faith in fundamental human rights, in the dignity and worth of the human person, in the equal rights of men and women and of nations large and small." Article 1 (3) of the Charter states that among the organization's aims are "encouraging respect for human rights and for fundamental freedoms for all without distinction as to race, sex, language or religion." Additionally, human rights is mentioned a few other times in the Charter. Articles 55 and 56 say that with the assistance of member states, the UN will promote "universal respect for human rights and fundamental freedoms for all without distinction as to race, sex, language or religion."

In Articles 62 and 68, the UN tasks ECOSOC as its organ to address human rights. Article 62 gives ECOSOC the power to "make recommendations for the purpose of promoting respect for, and the observance of, human rights and fundamental freedoms for all." Article 68 gives ECOSOC the authority to establish commissioning bodies for this purpose. The year after the Charter went into effect, ECOSOC created the Commission on Human Rights to play this role. Several decades later, in 1993, ECOSOC established the Office of the UN High Commissioner for Human Rights (OHCHR) to supplement the Commission on Human Rights in its efforts by providing a lead UN official to oversee and promote human rights in the UN system, as well as engage in such efforts with other IGOs, national governments, and NGOs.

Although the UN's inclusion of human rights in its mandate was revolutionary at its time, its commitment to this principle did exhibit some deficiencies. The first had to do with the fact that the Charter did not provide any guidance, let alone specificity, as to what constituted a human right or a fundamental freedom. The UN addressed this issue fairly soon; however, it was through a non-binding resolution in the form of the Universal Declaration of Human Rights (UDHR) rather than the legally binding provisions of the UN Charter. While the UN General Assembly joined ECOSOC as an active body in adopting resolutions regarding human rights, neither organ had the power to bind any states to obligations in these resolutions. UN bodies such as the Security Council and the International Court of Justice have authority to make binding decisions, but these organs did little to address human rights until after the Cold War. When they did make decisions based on human-rights-related issues, these decisions were based on circumstances involving humanitarian crises such as the brutal conflict in the former Yugoslavia in the early 1990s rather than human rights rulings per se (Karns and Mingst 2015).

In addition to a lack of specificity and power to make enforceable decisions, politics has been another factor in limiting the effectiveness of the UN in promoting human rights. Article 2 (7) of the Charter states that "nothing contained in the present Charter shall authorize the United Nations to intervene in matters which are essentially within the domestic jurisdiction of any state." Because human rights most frequently involves the treatment by national governments of its own citizens, this provision is problematic for the UN in trying to promote human rights on a global scale, while simultaneously protecting state sovereignty. The Commission on Human Rights was certainly constrained by this conflict. The commission was an intergovernmental body composed of representatives of member states rather than experts on human rights. Permanent members of the Security Council such as the United States, the Soviet Union/Russia, and China used their political leverage to protect their allies, while weaker states without powerful allies tended to be easy targets for condemnation of their activities. Authoritarian states, including those with poor human rights records, were also eligible to have representatives on the commission and often collaborated with one another to avoid the commission's scrutiny of their internal practices (Lauren 2007).

Criticism of the commission reached its peak in 2002 when Libya, then under the repressive dictatorship of Muammar Gaddafi, was elected to serve as chair of the commission. This selection caused the commission to lose much credibility in the international community. The political fallout led the General Assembly to pass a resolution in 2006 to replace the commission with the Human Rights Council. This replacement body would be a subsidiary organ to the General Assembly rather than to ECOSOC. Additionally, the forty-seven members of the Human Rights Council would be subject to review their human rights record, and the General Assembly could suspend any member of the council for human rights violations with a two-thirds vote (United Nations General Assembly 2006a). Although the Human Rights Council was designed to create a profile for human rights in international politics, some weaknesses from the commission continue to remain. It is still an intergovernmental body where all member states, regardless of their political openness, are eligible to serve. The decision-making process is still based on non-binding recommendations without any enforcement authority.

The Universal Declaration of Human Rights

The high point for the UN's Commission on Human Rights was its drafting of the UDHR, which was adopted by the UN General Assembly by a resolution in 1948. As noted, as a General Assembly resolution, the UDHR was a non-binding document. It has been argued, however, that some of the principles of the UDHR pose binding obligations because they are based on the human rights provisions of the UN Charter, as well as qualifying as customary international law (Gostin 2014). The UDHR contained thirty articles, which asserted a number of human rights. Among them, Articles 3–10 state that everyone has rights to life, liberty, and security; freedom from slavery, torture, arbitrary arrest and detention; and equal protection of the law as well as a fair and public hearing if charged with criminal penalties. Other significant rights in the UDHR include the right to marry, own property, freedoms of thought, religion, and expression; the right to social security, the right to work under favorable conditions, and the right to education. The provisions in the UDHR include a split between civil and political rights (such as the prohibitions against slavery, torture, and arbitrary arrest) and economic and social rights (such as the right to work, education, protection against unemployment, and an adequate standard of living).

The split between these two different kinds of rights created some contentious negotiations during the drafting of UDHR. The political and civil rights were considered to be the "old" rights derived from the eighteenth century and connected to the natural rights philosophy. The "new" economic and social rights were products of the nineteenth century and were influenced by the work of Karl Marx and Friedrich Engels. These "new" rights were supported by Latin American states as well as communist states such as the Soviet Union and Yugoslavia. The United States and the United Kingdom were, for the most part, opposed to these rights, because they were not consistent with their constitutions (Morsink 1999). Small states from Latin America, Asia, and the Middle East, however, joined with the Soviet Union and some NGOs to push for many of these socioeconomic rights to be included in the final draft of the UHDR (Waltz 2001). Nevertheless, the United States and the United Kingdom both consented to the inclusion of these "new" rights by being among the forty-eight states to vote in favor of adopting the resolution.

The UHDR may have passed the General Assembly with overwhelming support, however, it was widely acknowledged that it did not require legal obligations for member states, and it was within the discretion of national governments on whether to implement any of its principles. By the end of the 1950s, only prohibitions against genocide and slavery were covered as accepted human rights principles under international law (Freeman 2011). The establishment of the "new" rights covering economic and social objectives was especially contentious in moving from the UHDR to an international treaty. Scholars have made different arguments as to the position of Western states, especially the United States, in regard to these rights. Whelan and Donnelly (2007) have supported the view that these rights, as included in the UDHR, were reconcilable with the interests of the United States. They point out that none of the Western states, including the United States, demanded that economic and social rights be removed from the declaration (Whelan and Donnelly 2007: 917). In addition, these rights were also compatible with the goals for the United States in developing a welfare state as a plan for economic reform following the experience of the Great Depression of the 1930s. Kirkup and Evans (2009: 231), however, have argued that the U.S. acceptance of economic and social rights in the UDHR was primarily motivated by concerns that it might lose its "moral authority" at the UN. They also state that "indeed contrary to Whelan and Donnelly's claim that historically the United States has always embraced economic and social rights, the record shows that every effort was made to reject this class of rights" (Kirkup and Evans 2009: 232).

The International Bill of Rights

In the process of transforming the rights enumerated in the UDHR into binding international law, it was decided by the General Assembly, in a close vote of twenty-seven in favor, twenty in opposition, and three abstentions, to develop two separate treaties instead of a single document in 1952 (Whelan and Donnelly 2007: 930). Competing explanations have also been made to account for this decision. Whelan and Donnelly (2007) offered the view that it was motivated by the concerns on the differences between implementing civil and political rights compared to economic and social rights into domestic law. Most states at this time viewed themselves as better equipped to incorporate civil and political rights, and so it was deemed necessary to divide the "old" rights and the "new" rights into two treaties because each set would require different procedures for implementation. The counter claim, as advocated by Kirkup and Evans (2009), has been that the United States, the United Kingdom, and other North Atlantic states did not wish to recognize economic and social rights as binding international law. Dividing human rights into separate conventions suited the interest of the American government to promote civil and political rights (many of which were also reflected in the U.S. constitution) globally, while only rhetorically giving support to economic and social rights by not opposing a treaty covering these rights but also not intending to accept it.

After well over a decade of negotiations, the International Covenant on Civil and Political Rights (ICCPR) and the International Covenant on Economic, Social, and Cultural Rights (ICESCR) became adopted in 1966 and then entered into force in 1976. These two treaties, along with the UDHR became known as the International Bill of Rights. As of January 2018, the ICCPR had 169 parties, while ICESCR had 166 (United Nations Treaty Collection 2018). Although these numbers indicate that these treaties may not be universal, they are obligations accepted by the vast majority of UN member states. Notably, the United States did sign ICESCR in 1977 but has not yet chosen to ratify the agreement. These treaties, along with other major human rights agreements adopted since the end of World War II can be found in table 7.1.

ICCPR included many of the rights from the first half of the UDHR. Among the comprehensive list of rights provided in the treaty were self-determination; life; freedom from torture; freedom from slavery; liberty; a trial in a reasonable time if charged with a crime; freedom from arbitrary arrest; peaceful assembly; marriage; access to public service; equal protection of the law; and freedom of religion, culture, and language. A notable difference with UDHR was that the ICCPR did not include a right to own property or right to asylum, although self-determination was a right in the ICCPR that was not specified in UDHR. In addition to enumerating these rights, the treaty also establishes a Human Rights Committee to oversee implementation of these rights. Article 40 of the ICCPR obligates states to submit reports on their efforts to implement the treaty's rights to the committee for its evaluation. Article 41 also allows a member state to request that the Human Rights Committee investigate the possibility that another state has breached the treaty, as long as both states agree to give the authority to the committee to do so. The Human Rights Committee, however, is constrained primarily in that in all cases it may only offer non-binding recommendations in its review.

Table 7.1. Selected Human Rights Agreements in Global Governance

Agreement	*Adoption*
Charter of the United Nations	June 26, 1945
Convention on the Prevention and Punishment of the Crime of Genocide	December 9, 1948
Universal Declaration of Human Rights	December 10, 1948
International Covenant on the Elimination of All Forms of Racial Discrimination	December 21, 1965
International Covenant on Civil and Political Rights	December 16, 1966
International Covenant on Economic, Social, and Cultural Rights	December 16, 1966
Convention on the Elimination of All Forms of Discrimination against Women	December 18, 1979
Convention against Torture and Other Cruel, Inhuman or Degrading Treatment or Punishment	December 10, 1984
Convention of the Rights of the Child	November 10, 1989
International Convention on the Protection of the Rights of All Migrant Workers and Members of Their Families	December 18, 1990
Convention on the Rights of Persons with Disabilities	December 13, 2006
International Convention for the Protection of All Persons from Enforced Disappearance	December 20, 2006

The ICCPR was also supplemented by an Optional Protocol, adopted in 1966, which provided procedures for individuals to submit complaints to the committee about alleged treaty violations. In 1989, a Second Optional Protocol to the treaty was adopted, which addressed elimination of the death penalty. The design of the ICCPR certainly leads to the conclusion that its heavy emphasis on voluntary compliance functionally makes it very protective of state sovereignty (Keith 1999). A study by Keith (1999) analyzing 178 different countries from 1976 to 1993 supported this conclusion by finding that being a party to the agreement did not produce a noticeable impact on a state's human rights practices. Another study also discovered that repressive states who joined the ICCPR, as well as the International Convention against Torture and Other Cruel, Inhuman or Degrading Treatment or Punishment, did not improve the treatment of their citizens even with their commitments to these obligations (Hafner-Burton and Tsutsui 2007).

ICESCR's coverage incorporated many of the rights listed toward the end of the UDHR. Articles 1 and 2 address the right of self-determination and the obligation of states to provide economic, social, and cultural rights to its citizens. Article 4 provides a limitation, which allows the government to put limits on the enjoyment of these rights for protection of other citizens as well as for the overall good of society. Articles 6–15 enumerate the rights provided by the ICESCR. These rights include the right to work, just and favorable working conditions, right to form and join trade unions, right to social security, protection of mothers and children, right to an adequate standard of living, freedom from hunger, physical and mental health, education, right to take part in culture, and enjoyment of advances from science. Articles 16–25 address the states' reporting requirements for their measures in implementing the ICESCR.

Unlike the ICCPR, the ICESCR did not include a body to monitor the treaty. This omission was addressed by a resolution passed by ECOSOC in 1985 to create a Committee on Economic, Social, and Cultural Rights (CESCR) to review reports and make recommendations on the states' efforts to implement the treaty. As with the ICCPR's Human Rights Committee, CESCR's recommendations are not binding. An Optional Protocol to ICESCR was adopted in 2008 by the General Assembly. The primary purposes of this agreement were to permit complaints by individuals (as long as they were serious violations and the individual had exhausted all remedies with the state) and permitting CESCR to confidentially investigate allegations of serious violations. The most distinctive provision of the ICESCR is covered in Article 2 (1):

> Each State Party to the present Covenant undertakes to take steps, individually and through international assistance and co-operation, especially economic and technical, to the maximum of its available resources, with a view to achieving progressively the full realization of the rights recognized in the present Covenant by all appropriate means, including particularly the adoption of legislative measures.

This provision demonstrates a key difference between states' obligation under the ICCPR and the ICESCR. Their obligation under the ICCPR is to directly adopt the treaty's specified rights into their domestic legal system. On the other hand, the obligation in the ICESCR is adoption contingent upon each state's "maximum available resources" and "progressive realization" of these rights rather than direct adoption. This language is symptomatic of the view that while civil and political rights are relatively clear and can be readily applied, protected, and enforced by the legal system, economic and social rights are vague and unmanageable (Alston and Quinn 1987). As Chapman (1996) argues, "progressive realization" subject to "maximum available resources" makes monitoring violations of the ICESCR to be very challenging. It creates a process based on an ad hoc evaluation of each state's measures rather than a uniform standard. This process requires a tremendous amount of data, as well as an abstract determination by CESCR to determine whether or a not a state is breaching the treaty. She has proposed an alternative framework for monitoring, in which, violations of the treaty would be based directly on the rights included in the ICESCR without the "progressive realization" measure. In addition to the challenge of interpreting Article (1), CESCR also faces an issue in that it does not have nearly as much guidance by the decisions of national courts on economic and social rights as the Human Rights Committee does in evaluating civil and political rights (Craven 1995).

In addition to the International Bill of Rights and the human rights agreements listed in table 7.1, regional systems for human rights exist in Europe, Africa, and the Americas. The European system includes the European Convention on Human Rights, which covers on civil and political rights, and the European Social Charter, which addresses economic and social rights. It also features the European Court of Human Rights to address potential violations of the European Convention on Human Rights. Africa also has a regional treaty, the African Charter on Human and People's Rights, as well as the African Commission on Human and People's Rights, to protect, promote, and interpret that treaty. The African Court on Human and People's Rights was established in 2006 to assist the commission in its functions. The Americas features a similar system with a human rights convention, which has only been ratified by Mexico, Caribbean, and Latin American states, complemented by a commission and a regional court. Of the three systems, Europe has been the most robust. Moravscik (1995) has credited the greater development of pre-existing norms on human rights and the establishment of more mature democracies in Europe, rather than its regional institutions, to account for its superior record on implementation and compliance.

THE RIGHT TO HEALTH

Although health did not become associated with human rights as a legal principle until after World War II, public health and the state's treatment of its citizens have long been connected. From the late middle ages to the early twentieth century, states would periodically issue quarantines as a primary response to combating the spread of infectious diseases. While these states had an interest in protecting the public from these threats, some individuals were faced with ill treatment, such as arbitrary arrest and detention by the state in the process. As noted, because human rights did not become adopted as an international legal principle until the 1940s, public health emergencies trumped individual rights. This practice occurred even in liberal democracies such as the United States during this time (Fidler 1999: 172). While public health emergencies could cause injury to individual liberties, efforts by Britain in the nineteenth century to develop less stringent measures for disease control contributed to an evolving norm that governments had a responsibility for the health of their citizens (Fidler 1999).

The first step in health emerging as a principle of human rights was the adoption of the Constitution of the World Health Organization (WHO) in 1946. Its preamble states, "The enjoyment of the highest attainable standard of health is one of the fundamental rights of every human being without distinction of race, religion, political belief, economic or social condition" (Constitution of the World Health Organization 1946). Additionally, the preamble goes on to say that "governments have a responsibility for the health of their peoples, which can be fulfilled only by the provision of adequate health and social services" (Constitution of the World Health Organization 1946). By agreeing to include these provisions, it was not the intent of WHO negotiators to guarantee an individual's health (Tobin 2012). It did, however, serve as an acknowledgment of health as a human right, as well as the state's obligation to provide it. Nevertheless, because these rights are in the preamble rather than text of the agreement, they are designated as non-binding principles.

Around this time, the UDHR was also in the process of being drafted. In its enumeration of human rights, the UDHR also included a provision for health. Article 25 states, "Everyone has the right to a standard of living adequate for the health and wellbeing of himself and of his family, including food, clothing, housing and medical care." While this language is not as precise as the WHO Constitution in declaring health as a right, it still serves an expression of acceptance of this norm.

According to Meier (2010), when the WHO was created, it intended to pursue policies based on technical work promoting international cooperation in health as well as a rights-based approach to promote the norm of health as a human right. The roots of this dual approach can even be traced to the definition of health in the WHO Constitution, which says that "health is a state of complete physical, mental, and social well-being and not merely the absence of disease or infirmity" (Constitution of the World Health Organization 1946). This definition of health, although fairly ambiguous, does indicate an intent that health be viewed as beyond a biomedical interpretation of the concept. During the 1950s, the WHO played a significant role in the efforts to draft the health provision of the UDHR into an international treaty. From the mid-1950s to the early 1970s, however, the WHO retreated its efforts for rights-based policies to focus more on technical cooperation based upon a biomedical approach to health, especially in regard to the eradication of specific diseases (Meier 2010). Advancements in science, rather than politics and socio-economic factors, were viewed as the most effective remedy for global health problems. By the time ICECSR was adopted in 1966, the WHO effectively abandoned its promotion of health as a human right.

While the WHO began to withdraw its involvement from the ICESCR negotiations, health was included as one of its economic, social, and cultural rights, and the treaty's health clause did adopt the "highest attainable standard of health" language from the preamble of the WHO Constitution, making the clause closer to the WHO's standard than the language in the UDHR. The health clause is in Article 12 (1) of the ICESCR, which says, "The States Parties to the present Covenant recognize the right of everyone to the enjoyment of the highest attainable standard of physical and mental health" (International Covenant on Economic, Social, and Cultural Rights 1966). The article then specifically mentions reduction of infant mortality; improvement of environmental and industrial hygiene; prevention, treatment, and control of diseases; and creation of conditions to assure medical services to all as obligations of the states. The ICCPR does not mention health per se, but it does include the right to life, which in a non-binding interpretation by the Human Rights Committee means that it would be desirable for states to reduce infant mortality and make efforts to increase life expectancy, "especially in adopting measures to eliminate malnutrition and epidemics" (Human Rights Committee 1982). While this view is certainly not a strong endorsement of health as a human right, it is an implicit acknowledgment that health is relevant to civil and political rights even though health is not specified in the treaty.

The WHO gravitated back toward human rights in the mid-1970s following the initiation of the primary health care movement and the selection of Halfden Mahler as Director-General. Mahler began the Health for All by 2000 campaign. These events culminated in the crowning achievement of the primary health care movement, the 1978 Declaration of Alma-Ata on Primary Health Care. This declaration reaffirmed the definition of health as well as the fundamental right to the "highest attainable" standard of health in the preamble of the WHO Constitution. It also stipulated that governments had a responsibility to provide for all, and all people should achieve a standard of health sufficient to live a "socially and economically productive life" (World Health Organization 1978). Primary health care would provide the means of meeting the objective of health for all by 2000. In 1979, the UN General Assembly even followed this lead by adopting a resolution endorsing the Alma-Ata Declaration and the Health for All strategy (United Nations General Assembly 1979).

Despite the enthusiasm in the WHO and the UN for the Health for All strategy,it received a fair amount of criticism for being too idealistic with an impractical timetable (Cueto 2004). A counter-movement soon began emphasizing an alternative approach of selective primary health care, which would be aimed at alleviating some of the more serious global health problems rather than a health for all objective. Proponents of primary health care believed that selective primary health care was a return to a biomedical approach to health.

Such a program would mitigate the rights-based approach to health as well as deemphasize the impact of socioeconomic causes of health. The short-term focus and cost-effectiveness of selective health primary care, however, made it the more attractive option for most states (Cueto 2004).

The Alma-Ata Declaration, at least in terms of its means and its objective of health for all by 2000, proved unsuccessful. In addition to the rising support for selective health care during the 1980s, other factors also contributed to its declining support. One factor was the shift toward neoliberalism as a growing norm in the global economy. The Alma-Ata Declaration fit with the political climate of the 1970s. During the 1970s, developing states began to increase their political power in the UN General Assembly as their numbers gradually grew following the post-World War II wave of decolonization. These states promoted a New International Economic Order (NIEO) as a common policy objective. This strategy called for such reforms as changes in international trade to provide more equitable prices for raw materials, greater influence over control of natural resources, foreign investment, and multinational corporations (Karns and Mingst 2015). Its principal aim was to reduce global economic inequality, and the Alma-Ata Declaration aligned with the spirit of this purpose, which was to provide good health to all people regardless of their nationality. The UN was used as the primary mechanism to promote the NIEO objectives. The adoption of neoliberal economic policies by the United States and United Kingdom in the early 1980s became a formidable challenge for the NIEO. These policies were endorsed by the major global economic institutions, the World Bank and the International Monetary Fund, and their power to provide funding for neoliberal economic reforms prevailed over the UN's normative influence. Because neoliberalism emphasized the market over the state, the provision of health became increasingly more of a product of the market (i.e., the private sector) rather than a public good offered by the state (Thomas and Webber 2004).

In addition to the emergence of neoliberalism, Meier (2010) found that the loss of the WHO's credibility in supporting health as a human right prior to the Alma-Ata Declaration was detrimental to the cause. He suggests that states did not view the WHO as a legitimate actor in human rights because it did not consistently promote the idea that health was such a right. Additionally, Meier (2010) argues that WHO erred by not promoting the "health for all" objective as a legal obligation. Rather than try to link "health for all" to Article 12 of the ICESCR, which was part of a legally binding treaty, the WHO let the non-binding recommendation of the Alma-Ata Declaration stand on its own. As a result, it was much easier for states to support its objective in principle but not be compelled to implement it as policy.

The idea of health as a human right, however, continued well after Alma-Ata. Its influence was indicated in the Convention on the Rights of the Child

(CRC), which was adopted in 1989. Article 24 of the CRC provided that "States Parties recognize the right of the child to the enjoyment of the highest attainable standard of health and to facilities for the treatment of illness and rehabilitation of health" (United Nations 1989). This treaty, which maintains the "highest attainable standard of health" language is fairly universal in scope. Currently, 195 states have ratified the convention, with Somalia and the United States as the only states to sign but not ratify the agreement. The 2006 Convention on the Rights of Persons with Disabilities, which has also been ratified by most states but not the United States as of March 2018, additionally contains the "highest attainable standard of health" language for disabled individuals.

The WHO attempted to revive Alma-Ata with a "Health for All in the 21st Century" campaign in the late 1990s. This movement, however, was fairly constrained by the pervasiveness of neoliberal economic policies and the rise of the World Bank as a leader in global health in the 1990s and 2000s (Thomas and Weber 2004). Nevertheless, the UN's Millennium Development Goals (MDGs) included a "health for all"–related target by calling for universal access for HIV/AIDS treatment to all who needed it by 2015, indicating that this movement generated some momentum in global governance, at least in the context of HIV/AIDS. The Sustainable Development Goals (SDGs) adopted in 2015 went much further by having a target to achieve universal health coverage, access to quality essential health care services, and access to affordable essential medicines and vaccines for all by 2030. The SDGs are consistent with the WHO's report in 2008 titled "Primary Health Care: Now More than Ever," based on addressing health problems exacerbated by growing economic inequality, selective primary health care and specialization, as well as increasing commercialization of health care (World Health Organization 2008c). Although the report suggests recommendations for reforms to institute primary health care, it, along with the MDGS and the SDGs, does not create any legal obligation. So, while the Alma-Ata Declaration remains very much alive as a normative principle in global health governance, its status as a legal right is much less clear.

IS THERE AN INTERNATIONAL RIGHT TO HEALTH?

As discussed, health as a human right has had much normative support in post–World War II global governance as demonstrated by its inclusion in the UDHR, the preamble of the WHO Constitution, the ICESCR, and the Alma-Ata Declaration. The CRC provides it as a right to children, and the Convention on the Rights of Persons with Disabilities provides for it as a right for the disabled. Additionally, the International Convention on the Elimination of

All Forms of Racial Discrimination and the Convention on the Elimination of All Forms of Discrimination Against Women provide that neither race nor sex can serve as basis for excluding the right to health. Of these agreements, ICESCR and in particular its Article 12 provide the strongest legal basis for an international right to health. Neither the preamble of the WHO Constitution nor the Alma-Ata Declaration pose legal obligations, and the other human rights treaties protect certain classes of people rather than establish health as a universal human right. It is debatable whether the UDHR is legally binding. Furthermore, the ICCPR may include a health dimension with its "right to life" provision, but its language may be too imprecise to create a legal obligation for health.

The main question, of course, is what exactly is the legal obligation of national governments under Article 12 of the ICESCR? The most definitive, although not binding, interpretation of Article 12 comes from the CESCR's General Comment 14 issued in 2000. This statement elaborates many key points of the article. First, while it does recognize that health is a fundamental human right, it also specifies that the right to health does not mean that everyone has a right to be healthy (Committee on Economic, Social, and Cultural Rights 2000). It acknowledges that genetics and behavior can compromise the quality of a person's health. The obligation of the states is not to guarantee that its nationals will be healthy, but it is to provide the resources necessary for the "highest attainable standard of health" to be available and accessible to all people within its jurisdiction without discrimination. Additionally, CESCR has interpreted Article 12 in light of Article 2 (1)'s "progressive realization" standard for treaty obligations. CESCR says that in terms of fulfilling this standard, "such steps must be deliberate, concrete and targeted towards the full realization of the right to health" (Committee on Economic, Social, and Cultural Rights 2000). CESCR also considers food, housing, education, sanitation, and other social determinants to be part of the right. On the basis of CESCR's interpretation of Article 12, parties to the agreement are obligated to recognize a right for everyone to have access to high-quality health care facilities and services. States, however, are not obligated to provide the best health care possible, but they must make their best efforts to do so.

In addition to the global agreements, some states have also committed to a right to health through regional accords. These instruments include the European Social Charter and the African Charter on Human and People's Rights. The American Convention on Human Rights mentions a right to health but does not require it as a state obligation. An addtional protocol to the convention adopted in 1988, however, does provide for a right to health. The Revised Arab Charter on Human Rights, which was adopted in 2004, also recognizes a right to the "highest attainable standard" of health.

Currently over 130 states include health rights in their national constitutions (Gostin 2014). States, however, vary in their legal protections for health, as well as implementation. An example of a national constitution that has expressly incorporated a right to health is Brazil in its 1988 constitution. A unified national health care system was also created to support this right. Brazil, however, has had mixed success in providing health for all. On one hand, Brazilian courts have recognized a legally enforceable right to health for Brazilian citizens. Access to primary health care has also improved significantly under the creation of the unified national health care system. In fact, 93 percent of Brazilians who sought health care in 2008 were able to receive it (Paim et al. 2011). On the other hand, despite constitutional protection for health, the Brazilian government spends less on health than smaller South American economies such as Argentina, Chile, and Uruguay (Filho 2013). One of the issues is a Brazilian law based on fiscal responsibility, which requires a limit of 53 percent of the budget for spending on public administration (Filho 2013: 178). Quality of public health care has also been an issue. According to Paim et al. (2011: 1787), "People with private health plans or insurance policies report having better access to preventive services and higher health-care use rates than do those without such plans or policies." Because Brazilians in the upper and middle classes have this kind of private care, it seems that the underfunding of the public system creates some inequality in Brazil despite its right to health mandate.

South Africa's Constitution, which was adopted in 1996, provides rights of access to health care services, adequate housing, sufficient food and water, and social security. Unlike Brazil, however, the right to health care is subject to a standard of "progressive realization" to potentially mitigate the government's obligation. A major problem for South Africa has been the inequalities in health between white and black South Africans, as whites have much lower rates of infant mortality, incidence of disease, and much higher life expectancies (Coovadia et al. 2009). The South African government has made efforts to support the constitution through legislation such as the 2003 National Health Care Act to establish a national health system, but implementing access to a high-quality health system for all South African nationals has been slow to develop (Ngwena et al. 2013).

In contrast, India, another developing country, does not have a specific right to health in its constitution. The government, however, has a constitutional obligation to improve public health. To supplement this provision, India has ratified ICESCR and other international treaties establishing a right to health. Nevertheless, India spends less than 1 percent of its gross domestic product on public health, among the lowest in Asia. In addition, CESCR found India to have "alarmingly high" infant and maternal mortality rates, and many Indians lack access to even "basic health services" (Committee on Economic, Social and Cultural Rights 2008). India also lacks a unified national health care system, and features an expensive and largely unregulated private system of health care that has "a virtual monopoly of ambulatory curative services in both rural and urban areas, and more than half of hospital care is run by the private sector" (Duggal 2013: 119).

In comparison to both developed and developing countries, the United States stands as an exceptional state on the issue of a right to health. First, the United States is one of the minority of states in the world that does not mention health in its constitution. The United States also does not have any domestic legislation conferring health as a right. Second, the United States is one the very few countries in the world that has not ratified the ICESCR or any other international treaties that provide for a general right to health. The United States is also not a party to the American Convention on Human Rights. Nevertheless, the United States has not completely disavowed a right to health. It has ratified the WHO Constitution; the International Convention on the Elimination of All Forms of Racial Discrimination, which prohibits racial discrimination to a right to health; and the ICCPR, which includes a right to life provision. The United States has also signed the UDHR and the ICESCR. Interestingly, despite its ambivalence about the legal status of health, the United States spends far more on health care than any other state. In 2016, for example, the United States spent US$9,892 per capita; the country that is second most to the United States was Switzerland with US$7,919 (Organization of Economic Cooperation and Development 2017).

While the United States is known for well-trained physicians and high-quality health care, in addition to its high level of spending, the primary issue with health has to do with its insurance system. The government provides protection for the elderly and the poor, but most Americans depend on private health insurance, and many are uninsured (Yamin and Carmalt 2013). In 2010, President Barack Obama signed the Patient Protection and Affordable Health Care Act (ACA) to provide less expensive options for insurance and make it more available to the uninsured. In terms of its operational objective, this legislation has had some success as 11 million Americans obtained health insurance during the Act's first five years (Associated Press 2015). However, as Yamin and Carmult (2013: 233) argue, the ACA "fails to treat health and healthcare as a basic right, as opposed to a market commodity, and as a consequence, perpetuates the current structural failure to address the underlying causes of inequalities in the system." The act addresses a functional need in the United States but does not incorporate a principle of health as a right. The fact that the ACA has been a political battleground and has underwent intense constitutional scrutiny indicates that a norm of health as a fundamental right is not particularly strong in the United States. The election of Donald Trump as president of the United States in 2016 and his goal, along with many in the

U.S. Congress, to repeal this health care legislation and replace it with a more market-based solution are additional evidence to support this point.

Although health as a right may be a legal principle included in international treaties and some national constitutions, the political support and operational value remain questionable. Evans (2002), for instance, made the claim that neoliberalism, which has a strong foothold in Western states and international economic institutions, has mitigated the influence of health as well as other economic and social rights in political affairs. In this context, political and civil rights are viewed as legitimate human rights. As he puts it, "For liberals, socioeconomic claims are legitimate aspirations, but never rights" (Evans 2002: 201). Neoliberals often argue that extensive implementation of economic and social rights, as opposed to political and civil rights, will require too much intervention by the state into the marketplace. Such intervention would be detrimental to economic prosperity and reduce the quality of life for all. While the United States clearly represents a case where economic and social rights have not developed a strong normative basis, this conflict between a rights-based approach and neoliberalism is also present in Brazil, a state that has made commitments to health has a right both domestically and internationally. As Filho (2013) maintains, neoliberal political coalitions have used legislation to limit spending on health despite its constitutional status in that country. It seems that implementation of effective access to high-quality health care for all continues to be a challenging goal whether it is due to ideology, limited resources, or weak institutions.

BOX 7.1 THE COMPATIBILITY BETWEEN HUMAN RIGHTS AND ECONOMIC DEVELOPMENT

An important issue in implementing human rights as a practice has to do with its relationship with economic development and growth. In terms of a potential conflict between the two, on one hand, it could be argued that significant implementation of human rights, especially economic and social, are too idealistic and would require impractical economic policies with possibly excessive government regulation of the market that may stifle economic growth. On the other hand, it could also be argued that prioritizing market interests over human rights is not only unethical but morally unjust. A study by the World Bank (2012) found that although a tension exists between human rights and economics, they are, for the most part, complementary. Included in the number of ways they may complement each other are the following: (1) human rights may help frame economic development in such a manner to improve equity in economic development and lead to greater economic growth, (2) human rights may be an effective means to reduce poverty, and (3) human rights may help promote a more educated and inclusive citizenry that could deter or constrain state corruption and its related economic costs.

A right to health certainly has benefits for economic development. A state with a population that is relatively free from the burdens of infectious and non-communicable diseases has the potential to be much more economically productive than a state with an unhealthy population. A healthy population also significantly reduces the financial burden of health care costs both on the individuals and the government. Although a right to health and economics has similar tensions as human rights, more generally, and economics, there is also great potential for these goals to mutually benefit each other.

HIV/AIDS AND HUMAN RIGHTS

As discussed in chapter 4, HIV/AIDS is a relatively new disease that was first discovered in the United States during the early 1980s. The HIV/AIDS pandemic proved to be a critical step in promoting a norm of health as a human right. While this pandemic occurred decades after the UDHR and a few years before ICESCR went into force, the right to health was still more of an idea than an enforceable right prior to the outbreak. HIV/AIDS brought health forward as an issue in political and civil rights as well as in economic and social rights. In terms of political and civil rights, one significant problem was discrimination. As carriers of a potentially deadly virus with no known cure, people with HIV faced the prospects of possible job loss, segregated housing, and isolation due to their condition. Additionally, prospects for discrimination against people with HIV/AIDS were exacerbated as the condition became associated with homosexuals, intravenous drug users, and prostitutes, groups that were not held in high esteem by much of society. In the early 1980s, HIV/AIDS was often associated with a promiscuous gay lifestyle, which brought some moral condemnation to individuals who had the disease (Wolff 2012). As a result, carriers of the HIV virus faced an even greater social stigma than persons suffering from other infectious diseases. The economic and social issues involved the right to health, specifically the right to high-quality treatment for the HIV/AIDS virus. Advancements in research during the 1990s made HIV a much easier disease to treat. These treatments, however, were fairly expensive, creating a potential financial obstacle for those that needed it.

In some states, during the first decade of the pandemic, individuals with HIV faced much greater sanctions than a social stigma. Fear and ignorance about how the disease spread contributed to some coercive national policies. According to Gostin and Lazzarini (1997: 102–103), "At least seventeen countries have adopted legal measures to isolate, quarantine, or confine people with HIV infection or AIDS." These practices developed despite the fact that the WHO maintained that these measures were not justified against individuals who were being detained only because they carried the virus (Gostin and Lazzarini 1997). Included in this acknowledgment was a resolution passed by the WHA in 1988, which called for non-discrimination against persons with HIV in regard to employment, services, and travel. Additionally, countries such as China, Japan, Mexico, South Korea, and the Soviet Union put individuals suspected of having HIV/AIDS under surveillance (Tomasevski et al. 1992). Although both the UDHR and the ICCPR rights permit the state to restrict individual rights to protect public health, Gostin and Lazzarini (1997: 104), however, pointed out that detention of infected individuals "substantially burdens human rights and yields little to no public health benefit, because it confines persons who pose a minimal risk of infection to others." If an individual runs a major risk to spreading the virus, detention may be warranted after such a determination is made under due process.

Two factors, in particular, can account for why HIV/AIDS was the issue that began to transform health as a right from a legal principle to a practical right. First, as pointed out by Tomasevski et al. (1992), HIV/AIDS was the first disease to develop into a global pandemic in the post–World War II era of human rights. As noted earlier, in previous centuries, it was generally accepted that individuals with infectious diseases could be recipients of ill treatment by the government in order to protect public health. By the late twentieth century, however, when the HIV/AIDS pandemic began, a number of national legislative measures and court decisions, as well as UN resolutions and international treaties, had developed to provide stronger protection of individual rights than ever before. The norm of non-discrimination was fairly strong in the 1980s and has become more powerful only by the beginning of the twenty-first century. Second, mobilization efforts were taken by the gay community in the United States, especially in the two cities that were greatly burdened by the AIDS epidemic in the 1980s, New York and San Francisco (Wolff 2012). The gay rights movement had already been increasing momentum in the 1970s, and because HIV/AIDS disproportionately affected the gay community, the disease became effectively linked to a pre-existing and viable human rights movement. As a consequence, for the first time, a health issue was gaining traction as a political right. HIV/AIDS activists were successful in convincing the U.S. Congress to pass the Ryan White Comprehensive AIDS Resources Emergency Act in 1990. Ryan White was an Indiana teenager who contracted HIV from a blood transfusion in the 1980, and received excessive discriminatory treatment in his community prior to his death from the disease (Gostin 2014). This legislation called on the U.S. government to provide funding for medical care and treatment for low-income or uninsured individuals with the HIV virus.

Internationally, much credit in the effort to mobilize political support for linking HIV/AIDS and human rights goes to Jonathan Mann, who was the first director of the WHO's Global Programme on AIDS. Mann's key contribution was advocating that HIV/AIDS, as well as health in general, was as much of a social problem as it was a biomedical problem. He suggested that HIV disproportionately affected the poor and other socially marginalized groups that were already subjected to a fair amount of discrimination. This social practice of discrimination would actually obstruct efforts to combat the disease. Individuals who had HIV, or suspected that they might have HIV, would avoid testing and treatment due to fear of discrimination and social stigma that was associated with the disease. He also viewed HIV/AIDS flourishing in areas of social inequality where there was a lack of education about the transmission of the disease, high incidences of intravenous drug use, and poor health care systems (Mann 1999). Due to these findings, he advocated a rights-based approach as a necessary component to an effective anti-HIV/AIDS campaign. His efforts proved to be persuasive in the WHA's 1988 resolution for non-discrimination against individuals with HIV. Mann's position within the WHO, however, did not last long as he clashed with the new WHO Director-General Hiroshi Nakajima in 1988 over WHO policy. In particular, Nakajima wanted to de-emphasize both AIDS and human rights as part of the organization's agenda. Mann resigned in 1990 due to this conflict and his loss of support (Fee and Parry 2008). Subsequently, the WHO began to retract its rights-based approach to addressing HIV/AIDS and was replaced by UNAIDS as the leading international institution for HIV/AIDS by 1996.

Despite this change, human rights still continued to be part of the response of global health governance to HIV/AIDS. In 1996, the Commission on Human Rights recommended that the OHCHR collaborate with UNAIDS, NGOs, and persons infected with HIV to establish a set of international guidelines for human rights to protect individuals with the virus. These guidelines were issued in 1998. Its purpose was to provide a reference for states to follow a rights-based approach in addressing HIV/AIDS. Among the guidelines included were the protection of individuals with HIV/AIDS from discrimination; widespread availability of quality information, goods, and services for HIV prevention, treatment, and support; and legal support for HIV individuals to educate them about their rights and assisting these individuals in enforcing their rights (Office of the United Nations High

Commissioner for Human Rights and the Joint United Nations Programme on HIV/AIDS 2006).

The international political profile of HIV/AIDS grew in the 2000s as the issue began to receive more attention from the UN General Assembly. As noted, reduction of HIV/AIDS was included as a Millennium Development Goal. Additionally, in June 2001, the General Assembly conducted a special session to specifically address HIV/AIDS. This conference produced a declaration, which went further than the MDGs, by including active promotion and protection of human rights particularly in regard to the non-discrimination against persons with HIV/AIDS, non-discriminatory access to medical goods and services, and a need to reduce the costs of drugs used to treat the disease (United Nations General Assembly 2001). Despite the supportive language in the declaration, politics and social stigma continued to play a role in its drafting. The United States and some Middle Eastern states did not want the language in the declaration that singled out sex workers, drug users, and men who had sex with men as vulnerable groups that needed more protections (Csete 2007).

The UN General Assembly held a conference on HIV/AIDS in 2006, which resulted in another declaration that also did not specify these groups of individuals. The 2006 declaration did acknowledge that human rights is "an essential element in the global response to the HIV/AIDS pandemic, including in the areas of prevention, treatment, care and support, and recognize that addressing stigma and discrimination is also a critical element in combating the global HIV/AIDS pandemic" (United Nations General Assembly 2006b). The declaration also established a commitment by member states to eliminate gender inequities in protecting women and girls from risk of the disease through legal measures, in addition to education and health care.

The General Assembly followed with an additional resolution on HIV/AIDS in 2011, which was thirty years after the first AIDS case was discovered, and ten years after its first resolution on HIV/AIDS. In addition to reaffirming the provisions of the 2002 and 2006 declarations, the 2011 resolution specifically identified drug users, sex workers, and men who have sex with men as high-risk groups that needed more attention from national HIV programs (United Nations General Assembly 2011). The Security Council also noted a link between HIV/AIDS and human rights in a 2011 resolution. It mentioned both the problem of gender inequality with the burden the of HIV/AIDS on women and the "importance of strong support by United Nations mission civilian and military leadership for HIV and AIDS prevention, treatment, care and support, as a factor for reducing the stigma and discrimination associated with HIV and AIDS" (United Nations Security Council 2011).

The right to health, especially in terms of access to medicines, has also received growing political support from the HIV/AIDS movement. While discrimination was the primary human rights component of HIV/AIDS in the 1980s, the development of antiretroviral drugs (ARVs) during the 1990s made the issue of access to high-quality medical treatment another major human rights issue. As discussed in chapter 4, the cost of ARV treatment was very expensive, initially costing about US$10,000 per person on an annual basis (Mukherjee 2013). Because of those infected with HIV globally were disproportionately poor and lived in developing countries, ARV treatment was effectively prohibited to many due to its economic cost. Efforts by civil society and NGOs, however, have been fairly successful in persuading states and major institutions in global governance to support a right of access to essential medicines to treat HIV/AIDS patients.

Since the MDGs included an objective of the achievement of universal access to treatment for HIV/AIDS, the UN General Assembly has passed three resolutions affirming this goal. In terms of issue with intellectual property protection for these drugs, the Doha Declaration was passed in 2001 by the World Trade Organization's Ministerial Conference allowed for members to grant compulsory licenses to produce or import a lower cost generic drug without having to obtain consent from the drug's patent holder subject to some conditions (Gostin 2014). Activism in civil society on this issue was significant enough to convince government donors to participate with the private sector to form the Global Fund to Fight AIDS, Tuberculosis, and Malaria in 2002 to assist in reducing the financial burden of ARV treatment. National courts have also been supporting this principle. A study by Hogerzeil et al. (2006) revealed that in fifty-nine cases, mostly in Latin America, courts enforced access to medicines as a national right. They found that successful litigation was most likely to occur in states that included health rights in their constitution, although a court in Argentina recognized the right without a constitutional provision based on the government's international treaty commitments.

HIV/AIDS, for the most part, has been a successful case for advancing the principle of health as a human right. Some obstacles, however, still remain. One issue is that the cause of HIV/AIDS has been much more successful than other health issues in receiving human rights promotion and protection from the various actors in global health governance. This practice could lead to the possibility of "AIDS exceptionalism" in the area of human rights, where a right to health may be viewed as a more viable right in the case of HIV/AIDS than other diseases. Despite the efforts of global health governance, discrimination remains a problem for many people with HIV/AIDS. Homosexual acts continue to face criminal penalties in many countries, and sex workers also tend to face a high risk of criminal sanctions or discriminatory treatment. As a consequence, individuals associated with certain groups (i.e., men who have sex with men and sex workers) may be less likely to seek health care or receive promotion of treatment by their government (Baer et al. 2013). So, while the norm of non-discrimination against persons with HIV/AIDS may be strengthening, groups that are at high risk for contracting, or already having the virus, remain susceptible to a significant social stigma and prospects for discrimination in many countries. In regard to access to medicines, as discussed in chapter 2, bilateral trade agreements with TRIPS-plus provisions potentially mitigate the effect of the Doha Declaration in lowering drug prices by constraining the availability of generic drugs. Cost of medical treatment for HIV/AIDS remains fairly expensive, especially for the world's poor. Availability is also a factor for developing states. A study by Cameron et al. (2009) on medicine availability in thirty-six developing countries found that in the public sector, low-cost medicines tended to be in short supply. While the private sector consistently had more availability of these medicines, prices were also higher.

CHRONIC DISEASES AND HUMAN RIGHTS

Chronic or non-communicable diseases also have a fairly high profile on the agenda of global governance. In 2010, the UN General Assembly adopted a resolution on the prevention and control of non-communicable diseases (United Nations General Assembly 2010). A high- level UN meeting on non-communicable diseases followed in 2011, which was the first such meeting of the UN on a health topic other than HIV/AIDS. As discussed in chapter 6, the SDGs called for a significant reduction in premature deaths from these diseases by 2030. Chronic diseases, as is the case with HIV/AIDS, place a tremendous burden on the world's poor. In developed countries, poor populations face a much higher risk of death from these diseases than high-income groups. This problem is even more severe in developing countries, where 75 percent of deaths in the world from non-communicable diseases occur every year, because of lack of access to quality health care and treatment (Di Cesare et al. 2013). As also discussed in chapter 6, Tobacco control has received by far the most attention in efforts to combat chronic diseases. The Framework Convention on Tobacco Control (FCTC), which entered into force in 2005, is in fact currently the only international treaty that is specifically targeted at a public health issue besides the International Health Regulations. Diet and alcohol consumption, in the context of chronic disease prevention, have received more attention from the WHO over the past decade, but efforts in addressing those issues so far have only produced some general guidelines.

The FCTC does not include any language that directly references human rights. Cabrera and Gostin (2013), however, argue that some provisions of the FCTC are influenced by human rights considerations. In particular, they note that the preamble of the FCTC says that the parties to the convention "give priority to their right to protect the public's health" (World Health Organization 2003d). In terms of protection, the FCTC calls upon states to take measures to offer protection from tobacco smoke in public places. Additionally, they find that the FCTC's provisions on a right of access to information constitute a human right. Although these provisions may offer some support to a link between human rights and tobacco control, they are, nevertheless, limited in scope. The ICESCR may potentially contribute to a broader connection between the two through its Article 12 on the right for everyone to the "highest attainable standard of physical and mental health." In reference to CESCR's interpretation of Article 12, Dresler et al. (2013: 475) make the case that "protection from secondhand smoke, tobacco production regulation, marketing restrictions and efforts to decrease tobacco consumption are clearly covered by General Comment 14."

A major obstacle to establishing a legal principle that tobacco control is a human right comes from a counterclaim by the tobacco industry that such a right infringes on political and civil rights, such as freedom of speech. They have emphasized an individual rights approach based on the idea that smoking is an individual choice, and the freedom to make such a choice should not be obstructed by government interference. As Katz (2005: ii33) writes, "The epithet 'Health Nazi' was invented by the tobacco industry to discredit efforts to encourage public health." Tobacco companies have had some success challenging government regulations of their advertising on the basis of freedom of speech and commerce grounds (Crow 2005). Courts in Colombia and Peru, however, have supported legislation aimed at tobacco control on the basis that the public's right to health outweighed the protection of freedom claimed by the tobacco industry (Gostin 2014).

Similar arguments regarding the right to health versus the right of individual freedom can be made for regulation of unhealthy food and alcohol. Tobacco control, however, is a much better candidate for receiving human rights protection because it is a much stronger norm as evidenced by the adoption of the FCTC. But tobacco control falls far short of receiving the same kind of connection to human rights as HIV/AIDS. A couple of factors can account for this difference. First, HIV/AIDS has been associated with a human rights movement since the 1980s, while tobacco control has not sparked the same kind of activism in civil society. Second, tobacco control advocates face formidable opposition from the tobacco industry in promoting a rights-based approach. While the HIV/AIDS movement has had some challenges in its efforts to lower the cost of drug treatment from pharmaceutical companies, the tobacco industry has been much more vigorous in its contention, especially using rights-based arguments to defend itself. Tobacco control may someday gain similar political support in global governance to the extent that it is a right to health to the same degree as HIV/AIDS treatment, but it is a norm that is in a fairly early stage of development.

PROSPECTS FOR IMPLEMENTATION AND ENFORCEMENT OF A RIGHT TO HEALTH

A great deal of evidence suggests that as a legal principle, a right to health is recognized in global governance. The problem, however, is the implementation and enforcement of this right. Many of the international agreements providing for a right to health are non-binding. In those agreements that are binding, the right to health provisions are vague and lack coherence as to what exactly is the standard of health that is required for implementation by states. National courts, the CESCR, and academic scholars have all given interpretations of this standard, but at this point there is not a universal consensus in global governance as to what exactly the right to health entails. This issue is further complicated in that implementing the principle of right to health frequently comes into political conflict with the norm of neoliberalism, as well as powerful commercial interests. The theories of international relations covered in chapter 1, realism, neoliberal institutionalism, constructivism, and Marxism have different views for the prospects of health to be a right that can be effectively implemented and enforced.

Realism

As an historically dominant approach to understanding the nature of international relations, realism can certainly account for why human rights, let alone a right to health, has only been a relatively recent part of international affairs. Realists assume that states are the dominant actors in global politics, and the national interest of the state is to promote its power, or in the case of neorealists, its security interests. Human rights does not fit well as a national interest. States wish to protect their own nationals, but protecting the treatment of non-nationals does not enhance the power or security of the state. Realists could point to the fact that it took a massive humanitarian tragedy for human rights to become an instrumental part of international law and diplomacy. Even then, the support for human rights is more in principle then a cause for state action. Realists would assume that states would be more likely to promote human rights when they can use it as an issue for political leverage to weaken the reputation of other states in the eyes of the international community. Human rights can be a useful tool of foreign policy, but it is of relatively low interest to the state.

Within the context of human rights, realists would argue that health would be a low priority in foreign relations. Powerful states, especially the United States, have consistently supported the importance of political and civil rights over economic and social rights for the agenda of global governance. Even European states, which have a fairly robust regional human rights system, do not guarantee health as a right in the European Convention on Human Rights. Realists would attribute the progress of HIV/AIDS treatment as a human right as a result of the fact that it is an incurable infectious disease that could potentially emerge as a security threat to the state if it becomes widely transmitted. Because this concern is related to HIV/AIDS and other emerging infectious diseases, it is an exceptional health issue that is of interest to states. In the case of other health issues, or a right to health generally, powerful states do not have a great deal of interest in advancing these causes as part of their main foreign policy interests. As a consequence, realists would assume that an international right to health place in global governance would not go much more beyond an agreement in principle, as exemplified by the outcome of the Alma-Ata declaration and the ambiguity of the right to health in the ICESCR.

Neoliberal Institutionalism

Neoliberal institutionalists, in contrast, would point to the progress that both human rights and the idea of health as a human right have made as issues in global governance over the past several decades. States have more of an incentive to cooperate in this area than realists suggest. This benefit is not only that an international right to health could reduce the burden of transnational infectious diseases. It could both serve a humanitarian purpose and contribute to healthier populations that would be more productive as labor and consumers in the global economy. The most notable accomplishments would be the ICCPR and ICESCR, two international treaties covering human rights, including the right to health, which have received almost universal acceptance from national governments around the world. The weakness of establishing health as a functional, effective right, however, has to do with ambiguity and the progressive realization and maximum available resources standards in the ICESCR that limit the provision's influence on national policy. For health to continue to evolve as an international human right, either the ICESCR would need to be amended to clarify the nature and obligation of the right or another international agreement would need to be concluded to assert health as a human right with more clarity.

In order to strengthen the position of health as a human right in global governance, Friedman and Gostin (2012) have proposed such a means in the form of a Framework Convention on Global Health (FCGH). This proposal would serve to provide a number of mechanisms, which would commit states not only to an obligation of health as a human right but also to some measures for enforcement of this right. Under the FCGH, the right to health would be legally enforceable in national courts, and Friedman and Gostin (2012) put forward a proposition to be included in the FCGH that would create an obligation for states to contribute to a database on legal cases around the world and participate in a process of enhanced monitoring of the implementation of the right to health by national governments that are parties to this agreement. In addition, transparency of government practices would be reinforced by a requirement in the FCGH for civil society, especially marginalized and vulnerable populations to be included as participatory partners in efforts to implement this right. The FCGH would also feature a funding mechanism that states would be obligated to support. This funding mechanism could be used to assist poor states in implementing health care and addressing other causes related to ill health (i.e., water and sanitation), as financing assistance to health-related NGOs, and as a financial incentive for states to comply with the provisions of the FCGH. They also recommend that a FCGH should also include the possibility of sanctions for non-compliance such as suspension from the WHO Executive Board and the Human Rights Council.

While neoliberal institutionalists would find that a comprehensive agreement such as the FCGH could offer an effective means to provide good health at the global level, the main problem would be sufficient political will to conclude the agreement. The FCGH imposes some significant obligations on states, much more so than the ICESCR, the WHO, or other health treaties such as the FCTC and the 2005 International Health Regulations. Realists, in particular, would be highly skeptical that such a demanding agreement would receive support by an international consensus of states. Neoliberal institutionalists would be more optimistic about such prospects, but they would suggest that it would be dependent on whether a substantial number of national governments find that the benefits of the FCGH outweigh the costs of its obligations. Given that global health has tended to not be considered as major national interest for many states, such a calculus would be a significant challenge.

Constructivism

Constructivists would base their assessment of health as a right in international politics on the strength of the norm and its status as part of states' identity. Health as a right has clearly been emerging as a norm after the ICESCR went into force. It has been included in subsequent treaties such as the CRC and the Convention on the Rights of Persons with Disabilities. Several national constitutions have even incorporated health rights without an international obligation to do so. For health to evolve into an effective human right, it is not necessarily required to become part of a precise, obligatory international treaty, but it does eventually need to become internalized as a standard practice of national governments.

In terms of human rights, Risse and Sikkink (1999) have developed a constructivist framework for understanding how human rights can become effectively implemented. The first stage in the model is repression. States that try to repress human rights decide to conceal repressive practices and deny that certain practices even violate legitimate human rights. The second stage is based on the material and normative pressure that outside actors, such as other states, as well as IGOs and NGOs, place on repressive governments to change their practices. This stage could include some form of economic or diplomatic sanction. It could also include "naming and shaming" the repressive state as a deviant in the international community. Stage three involves tactical concessions and dialogue. In this stage, domestic NGOs in the repressive state work with outside actors to advance the issue within the state's civil society, which creates both internal and external pressure on the state to change its policy. The fourth stage refers to a point where the government agrees to give "lip service" to the right although it may not be consistently implemented or protected. In the final stage, the right becomes internalized and becomes accepted as part of the state's identity.

This model demonstrates the potential process that the idea of health as a human right would follow to become an effective and enforceable right. The main issue, however, is that as a prospective norm it would need to be sufficiently strong to follow through all five stages of the model. As the analysis in this chapter indicates, even though the right to health is emerging as a norm, it does not yet seem to be sufficiently accepted to even reach stage two of this model involving pressure by outside actors. It lags well behind civil and political rights as part of global governance's human rights agenda. It is also constrained by the fact that the world's lead agency for global health and potentially powerful norm entrepreneur, the WHO, has been inconsistent and often reluctant to promote health as a human right. Powerful states have also not demonstrated much support for health as a human rights priority, let alone a foreign policy interest. Until the idea of health as a human right gains more widespread political acceptance, it cannot be considered a particularly viable right, especially outside of the HIV/AIDS context.

Marxism

Marxist and neo-Marxist approaches would find that the movement for health as a human right is constrained by the dominance of the market in international politics. In many ways, a universal health care system is at odds with the dynamics of the marketplace. A free market economy dictates that health is a commodity rather than a right. In this kind of system, wealthier individuals will have much better access to high-quality health care. Marxists would suggest that this dynamic can account for much of inequality of health and life expectancy between the rich and the poor in terms of both states and people. Difficulties related to providing access to medicines and control of tobacco, alcohol, and unhealthy food are all related to the market. The dissemination of drugs to the poor is constrained by their high costs. Unhealthy products have both a high consumer demand and support by wealthy and powerful multinational corporations.

For health to become a practical human right, Marxists would suggest that fundamental changes must occur in global governance to de-emphasize the role of the market in international politics. The institutions of global governance would need to promote a greater role of state regulation over the market. In addition, these institutions would also need to promote a norm of equality and rein in neoliberalism. Marxist perspectives assume that economic interests ultimately override humanitarian motives. It is dependent on the state to overcome these interests and provide quality health to all. As neo-Marxists have often found, however, ideological support of capitalism is deeply entrenched in powerful states and influential international institutions. Consequently, the dominance of the market in global governance will make the transformation of health as a human right from a principle to a practical right very problematic.

CONCLUSION

Due to the historical legacy of state sovereignty, human rights are a relatively recent addition to the practice of international politics. After human rights became entrenched as part of global governance following the atrocities of World War II, some debate has taken place as to what exactly constitutes a human right? Health has been an issue that has been caught in this debate. While health as a right has received some political support in global governance by means of the Universal Declaration of Human Rights, the World Health Organization's Constitution, and the International Covenant on Economic, Social, and Cultural Rights, its influence has been constrained by a lack of both obligation and precision of meaning at the international level. The fact that health has been considered to be an economic and social right rather than a political or civil right has also to some extent relegated it to a secondary human right.

In terms of health issues, HIV/AIDS stands out as the most successful case for health to receive recognition as human rights. In comparison to other health issues, however, it benefited from both its visible political profile and its connection to a broader human rights movement. Realists are very skeptical about the prospects for health to become an effective human right. They would find that it does not fit as a foreign policy priority for powerful states. Neoliberal institutionalists may be more optimistic, but they suggest that the idea of health as a human right would require stronger support and commitment by international institutions to become viable. Constructivists would view health as a human right as an emerging international norm that needs greater acceptance by both domestic and international actors. Marxist approaches are perhaps the most pessimistic about health as a human right. They find the idea to be at odds with capitalism, which they consider to be the dominant force in contemporary international politics. Underpinning all of these approaches is the requirement that political will is necessary to advance the cause of health as a human right. Whether this movement is constrained by other more pressing national interests, weak and unresponsive international institutions, or the market and neoliberal economics, the obstacles must be overcome for it to become a robust aspect of global health governance.

DISCUSSION QUESTIONS

1. Why are human rights such a complex and controversial issue in international politics?
2. What are the main differences between the International Covenant on Civil and Political Rights (ICCPR) and the International Covenant on Economic, Social, and Cultural Rights (ICESCR)? Why have the rights from ICESCR been more difficult to implement?
3. How did health become associated with human rights? What has been the World Health Organization's experience with a rights-based approach?
4. What are the political challenges that health faces, both domestically and internationally, to be recognized as a fundamental human right?

SUGGESTED READINGS

Freeman, Michael. 2011. *Human Rights: An Interdisciplinary Approach*. Second Edition. Cambridge, UK: Polity.

Provides a good background on human rights in both theory and practice.

Tobin, John. 2012. *The Right to Health in International Law*. New York: Oxford University Press.

Very good overview on the status of the right to health in international law.

Wolff, Jonathan. 2012. *The Human Right to Health*. New York: W. W. Norton.

Covers and analyzes the difficulty to establish a right to health in practice.

Chapter 8

Global Health and the Environment

The World Health Organization (WHO) estimates that environmental hazards account for 80 percent of all infectious and chronic diseases that it monitors (World Health Organization 2011). A number of different factors constitute these hazards. The first and the most high-profile factor in global health governance is the problem of climate change. As the temperature of the Earth increases, the likelihood of poor air quality, floods and droughts, less access to drinkable water, and greater frequency and intensity of natural disasters pose a threat to the quality of human health. Pollution, both in terms of outdoor and indoor air pollution and water pollution, is also a significant environmental hazard, as is poor sanitation and exposure to chemical and other toxic materials.

In 2016, the WHO issued a report, *Preventing Disease through Healthy Environments*, to provide an estimate of the impact that the environment places on the prospect for the global spread of disease. This report found that 22 percent of the global disease burden, which would account for loss of healthy life years, and 23 percent of all premature deaths were due to the environment. Most of this burden fell on developing states, which had the highest fraction of deaths and disease attributable to the environment (World Health Organization 2016d). The diseases most closely associated with the environment are diarrhea (poor water quality and sanitation), lower respiratory infections (indoor and outdoor air pollution), workplace hazards (exposure to chemical and toxic materials), malaria (land use, deforestation, and water management), and chronic obstructive pulmonary disease (exposure to chemicals and air pollution). According to the WHO even 20 percent of all global cases of cancer could be attributed to the environment.

Although many of the world's health problems are caused by environmental factors, the actors of global health governance have not placed much emphasis on the relationship between the two in promoting global health. This issue began to receive more attention in recent years with the United Nation's (UN) Millennium Development Goal (MDG) Number 7, which was directed at ensuring environmental sustainability. Included in the target for this goal was a 50 percent reduction in the number of people worldwide who did not have access to safe drinking water and basic sanitation. The Sustainable Development Goals (SDGs) in 2015 went further by considering the impact of pollution as part of its goal Number 3 of good health and well-being by targeting a significant reduction in the hazards of air, water, and soil pollution by 2030. The World Health Assembly (WHA) has followed suit in the 2000s as evidenced by its passing a resolution in 2008 addressing climate change and a resolution in 2015 directed at air pollution. Nevertheless, as Wiley (2010) argues, international cooperation on global health has been largely guided by approaches based on medical treatment or security approaches to resolve health problems. In terms of treatment, actors in global health governance have emphasized such measures as greater access to health care and essential medicines, as well as greater distribution of vaccines and more research and development for pharmaceuticals. The security component is primarily aimed at infectious diseases, particularly in terms of surveillance and the dissemination of information. In comparison, an environmentally based approach to health has not received the same kind of support by the actors of global health governance.

The purpose of this chapter is to analyze key environmental issues in the context of global governance. The first step is an overview of the general role of environmental politics in international affairs and global governance. Second, three environmental issues that have a significant impact on health, climate change, the depletion of the ozone layer, and air pollution, will be analyzed. In conclusion, these issues and international environmental politics in general, will be examined based on the international relations theories of realism, neoliberal institutionalism, constructivism, and Marxism discussed in chapter 1. Some important questions to consider in this chapter are the following: What is the status of the environment in the agenda of global governance? How are global environmental problems related to global health? Are global environmental problems adequately addressed by the actors and institutions of global governance?

ENVIRONMENTAL POLITICS AND GLOBAL GOVERNANCE

Similar to human rights, the environment is a relatively recent addition to global governance. As discussed in chapter 7, while human rights did not emerge as an issue in international affairs until the mid-1940s, it was not until the late 1960s when the environment, at least as it pertains to human health, began to attract attention as an international issue. The environment, as was the case with human rights, was long viewed as an issue that was primarily connected with state sovereignty. Traditionally, it was considered to be a local problem rather than a transnational one. As described by Bodansky (2010a), the emergence of the environment in international law occurred in three waves, which all continue to run concurrently. The first wave was based on conservation, with a focus on the protection of animal populations. It was the dominant emphasis in international environmental politics in late nineteenth century through the first decades of the twentieth century. The second wave, which began in the late 1960s added climate change and pollution to the international agenda. The mid-1980s brought the third wave, based on sustainable development, which sought to merge environmental protection with the need for continued economic growth and development.

As conservation dominated environmental concerns during the first half of the twentieth century, unlike human rights, the issue of the environment was not included in the United Nations (UN) Charter, which was signed and went into force in 1945. In addition, no UN-affiliated intergovernmental organizations (IGOs) were established to address environmental issues. While human rights were able to transcend state sovereignty by the atrocities of World War II, the environment, with the exception of the conservation treaties, was considered to be almost strictly an issue of national concern. Among environmental issues, conservation was the strongest international norm and as such was the first issue to make successful inroads on the agenda of post–World War II global governance. In 1946, the International Convention for the Regulation of Whaling was signed for the purpose of conserving whale stocks. This treaty included an international commission authorized to study whaling activities, collect data on whale stocks, and to oversee the schedule of the convention, which sets out specific measures for regulating whaling such as limits on the catch of certain species as well as hunting methods. Without any other IGO beside the International Whaling Commission, conservationists, with the support of some national governments and NGOs, were able to form the International Union for the Conservation of Nature, a public-private partnership dedicated to protect wildlife and preserve natural resources (Sands and Peel 2012).

Although the environment does not fall under the purview of any UN agencies, conservationists had success working through the UN's Economic and Social Council (ECOSOC) as evidenced by its resolution in 1949 to assemble the UN Conference on the Conservation and Utilization of Resources. In this resolution, ECOSOC emphasized the importance of managing natural resources as part of economic development. It served as the first step for the

UN to begin to assert itself as an actor in environmental politics (Sands and Peel 2012). Water pollution began to make some progress on the agenda of global governance in the 1950s. The International Maritime Organization (IMO) adopted the International Convention for Prevention of Pollution by Oil in 1954 at a conference in London. This agreement provided regulations for the discharge of oil by tankers. With a few exceptions, it prohibited discharge of oil in sea areas located fifty miles away from land. The 1958 Geneva Convention on the High Seas, which obligated member states to establish regulations to prevent oil discharge by ships and pipelines as well as refraining from dumping radioactive waste into the sea, was added to strengthen international management of pollution of the sea.

Despite these advancements, the issue of the international environment had little connection to human health. The second wave of environmentalism, however, successfully developed this link and created more motivation for states, especially developed states, to make environmental issues a greater priority in their foreign policy. Public opinion in developed states began to develop more support for environmental regulation following the publication of the book *The Silent Spring* by Rachel Carson in 1962 (Griswold 2012). In her book, Carson used a scientific analysis to explore how pesticides, in particular DDT, had moved from killing insects to affecting birds and fish and then threaten the health of human beings. It provided a scientific demonstration that human activity was damaging nature, which in turn, could be a threat to human well-being. The book gained so much attention that Carson testified before a U.S. Senate subcommittee the year after it was published (Griswold 2012). The oil tanker disaster in 1967 that occurred off the coast of the United Kingdom and the media coverage of that event further galvanized civil society to push for environmental protection at the national and international levels (Kiss and Shelton 2007).

A global conference on the environment soon followed. This conference, the Intergovernmental Conference for Rational Use and Conservation of the Biosphere, was sponsored by the United Nations Educational, Scientific, and Cultural Organization (UNESCO) in 1968. It provided discussion of the effects of human activity on the biosphere such as air and water pollution, overgrazing, and deforestation. It produced several recommendations including improvements in research, new approaches to education about the environment, and the need for the planning of development projects to take potential impact on the environment into account (McCormick 1991).

The Stockholm Conference and the Human Environment

Although the 1968 Biosphere conference was a notable achievement, it was soon to be overshadowed four years later by the much larger and high-profile

United Nations Conference on the Human Environment (also known as the Stockholm conference) in 1972. This conference and its outcome served as the first major step toward recognition of the link between human health and the environment in global governance. The origin of this conference was based on the concern of Sweden about the growing increase in acid rain affecting the country. Sweden promoted a resolution in ECOSOC, which was later adopted by the UN General Assembly, for the UN to establish an international conference to develop a framework for the UN to promote international cooperation to address the world's environmental problems (McCormick 1991). Stockholm, Sweden, played host to the conference, which included representatives from 113 states, major IGOs, 400 non-governmental organizations (NGOs), and 1,500 journalists (Kiss and Shelton 2007: 34). The conference provided an open format of discussion where both developed and developing states as well as civil society were able to express their views. A notable feature of this conference was the relationship between developed and developing countries. Prior to the Stockholm conference, the global environment was considered to be a problem for post-industrial societies or "rich countries" whose citizens were demanding government action for altruistic purposes. Developing states were inclined to see environmental protection as more of a luxury interest and were more willing to bargain on the issue as long as developed states were willing to offer technology and financial assistance in return for their cooperation (Brenton 1994).

Negotiations at the conference concluded with the Stockholm Declaration composed of twenty-six general environmental principles and an action plan of 109 recommendations. While both of these instruments were not legally binding, they were the first substantial proclamations regarding protection of the environment that were agreed upon by much of the international community (Kiss and Shelton 2007). In the declaration, an important obligation was that natural resources including air, water, and flora needed to be protected for current and future generations. Health was also mentioned in Principle 7 of the declaration, in regard to committing states to prevent pollution of the seas with substances that could pose harm to human health. The interests of developing states were also acknowledged in Principle 11 that said, "The environmental policies of all States should enhance and not adversely affect the present or future development potential of developing countries, nor should they hamper the attainment of better living conditions for all" (Declaration of the United Nations Conference on the Human Environment 1972). The most significant legal provisions in the declaration were the right of states to exploit their own natural resources and a responsibility not to harm the environment of other states, an obligation for states to develop international environmental law, and a request that states should make cooperative arrangements to manage or eliminate activities that harm the environment while taking account of national interests and state sovereignty (Sands and Peel 2012).

According to Sands and Peel (2012), the Stockholm Conference shaped international action for the environment directly and indirectly. A significant achievement of the conference was the establishment of the United Nations Environment Programme (UNEP) as the first institution for the environment in the UN system. UNEP was tasked by the UN General Assembly to perform various functions such as promoting international cooperation on the environment, acquiring and assessing information and data about the environment, providing policy guidance on the environment in the UN system, and to review national and international environmental policies (United Nations General Assembly 1972).

The primary political debate regarding the creation of UNEP was whether to establish it as an IGO that would be a specialized agency within the UN system such as the WHO, to place it as a unit within the UN Secretariat, or to place it as a program in ECOSOC. A position as an IGO was the most prestigious option and would give it more independence, but this choice was rejected because other UN-affiliated organizations such as the WHO, the World Meteorological Organization (WMO), and the Food and Agriculture Organization (FAO) were already performing various activities related to the environment, and it was an area that was viewed as involving work of several organizations rather than one that required a leading agency. Additionally, a fair amount of dissatisfaction with UN organizations had taken root by the 1970s, especially by the United States (Ivanova 2010). As a result, it was designated as a subsidiary body to the General Assembly and ECOSOC rather than an autonomous organization. According to Ivanova (2010: 153), although the choice to relegate UNEP to this role was not "intended to diminish UNEP's authority, the decision to constitute it as a program rather than a specialized agency has negatively impacted its clout and ability to fulfill its functions over the years." Most significantly, it has had difficulty in demonstrating leadership and political support in the UN system for environmental issues. Despite its institutional weakness, UNEP is still regarded as the lead authority for the global environment (United Nations Environmental Programme 2015).

The post-Stockholm era brought forth a significant increase in international environmental treaties. These new laws, however, were directed at specific sectors such as marine waters, the atmosphere, and protection of wildlife rather than the environment per se (Kiss and Shelton 2007). By the mid-1980s multilateral treaties had been established to address air pollution and the ozone layer. The UN General Assembly also took an active role in addressing the environment by adopting the World Charter for Nature in 1982. This agreement, which, like the Stockholm Declaration, was not binding, provided for the safety of habitats, conservation of both land and sea, and a general protection of nature. It received a more favorable reception by developing states than the negotiations in Stockholm a decade earlier (Sands and Peel 2012).

Another major achievement of the General Assembly was its establishment of the World Commission on Environment and Development, which became known as the Brundtland Commission after its leader, a future Director-General of the WHO, Gro Harlem Brundtland. This commission's 1987 report (also known the Brundtland Report) advocated for the idea of sustainable development to be a guiding principle in international environmental politics. The report defined sustainable development as "meeting needs of the present without compromising the ability of future generations to meet their own needs" (World Commission on Environment and Development 1987: 8). The report also mentions the idea that poverty can be a cause of environmental degradation. By including a social condition, and not just human activity relating to economic growth, as a factor in maintaining environmental quality, the link between health and the environment acquired another dimension in global health governance through this concept of sustainable development.

The Rio Conference and Sustainable Development

The UN General Assembly not only adopted the Brundtland Report but also decided to convene another UN conference on the environment to expand the idea of sustainable development further into the international community. The conference was to be held twenty years after the previous UN conference in Stockholm. It was titled the United Nations Conference on Environment and Development (UNCED) due to the request of developing states to separate the issue of environmental protection from development (Bodansky 2010a). UNCED was staged in Rio de Janeiro, Brazil, in June 1992. In addition to its official title, it was also known as the Rio Conference, as well as the Earth Summit. The Rio Conference was even larger than Stockholm Conference, in fact it was the largest UN conference ever at that time. It featured representatives from 176 states, which constituted almost every member of the UN. Some 114 heads of state attended along with almost 10,000 national delegates, while 1,400 NGOs were invited to the conference along with 9,000 journalists (Kiss and Shelton 2007). This conference paved the way for global environmental governance in the next millennium by establishing sustainable development as a cornerstone of international environmental politics and providing the first international agreement on climate change.

Five instruments emerged from the negotiations at Rio. Three of which were non-binding. One of the non-binding documents was the Rio Declaration on the Environment and Development (Rio Declaration). This instrument reaffirms some of the principles of the Stockholm Declaration (such as the right of states to exploit their natural resources with the added qualification to do so in accordance with developmental policies to go along with environmental policies mentioned in the Stockholm Declaration, duty to make information widely available, and an obligation to develop laws for liability and compensation of pollution victims). It also evolves beyond Stockholm Declaration to include new principles (such as a duty to eradicate poverty as a condition for sustainable development and an obligation for states to conduct an environmental impact assessment for activities that are likely to have significant on the environment). Another of the non-binding instruments from the Rio Conference was Agenda 21, a document that covered over 100 topics covering socioeconomic dimensions of environmental cooperation (including health), conservation and resource management (i.e., atmosphere, water), strengthening the role of NGOs in environmental policy, and means of implementation (i.e., financing, legal instruments). The third non-legally binding instrument from Rio was related to the failure to successfully conclude a binding treaty on forests. As an alternative, the instrument Non-Legally Binding Authoritative Statement of Principles for a Global Consensus on the Management, Conservation, and Sustainable Development of All Types of Forests, also known as the Rio Forest Principles, was adopted. The binding legal instruments produced at Rio were the United Nations Framework Convention on Climate Change (UNFCCC) and the Convention on Biological Diversity.

While much of the outcome of the Rio Conference was based on the agreement of non-binding principles, an international institution was added to global governance in the form of the United Nations Commission on Sustainable Development to monitor states' compliance with the Rio Declaration and Agenda 21. As with UNEP, however, this institution was also granted little power. It can give policy recommendations on sustainable development issues, and it receives and disseminates reports from states, IGOs, and NGOs. Yet, its recommendations are based on non-binding principles, and state's environmental reports are not only voluntary, but also their content is determined by national environmental ministries. The commission has experienced some success with agenda-setting and promoting dialogue, but it has been much weaker in policy guidance. Much of its mixed record of effectiveness can be attributed to its institutional setting as a soft forum, lack of entrepreneurial leadership, and the influence of developing states, as well as the actions of both the United States and China in slowing down its decision-making process (Kaasa 2007).

The emergence of the environmental norm through sustainable development in the 1990s was also evident in international economic institutions, which had received some criticism from civil society groups for neglecting the environment in pursuit of economic growth. The World Bank established a program known as the Global Environment Facility (GEF) in 1991 to serve as a funding mechanism for developing states, NGOs, and the private sector to assist these actors in addressing environmental problems. Major sources of funding have included actions related to climate change (i.e., solar power technology), polluted international waters, biodiversity, and sustainable land and water management. Since its inception, GEF has provided US$17 billion in grants and helped obtain US$88 billion in co-financing for 4,000 projects in 170 developing states (Global Environment Facility 2018).

When the World Trade Organization (WTO) was established in 1994, its founding document, the Marrakesh Agreement Establishing the World Trade Organization, included sustainable development in its preamble. The 1994 General Agreement on Tariffs and Trade's Article XX, which is incorporated in the WTO, provides "the conservation of exhaustible natural resources" as one of the exceptions to non-discrimination in the trade of goods. Although the preamble is by itself not legally binding and the natural resource provision is rather vague, the WTO's Appellate Body did decide in a 1998 dispute between the United States and a group of India and other Asian countries over shrimp imports that the principle of sustainable development was applicable to that case (Ramlogan 2011).

Post-Rio Developments: Has International Cooperation on the Environment Peaked?

In 1997, a special session of the UN General Assembly, known as Rio+5 or Earth Summit+5, was conducted to review the progress of the implementation of the Rio agreements. Although progress had been made in implementing the Rio principles, it was noted at the Rio+5 meeting that the condition of the global environment continued to worsen. Sustainable development was still continued to be viewed as the appropriate strategy, but the report of the conference emphasized that the Rio principles and Agenda 21 provisions would need to be implemented much more rapidly to prevent further degradation of the environment (Galizzi 2005). Despite this warning, the environment did not initially receive much attention on the setting of agenda for the UN General Assembly's Millennium Summit in 2000. UN Secretary-General Kofi Annan, however, was able to persuade member states to include it in the Millennium Declaration with respect for nature constituting one of its fundamental values for international relations in the twenty-first century (Galizzi 2005). In addition, sustainable development was included as one of the MDGs.

To commemorate the tenth anniversary of the Rio Conference (and the thirtieth anniversary of the Stockholm conference), the UN moved forward with another Earth Summit meeting titled "The World Summit on Sustainable

Development" (also known as Rio+10) in Johannesburg, South Africa, in 2002. The politics in Johannesburg proved to be more contentious than the previous UN environmental conferences. The primary conflict was between developing states, who wanted the meeting to focus on development issues, wealth redistribution, and poverty eradication, and some developed states and environmental NGOs, who were concerned that environmental protection was becoming overshadowed by development (Galizzi 2005). Some states, especially the United States but also to a certain extent Canada, Japan, and Australia, were simply not interested in making any further commitments to international environmental cooperation (Pring 2002).

The negotiations in Johannesburg produced only two agreements: the Declaration on Sustainable Development (also known as the Johannesburg Declaration) and the Plan of Implementation of the World Summit on Sustainable Development, which was aimed at strengthening national implementation measures for Rio's Agenda 21 goals. The Johannesburg Declaration was another non-binding instrument, which reaffirmed political support of the Rio Declaration and Agenda 21. It did not provide any further obligations to the environment, and mainly focused on development issues. The Plan of Implementation also did not add anything new to global governance and environmental protection; however, it served as a commitment by the international community to maintain the terms and the objectives established by the Rio Conference a decade earlier (Kiss and Shelton 2007).

The marginalization of the environment in the development agenda continued during the UN General Assembly's 2005 World Summit to review the progress of the implementation of the MDGs. At the conclusion of the conference, member states agreed on the importance of promoting international conference in four areas: development, peace and collective security, human rights and the rule of law, and strengthening the UN. Environmental issues were included in the World Summit's Outcome Document, but it was added as a subset of development (Galizzi 2005). For the remainder of the decade, the UN General Assembly passed a series of resolutions calling for implementation of Agenda 21 and Johannesburg's Plan of Implementation. In December 2011, the General Assembly called for another conference, the United Nations Conference on Sustainable Development to be held in Rio de Janeiro in June 2012. This conference, of course, was scheduled to commemorate the twentieth anniversary of the Rio Conference and would also be known as Rio+20.

The UN Conference on Sustainable Development was the largest environment conference yet with almost 50,000 participants and 100 heads of state (Romero and Broder 2012). Due to the lack of progress in environmental cooperation during the 2000s, Rio+20 did not appear to be a promising forum for comprehensive reform. According to Bernstein (2013), the conference lacked an overall vision by both the General Assembly and the conference secretariat. As with Johannesburg and the 2005 World Summit, the goal for Rio+20 was more about promoting implementation of existing principles rather than addressing new themes or devising innovative strategies to global environmental problems. Despite low expectations, Rio+20 still produced mixed results. On one hand, the conference's outcome document was primarily reinforcing previous commitments, maintaining the guiding principle of sustainable development, and did not set forth any priorities or specific objectives. On the other hand, as noted by Ivanova (2013) the outcome document called for reform of international environmental institutions, agreement to establish a set of global sustainable development goals, and it acknowledged a desire for greater involvement by civil society in global environmental governance.

In terms of institutional reform, one change was to bolster the power of the UNEP. While it was not to receive the status of a UN specialized agency, its governing council expanded from fifty-eight states to universal membership granting it greater legitimacy as an actor (Ivanova 2013). Additionally, funding to UNEP was bolstered by a UN General Assembly resolution, which requested that the UN Secretary-General maintain the need for UNEP's resources through the UN's regular budget. Interestingly, while UNEP was empowered, the negotiations at Rio+20 also resulted in the end of the UN Commission on Sustainable Development. Disappointed in the commission's performance over the past twenty years, it was decided that the commission would be replaced by a high-level political forum to provide global leadership on sustainable development issues. This forum would be convened for heads of state in the General Assembly once every four years and on a yearly basis for ministers in ECOSOC.

The SDGs are a set of objectives for sustainable development that serve as a successor to the MDGs as part of the UN's post-2015 development agenda. While most of these goals were aimed at development issues, the environment received substantial attention by the proposals for goals calling for the availability and sustainable management of water and sanitation, ensuring sustainable production and consumption patterns, taking urgent action against climate change and its impact, conserving and sustainably using oceans, and developing sustainable cities and forms of development. The outcome document of Rio +20 also stressed the importance of participation of all states in the process of global environmental governance and the engagement with civil society actors in the process of both decision-making and implementation. The UN supported these recommendations by adopting the seventeen SDGs during a summit meeting in September 2015.

It remains to be seen what the long-term impact of Rio+20 and the SDGs will be on global health governance. The various negative impacts that the environment has on health will be influenced by the effectiveness of decision-making and implementation of rules regarding environmental protection by the actors and processes of global governance. The environment faces a number of challenges on the international community's agenda. Most notably, how to reconcile environmental protection with both developmental and neo-liberal economic policies. The next section of this chapter will look at efforts to address climate change, depletion of the ozone layer, and outdoor air and water pollution to analyze both the effect of these issues on health and efforts by global governance to mitigate their effect on human health.

CLIMATE CHANGE

Climate change, or global warming, can impact human health in a myriad of ways, including heat stress, water shortages, food insecurity, possible climate-induced spread of communicable diseases, and harm posed by an increased likelihood of extreme weather events. The WHO (2014d) estimates that climate change will contribute to 38,000 deaths from heat stress, 48,000 deaths from diarrhea, 60,000 deaths from malaria, and 95,000 deaths from childhood malnutrition by 2030. Overall, an additional 250,000 deaths worldwide are estimated to be attributed to climate change between 2030 and 2050 (World Health Organization 2014d). Vulnerable populations such as children, the elderly, and people living in low-income countries will face most of this burden. Despite the threat that climate change presents to global health, a commission of international medical experts has also suggested that "tackling climate change could be the greatest health opportunity of the 21st century" (Watts et al. 2015: 1861). The reason behind this statement is that although climate change does threaten to negate and even reverse, progress in improving health from economic growth, actions toward mitigation of climate change could also spill over to alleviate other social determinants of poor health such as poverty, economic inequality, and inadequate health care systems (Watts et al. 2015).

Climate change has been an issue at the top of agenda of global environmental governance since the early 1990s. According to a 2013 report by a working group of the Intergovernmental Panel on Climate Change (IPCC), an international scientific organization under the auspices of the UN, the past thirty years have likely been the warmest in the world's northern hemisphere in over 1,400 years. Additionally, the upper ocean (75 meters) has warmed by 0.11°C from 1971 to 2010. As a result of these trends, glaciers worldwide and the ice masses of Antarctica and Greenland have been deteriorating. A further consequence has been a consistent rise in sea level over the past century. To accompany these warming trends, concentrations of the greenhouse gases, carbon dioxide, methane, and nitrous oxide, which have increased since 1750, are now at the highest levels of concentration in 800,000 years (Intergovernmental Panel on Climate Change 2013). While some of the causes of global warming may be natural, the report also found clear evidence of human activity, especially in terms of the release of greenhouse gases, to be responsible. In fact, the report attributes more than half of the increase of global average surface temperature from 1951 to 2010 to such activity (Intergovernmental Panel on Climate Change 2013: 17).

The WHO has espoused both direct and indirect negative consequences of global warming on human health. It associated climate change with an increase in extreme heat contributing to more cases of cardiovascular and respiratory diseases, a rise in natural disasters such as floods, hurricanes, and other extreme weather events, and a lengthening of transmissions of diseases spread by insects such as dengue and malaria. Although climate change has a global impact, its effects are not spread evenly throughout the world. As Freeman and Guzman (2009) note, it will be developing states, particularly the poorest, who contribute the least to the world's greenhouse gas emissions that face the greatest danger. They attribute this outcome due to developing states lacking the capacity to respond to climate change; the fact the economies of these states are more dependent on agriculture, which is an industry that could face great harm from climate change; and because many of these countries are already located in warm climates, making the hazards of global warming even more intense than in northern states (Freeman and Guzman 2009).

Climate change first emerged on the radar of global governance in the late 1980s when UNEP and the WMO elected to establish the IPCC to facilitate scientific research on the phenomenon. The IPCC's first report in 1990 indicated with a great deal of certainty that greenhouse gas emissions from human activity were contributing to global warming. Despite lacking universal support, this finding was accepted by most of the international scientific community at that time (Breidenich et al. 1998). The first step in multilateral efforts to combat climate change was the UNFCCC, which as previously noted, was one the two international treaties emerging from the 1992 Rio Conference. Among the key commitments in the UNFCCC are obligations for parties to provide information regarding human-related greenhouse gas emissions and removal of gas sinks (i.e., forests, which can act to absorb carbon dioxide); take measures to mitigate greenhouse gas emissions; promote cooperation, including transfer of technology, to reduce greenhouse gases; and to consider the impact of climate change in regard to any social, economic, or environmental policy under consideration. The UNFCCC also further commits certain countries, mostly developed states, to adopt policies to reduce greenhouse gas emissions and protect gas sinks and report on implementation of these policies. Health was addressed in a couple of places in the UNFCCC. In particular, the agreement mentions the effect on public health as policy consideration for states in taking measures to adapt to climate change. For the most part, however, the relationship between climate change and health received little attention (Wiley 2010).

Kyoto Protocol

Although the UNFCCC was a political success in that it has become almost universally accepted with 195 states as parties to the convention, it still exhibited some fundamental limitations for achieving the objective of reducing greenhouse gas emissions. The first limitation was that the majority of the states (i.e., developing countries) were obligated only to report their activities, not to reduce their emissions. Reduction was an obligation only for more industrialized states. Even for these countries that had an obligation to reduce their emissions, the UNFCCC did not include any target or timetable for such reduction. As a consequence, it was decided rather early after the UNFCCC went into force that states needed to make stronger commitments for the agreement to have any impact on global warming (Breidenich et al. 1998). In 1997 at a climate change conference in Kyoto, Japan, it was decided by the international community to strengthen the terms of the UNFCCC with a supplementary agreement known as the Kyoto Protocol. This agreement added a number of different commitments and mechanisms to address climate change.

The most significant addition of the Kyoto Protocol was that those states identified by the UNFCCC as developed countries (referred to in the treaty as *Annex I parties*), were now obligated to reduce their greenhouse gas emissions to specific target levels. Some of these states (i.e., members of the European Union) were required to reduce their emissions by 8 percent from their levels in 1990 by the commitment period of 2008–2012. Other developed states, most notably Australia, Canada, Japan, Russia, and the United States, had lower targets, primarily between a 5 and 7 percent reduction from the 1990 levels during this time frame. Considering that climate change is a collective action problem and to create more flexibility for states in meeting these targets the Kyoto Protocol permitted emission credits for the development of gas sinks and also allowed states to trade portions of their assigned emissions targets to other states. In addition, developed states could gain emissions credits by investing in projects for the reduction of greenhouse gases in developing states (or non-Annex I countries) in what is known as the protocol's clean development mechanism.

In terms of omissions, however, the most significant was that developing countries were not obligated to reduce their emissions of greenhouse gases. As a result, China and India, which ranked first and third globally in carbon dioxide emissions, producing over 9 million and 2 million kilotons, respectively, by 2011, did not assume an international commitment to reduce their emissions by accepting the Kyoto Protocol (World Bank 2016c). Also, the United States, which was the world's second largest emitter of carbon dioxide, with over 5 million kilotons by 2011, signed the treaty but has not ratified it as of 2018. Former American president George W. Bush set forth the concerns that the United States had with the Kyoto Protocol or would have with any future agreement that would limit carbon dioxide emissions to be (1) the necessity to have developing countries also make binding commitments to reduce greenhouse gases, (2) uncertainty regarding the extent of the negative impact of climate change, and (3) a preference for voluntary rather than mandatory commitments for the reduction of greenhouse gas emissions (Schelling 2002). Despite these deficiencies, a sufficient number of states ratified the Kyoto Protocol for it to enter into force in 2005.

Under the terms of the Kyoto Protocol, the Conference of the Parties (COP), which includes representatives from all countries that have accepted the agreement, was designated as the supreme decision-making body. During the meeting of the COP in 2007, the Bali Action Plan was adopted to set a framework to address climate change following the expiration of Kyoto's commitment period in 2012. This plan was to establish "an agreed outcome" by 2009, which left open as to what legal form the COP decision would take (Rajamani 2009). The result of these negotiations was the Copenhagen Accord. In a brief document, which was only two and a half pages long, participating states agreed that greenhouse gas emission cuts were necessary to prevent the average global temperature from rising above 2°C from pre-industrial levels. Developed states agreed to define and adopt their own target level for emission reductions, while in a change from the Kyoto Protocol, developing states also made a similar pledge for self-defined emission reductions. As a concession, however, developed states agreed to spend US$30 billion from 2010 to 2012 followed by US$100 billion by 2020 to assist developing countries with their adaption and mitigation efforts.

Although 114 states agreed to the Copenhagen Accord, it was a political, rather than a legal commitment. Its main accomplishments were that it was the first agreement to establish a ceiling on acceptable global temperature rise and its funding pledge, and perhaps most significantly, the commitment to the international community by developing states to reduce their greenhouse gas emissions (Bodansky 2010b). Its critics, however, emphasized that in some ways it was a step back from Kyoto because now developed countries were not committing themselves a specific target for reduced emissions after 2012 and a lack of clarity as to whether the pledge of funds would be a new source of funds or if it was based upon preexisting commitments for funding climate change initiatives (Kohr 2010). U.S. president Barack Obama, who was more supportive of the principles of the Kyoto Protocol than his predecessor, accepted the accord. Nevertheless, its non-binding nature and its emphasis on volunteerism for emissions reductions were not indications of much of a change in American policy on this issue. The Cancun Agreements negotiated at the COP meeting in 2010 were more formal, much longer, and more detailed than the Copenhagen Accord but, for the most part, primarily reaffirmed the principles and commitments of Copenhagen.

During the COP's meeting in Doha, Qatar, in 2012, the Kyoto Protocol was amended to a new commitment period for developed countries (with the exception of Canada, Japan, New Zealand, Russia, and the United States) from 2012 to 2020. Not only did the Doha Amendment provide for this second commitment period for these developed countries, it also strengthened their emissions reduction requirements from 5 percent against 1990 levels by 2012 to 18 percent against 1990 levels by 2020. As of March 2018, however, the amendment has only been ratified by 109 states, and so it will not go into force until it has been ratified by 144 states.

This lack of an international commitment to climate change has carried over to a continued rise in the production of greenhouse gases based on human activity. According to the IPCC, anthropogenic greenhouse gas emissions were the highest in human history from 2000 to 2010. Additionally, the IPCC estimated that without improved efforts at reducing these emissions, it could be expected that the global temperature rise would be between 3.7°C and 4.8°C by 2100 from preindustrial levels (IPCC 2014). This expectation is well above what is considered to be the safe limit of 2°C, agreed upon in the Copenhagen Accord (Costello et al. 2011). Although it seems that some progress was made with global carbon dioxide emissions rising only 0.5 percent in 2014, it was still the warmest year on record until it was surpassed in 2015 (Olivier et al. 2015); 2016 proved to be even warmer, and although 2017 did not have quite as high of an average temperature as 2016, it was still the second hottest year ever recorded, and scientists do not foresee any trend toward cooler weather (Fountain et al. 2018).

Much of the lack of success of the Kyoto Protocol has been directed at the institutional design of the agreement. Rosen (2015) identified four weaknesses, in particular, that render it as an ineffective agreement for addressing global climate change. The first was the short time frame. Both the first and second commitment periods were five-year terms, leaving little time for policy implementation and research and development to assist states in meeting their emission targets. Second was the low target of a 5 percent reduction for developed states. Third was that the calculation of emissions and the clean development mechanism meant that some developed states could still comply with the agreement by increasing their emissions, as long as they supported emissions-reducing projects in developing countries. In addition, developed states could move industrial production to other countries as a way to lower their domestic emissions. The fourth weakness was the fact that the Kyoto Protocol provided for multiple commitment periods to be considered every few years rather than any long-term commitment to a reduction in greenhouse gas emissions.

Paris Agreement

The latest international effort to address the climate change problem was the conclusion of the Paris Agreement during the COP meeting in 2015. This agreement became the first that committed almost every state (195 countries) to lower greenhouse gas emissions. In order to achieve such a universal consensus, participants choose to model the agreement more on the Copenhagen Accord than the more restrictive Kyoto Protocol. Its obligations were based on volunteerism and self-regulation of member states rather than specific target levels required by a treaty. The agreement maintained the commitment to keep the average global temperature from rising above the 2°C threshold and pursue limiting the increase to 1.5°C. While members could set their own target levels for emission reduction, they were required to report their efforts on their progress in doing so. Member states were also obligated to meet every five years starting in 2023 to set more ambitious emissions reductions based on scientific evidence.

Developed countries also affirmed their pledge of US$100 billion per year from 2020 to 2025 to developing countries to assist them in undertaking climate action. The agreement entered into force in November 2016 once it was ratified by fifty-five states that produce 55 percent of the world's greenhouse gas emissions. Currently, 175 states have ratified it. The United States, China, India, and the European Union (EU) were the key actors in designing the agreement. The U.S. position, in particular, was significant as the United States made it clear that the emissions reduction requirements would need to be voluntary for it to make any kind of commitment. China was more amenable to pledging to reduce its enormous emissions as it was coping with growing diplomatic pressure from developing countries to do so. While the EU was more supportive of legally binding targets, it was willing to concede on this point due to the necessity of a universal binding agreement in the wake of the failures of Kyoto and Copenhagen. India and other developing states were more dissatisfied with the agreement because of the lack of legally binding commitment targets and their desire for more financial support for mitigation actions (Clemencon 2016). Nevertheless, these parties decided to accept the agreement.

While the Paris Agreement may be considered a political success with its universal acceptance, a substantial reduction of greenhouse gas emissions must take place to reach its objective. One study found that to achieve a 2°C standard, developed countries would need to reduce their emissions by 50 percent below 1990 levels by 2020 or a 13 to 18 percent reduction coupled with a 22 to 34 percent reduction of emissions by developing countries by 2020 (Den Elzen et al. 2013). Another study by Rogelj et al. (2015) suggested that net carbon emissions worldwide need to reach zero between 2045 and 2060 to keep the average global temperature below 2°C by the end of the twenty-first century. While the Paris Agreement has a heavy emphasis on transparency, its oversight comes from an expert committee without any sanctioning power. The agreement, as with previous international agreements on climate change, does not include a dispute settlement mechanism or any delegation of authority to a third-party organization. It is legally binding, but compliance is very much based on self-regulation by national governments and global peer pressure. Whether this system is sufficient for such an ambitious goal may be questionable. Another issue, as discussed in box 8.1, is the U.S. decision to leave the agreement.

WHO and Climate Change

Activity by the WHO and climate change began soon after the Rio Conference. The IPCC asked the WHO to participate in its report in 1993 to assist with addressing the health dimension to climate change. In addition, the WHO partnered with the WMO, UNEP, and other IGOs on a climate agenda to provide support for countries in addressing the effects of climate change (World Health Organization 1998b). Subsequently, the World Health Assembly (WHA) passed a resolution in 1998 that urged member states to consider the threat that climate change could pose to human health and supported WHO's participation with its partners in the climate agenda. A decade later, the WHA approved a more detailed resolution on health and climate change. In addition to asking the WHO to advocate for climate change awareness and continue to work on the climate agenda and assist member states with assessing and addressing the influence of climate change on health, it also urged member states to strengthen their health systems to monitor and minimize the effects that climate change may have on their populations and provide a plan to address the impact of climate change on health at the national level, as well as collaborate with the WHO and other international organizations addressing the issue of climate change.

World Bank and Climate Change

In regard to financing for climate change, the World Bank is a significant actor. The World Bank provides approximately US$10 billion per year for climate-related activities. It is also increasing its support as World Bank president Jim Yong Kim announced in October 2015 that the Bank could increase its financing for climate change action to about US$29 billion by 2020, which would mean that 28 percent of all World Bank financing could be related to climate change by this date (World Bank 2015). In addition, the Bank is a valuable partner in the fight against climate change by also promoting investment from the private sector, and conducting research and technical assistance on climate change initiatives. The Bank's International Finance Corporation (IFC) provided US$13 billion in investment financing between 2005 and 2015 for use in renewable energy such as solar and wind power projects, energy efficiency initiatives, sustainable agriculture, and climate adaptation strategies for the private sector. The sum provided in 2015 constituted about 21 percent of IFC's long-term financing (World Bank 2016b). In addition, the World Bank has commissioned a series of "Turn Down the Heat" reports since 2012 to analyze the risks associated with climate change. Even the International Monetary Fund has incorporated climate change into its agenda. In particular, it has been emphasizing carbon pricing, which is charge (i.e., tax) on carbon dioxide emissions, as part of its recommended macroeconomic policies (International Monetary Fund 2015).

Health and Climate Change

Although the relationship between health and climate change has been recognized, for the most part, climate change and its impact have been more central to environmental governance than health governance. The UNFCCC contains very little mention of health, no mention of health is found in the Kyoto Protocol, and the Paris Agreement mentions only "the right to health" in the preamble of the agreement. In fact, in preparing negotiations for the Copenhagen Accord in 2009, only four of forty-seven states even mentioned health as an issue in their position (McMichael et al. 2009). The WHO, the world's lead IGO for public health, has passed only a couple of resolutions associated with climate change and primarily acts in a partnership role with other scientific and environmental organizations. This position for the WHO is much more subdued compared to its activities addressing infectious diseases and tobacco. Even another significant actor in global health, the World Bank, has framed climate change as an economic development and poverty issue rather than a health issue.

Why has climate change, which has the potential to create a devastating impact on human health over the next century, played a secondary role in global health governance? A major factor has to do with the complexity of climate change and establishing a causal connection between climate change and the environment that can achieve political salience. As Watt et al. (2015: 1872) point out, "Most climate-related health impacts are mediated through complex ecological and social processes." Ecologically, warmer weather, rising sea levels, and changing weather patterns can contribute to the spread of infectious diseases by facilitating the transmission of malaria by mosquitoes and the spread of cholera from an increase in contaminated water sources created by extreme weather events. Heat stress and droughts may threaten the food supply by damaging crops and livestock. In terms of social factors, age, socioeconomic status, and health care quality may shape the impact of climate change on health (Watts et al. 2015). These mitigation factors make it difficult and more challenging for the WHO to frame climate change as a danger to human health in the same way as more direct threats such as HIV/AIDS or tobacco consumption. As covered in chapter 2, one of the most powerful legal tools for the WHO to influence national policy change is the International Health Regulations (IHR). The IHR, however, is focused on detecting and containing a particular event. But the impact of climate change on health does not occur as an event, such as an outbreak of avian influenza or the Ebola virus, rather it is a gradual intensification of existing processes rather than a novel disease (Wiley 2010).

Despite its secondary role in climate change policy, the global health community, however, may still have an important role in the political process. A study by Hulme (2009) identified the main obstacles to achieving an agreement on global climate change. These barriers include (1) the complexity of climate change and the difficulty in educating the public about its impact, (2) the abstract nature of climate change, which contributes to both misunderstanding and ignorance of the issue, (3) the strong connection between the use of greenhouse gas–producing fossil fuels and economic development, and (4) resistance by powerful interest groups who face a prospect of significant economic loss by reducing carbon emissions or are ideologically opposed to a greater intervention by the government in the market, which an effective climate change regime may require. As noted, however, by Watts et al. (2015: 1904),

> "By considering directly how climate change will impact human health, we are naturally drawn to the human component of climate impacts, rather than the environmental (flooding, forest fires) or more abstract (the economy, the climate). This supports a human framing of climate change, putting it in terms that may be more readily understood by the public."

Greater understanding of climate change by the public could, in turn, give the climate change issue sufficient political salience to convince policy-makers to commit and implement climate change objectives.

BOX 8.1 WHAT WILL BE THE EFFECT OF THE U.S. WITHDRAWAL FROM THE PARIS AGREEMENT ON CLIMATE CHANGE?

Less than two years after the Paris Agreement on climate change was adopted, the United States decided to withdraw from the agreement. Despite the voluntary nature of emissions reductions under the agreement, American president Donald Trump cited the agreement as unfair to the United States and would seek to negotiate an international climate change agreement to better suit U.S. interests (Shear 2017). The Paris agreement is almost universal in scope. As of January 2018, 197 states are parties to the agreement and 174 of these states have ratified it. Once the U.S. withdrawal becomes official, it will be the world's only recognized state to not be a party.

What impact will the withdrawal of the United States, the world's second largest emitter of greenhouse gases, have on climate change? A study by Zhang (2017) argued that even though the strong international consensus on climate change will mitigate some of the detrimental effects from the loss of the United States, in the long-term global environmental governance could see a negative impact as the United States may choose to reduce its spending on climate change research and its financial assistance for developing countries to address climate change issues. Nevertheless, other powerful states, especially China and the EU countries, have expressed continued support for the agreement. The leadership of these states, along with support by local governments and NGOs, may also temper the effect of the U.S. withdrawal.

DEPLETION OF THE OZONE LAYER

A more successful case of environmental cooperation in global governance has been addressing the depletion of the ozone layer. The ozone layer is a blanket of ozone gas in the Earth's upper atmosphere that shields the planet from ultraviolet radiation. This ozone gas, however, may be depleted by the release of some chemicals, especially chlorofluorocarbons (CFCs) into the atmosphere. CFCs are non-toxic chemicals that are used in aerosol sprays (i.e., insect repellant and hair spray) and refrigerants. The principal health threat from increased exposure to ultraviolet radiation is a rise in the incidence of cataracts and skin cancer in fair-skinned individuals. Additionally, concerns have been raised that such increased exposure could weaken the immune system, which may make humans more susceptible to infectious diseases (McMichael et al. 2003).

The attribution of the depletion of the ozone layer to CFCs was first hypothesized by two American chemists in 1974. Soon after, the U.S. National Academy of Sciences issued a report acknowledging significant depletion of the ozone layer. Whether or not this depletion was due to the release of CFCs was a debated issue. Politically, the CFC hypothesis was controversial. CFCs were produced only in sixteen countries with the United States leading the world in the production and consumption of these chemicals (Haas 1992). Industries that produced CFCs hired scientists to challenge evidence indicating that the ozone layer was depleting. Additionally, some scientists, particularly those in Europe, did not believe that the extent of ozone depletion was significant (Rowlands 1995). Despite the scientific debate in the 1970s and early 1980s, UNEP took a lead role in attempting to combat ozone depletion by promoting an international treaty on the issue as early as 1977. With surges in CFC production during this time, there was a sufficient international consensus for such a treaty in the form of the Vienna Convention for the Protection of the Ozone Layer, which was signed on March 22, 1985. This treaty called on states to cooperate with one another in regard to observations, research, and information about the effect of human activities on the ozone layer, as well as to take legal action to constrain those activities, which are found likely to have such an effect (Vienna Convention for the Protection of the Ozone Layer 1985). States, however, were not obligated to reduce CFCs or any other materials under the terms of the treaty. In fact, CFCs were mentioned only in the annex of the treaty as one of the chemicals that may possibly impact the ozone layer.

Another breakthrough event during this time to even more firmly place the ozone issue on the international agenda was the discovery of a significant hole in the ozone layer above Antarctica by scientists from the British Antarctic Survey in 1985. The ozone levels had dropped 30 percent during the spring in the Antarctic. This finding was later confirmed by American space satellites (Rowlands 1995). The following year, the United States and UNEP conducted a study that found a relationship between growing CFC use and an acceleration of ozone depletion. The U.S. Environmental Protection Agency even sponsored a project finding that the estimated growth in CFCs would lead to 40 million more cases of skin cancer in the United States over the next eighty-eight years than if CFC emissions remained at its 1986 level (Haas 1992). This report had a significant impact among the actors in global governance. Particularly striking was the response by the Dupont Corporation, which was a dominant actor in the production of CFCs in the United States, when it became supportive of an international agreement to limit emissions while requesting the U.S. government to subsidize the development of safer alternatives to CFCs (Haas 1992). Following the report of these scientific findings and Dupont's change in position, UNEP requested that national governments resume negotiations over the ozone layer at the end of 1986.

Despite this progress, negotiations during 1986–1987 were still fairly contentious. The Scandinavian countries had long been supporters of a binding treaty to decrease CFC emissions. They were joined by the United States and Canada in supporting significant reductions on the use of CFCs. West Germany, which had previously been reluctant to support binding reductions, decided to join this coalition by 1987. France, Italy, and the United Kingdom, which led the European Community bloc, and Japan, however, viewed drastic reductions of CFCs much less favorably. The Soviet Union was also reluctant to support major reductions, but it did not demonstrate a strong opposition to this objective (Sprinz and Vaahtoranta 1994).

During negotiations, an influential draft agreement was developed by UNEP executive director Mostafa Tolba. This proposal called for a freeze on the emission of CFCs within two years (which was soon changed to one year) after the agreement went into force, followed by a 20 percent reduction within four years. This objective was supported by Canada, Norway, and the United States, but these states wanted to go further by requiring an additional 30 percent reduction in six years. The baseline year for these emissions standards was 1986. In the final conference at Montreal, Argentina, Australia, Japan, Mexico, and Venezuela decided to back the extensive cuts proposed in the draft agreement. As an international consensus grew, the European Community decided to accept the proposed cut in exchange for clause to eventually eliminate all ozone-depleting chemicals to be moved to the agreement's non-binding preamble and a delay of each successive control measure by an additional six months (Benedick 1998). As a result, the Montreal Protocol on Substances that Deplete the Ozone Layer was signed by the parties on September 16, 1987, and received a sufficient number of ratification to enter into force on January 1, 1989.

Although a binding international treaty that mandated the reduction of ozone-depleting chemicals was a landmark achievement in global governance, it was not without some problems. Environmental NGOs such as Friends of the Earth International, Greenpeace International, and the National Resources Defense Council launched a public relations campaign against the Montreal Protocol and its proposed revisions by arguing it was of inadequate response to ozone layer depletion, especially the protocol's maximum requirement of a 50 percent reduction. This social movement, along with the adoption of even more rigid national measures on the emissions of these chemicals by some governments and new scientific evidence led many states to become more receptive to strengthening the Montreal Protocol at a meeting in London in 1990. Negotiations led to an agreement to reduce emissions by 85 percent of 1986 levels by 1997, followed by a commitment to phase out these chemicals by 2000 (Benedick 1998).

In retrospect, evidence indicates that the Montreal Protocol and its subsequent amendments have been quite successful in addressing the problem of the ozone layer. A report by UNEP (2014) credits these agreements for preventing 2 million additional deaths from skin cancer per year by 2030, as well as increased damage to human eyes and immune systems. Additionally, UNEP (2014) has identified the ozone layer as "on track" for full recovery by the 2050s. Some lingering issues that remain, however, are that some ozone-depleting substances continue to remain in the atmosphere and the possibility of future discovery of other chemicals that may contribute to ozone layer depletion. Additionally, some of the substitutes for CFC and other ozone-depleting substances act as greenhouse gases and may exacerbate climate change (UNEP 2014).

A number of factors have been cited to explain the political success for global governance's response to the ozone layer problem. Benedick (1998) credits the evolving scientific understanding and the close collaboration between scientists and government agencies as an important factor. Additionally, a well-informed public, the efforts of UNEP to inform public opinion and push negotiations forward, U.S. leadership in taking action to institute strong regulations nationally and offer global solutions, support by NGOs and industry, and the creation of a flexible and dynamic instrument in the form of the Montreal Protocol making its commitments adaptable to changing conditions were significant elements in achieving a successful outcome. Sprinz and Vaahtoranta (1994) emphasize how a convergence of national interest of each state eventually led to a consensus on the ozone layer. Strong supporters of CFC reduction such as Australia, Canada, Norway, and Sweden had a high proportion of light-skinned citizens and did not produce very much of these chemicals. Other supporters such as the United States and West Germany were high CFC producers, but they were proponents of the agreements due to advances in technology to develop economically suitable substitutes for CFCs. The strongest opponents, France, Italy, the United Kingdom, and Japan, were all high-level producers, and they were also concerned that the United States would gain an economic advantage if substitutes to CFCs were required because of its advanced research. Growing public pressure on these states, however, persuaded theses states to become more amendable to an agreement.

From a constructivist perspective, Haas (1992: 187) argues that it was the role of an epistemic community, "a knowledge-based networks of specialists who shared belief in cause-and-effect relations, validity tests, and underlying principled values and pursued common policy goals," which was a key factor in the political process. In the context of ozone layer diplomacy, the epistemic community was composed of scientists and policy-makers that supported their findings. In terms of explaining why certain states supported reduction of CFCs, Haas (1992) finds that their support was related to the epistemic community's influence on a particular country. For example, the reason why West Germany defected from the European Community's position was due to its government's relatively stronger pro-environment sentiment. In comparison, French scientists did little research on the ozone layer, and Japan, which did not feature much of a relationship between its scientists and policy-makers were more reluctant to accept a reduction policy (Haas 1992).

AIR POLLUTION

An environmental problem that has received much less attention by global governance, outside of its climate change and ozone layer implications, has been the issue of outdoor air pollution. The health risks posed by air pollution are significant. According to the WHO (2018c) 4.2 million deaths globally were attributed to outdoor air pollution in 2016. Of these deaths, 91 percent occurred in developing countries. The most common causes of death from exposure to outdoor air pollution were heart disease, stroke, chronic obstructive pulmonary disease, and lung cancer (World Health Organization 2014e). Based on this data, Maria Neira, the WHO's Director for Public Health, Environmental and Social Determinants of Health, stated that "the risks from air pollution are now far greater than previously thought or understood, particularly for heart disease and stroke" (World Health Organization 2014f). Populations in developing countries in Asia have been particularly vulnerable. According to the WHO (2016e), about thirteen of the world's twenty most polluted cities were located in India, with Delhi having the highest concentration of air pollution for a city of over 14 million people. Saudi Arabia, China, and Pakistan also had multiple cities listed among the world's top fifty cities for air pollution. Overall, 98 percent of cities with a population of over 100,000 in developing countries do not meet the WHO's air quality guidelines. At the same time, however, air pollution is not just a problem for developing countries, as 56 percent of these cities in developed states also do not meet the WHO standard (World Health Organization 2016e).

The primary reason why global governance has not regarded air pollution as a significant political issue to the same extent as climate change and the ozone layer is that most of the harm is caused by local air pollution rather than transnational activities. Although the WHO has air policy guidelines, these measures are not binding. Overall, outside of the EU context, international law has not addressed local air pollution (Fidler 1999). Addressing local air pollution through global governance is problematic for a couple of reasons. The first is the issue of sovereignty. Air pollution is generally framed as a local political problem and correspondingly, not one that states have been willing to attempt to remedy by international compacts. Second is the issue of a human right to a decent environment. Although a plausible principle with some legal basis, this is a right that has not yet received much attention or support in UN human rights institutions or in international environmental agreements (Boyle 2012).

An environmental area of greater international concern is transboundary air pollution. The first recognition of state responsibility under international law for damaging another state was during a dispute between Canada and the United States during the late 1930s. In the *Trail Smelter* arbitration decision, a tribunal found that sulfur dioxide emissions from a company in Canada was causing damage to crops and timber in the state of Washington. As a consequence the Canadian government was directed to compensate the United States for this action (Okowa 2009). This idea of state responsibility for environmental damage was also included as a principle in the non-binding 1972 Stockholm Declaration. Nevertheless, state responsibility for damage by air pollution has not been established by other court decisions, and it has been suggested that its prohibition has not been supported by state practice (Fidler 1999).

International law on transboundary air pollution has almost been exclusively based on a few bilateral and regional agreements. Much of the reason for this practice results from the difficulty in tracing the source and the extent of damage caused by pollution emanating from another states (Okowa 2009). Geographic proximity makes the cause more identifiable. Globally, the closest agreement is the United Nations Convention on the Law of the Sea, which requires member states to prevent air pollution to the marine environment and that atmosphere. This provision, however, in practice has not received a good deal of compliance from the parties to the treaty (Nanda and Pring 2013). Among bilateral agreements, the United States has established treaties with its neighbors, Canada and Mexico, regarding transboundary pollution.

The most significant regional agreement that addresses this problem is the 1979 Geneva Convention on Long-Range Transboundary Air Pollution (LRTAP). The parties to this agreement are mostly EU states, but it has also been ratified by Canada, United States, Russia, and many of the other states from the former Soviet Union. The original LRTAP treaty aimed at requiring its members to make efforts to limit air pollution and share information and research. Additional protocols to the agreement, since it went into force in 1983, strengthened the treaty's regulations that called for more specific reductions in sulfur emissions, nitrogen oxide, volatile organic compounds, heavy metal (i.e., lead and mercury) emissions, and persistent organic pollutants (i.e., pesticides). Although, it should be noted, some states that ratified LRTAP have not ratified these more demanding protocols. Overall, these regulations have demonstrated a positive impact on reducing transboundary air pollution (Okowa 2009). LRTAP is primarily directed at Europe, and many of its parties are developed states with relatively clean air. Air quality in EU states is further bolstered by EU legislation and regulations. The world's more polluted regions, Asia and the Middle East, do not have such legal protections. The Association of Southeast Asian Nations (ASEAN) did produce an Agreement on Transboundary Haze Pollution in 2002 following extensive forest fires in Indonesia during the late 1990s. Although a significant milestone for environmental cooperation in the region, the obligation in this agreement, however, is limited to controlling pollution emanating from land-based forest fires.

The issue of air pollution is beginning to receive more notice in global health governance. Following the release of the WHO's data, the WHA debated air pollution for the first time during its 2015 meeting (World Health Organization 2015c). It also passed its first resolution on the topic. The resolution urges states to monitor air quality, improve surveillance of the effects of air pollution on health, and improve cooperation in knowledge and technology directed at air pollution. Although this resolution served as a recommendation to national governments, rather than a mandate, it was still a significant step to incorporate air pollution into the global health arena.

ADDRESSING THE ENVIRONMENT'S IMPACT ON GLOBAL HEALTH

A considerable overlap exists between the environment and health. The world's most significant environmental problems all have deleterious impacts on the quality of human health. Despite this connection, environmental issues have largely been outside the area of global health governance. Global environmental governance is centered on UNEP, with the WHO playing a more limited partnership role. Nevertheless, successful resolution of environmental problems will greatly improve of the quality of global health. Realism, neoliberal institutionalism, constructivism, and Marxism all provide different understandings of the prospects of achieving such a successful resolution on these international environmental matters.

Realism

Due to neorealist's assumption that the national interest of the state is security, the environment has traditionally been viewed as an area of "low" politics, and one that is not generally a focus of global governance. International environmental regulations have not been viewed as desirable from realist perspectives because they constrain state sovereignty, and the abatement costs for climate change and air pollution could be harmful to a state's economic strength. This view appears to particularly influence developing states, especially those with high concentrations of air pollution, to be reluctant to accept reductions mandated by an international treaty. These states promote their interests in climate change negotiations based on fairness. They do not believe that their economic development should be constrained by environmental regulations that developed countries did not have to address during the time of their economic development. Additionally, they contend that developed states have a historic responsibility to accept a greater burden for greenhouse gas emissions because the effect of human activity on climate change was largely due to their economic activities (Soltau 2009).

While this perspective may have a moralist foundation, it fits with a realist perspective on international environmental negotiations. The global environment is a collective action problem that affects everyone. By shirking responsibility and shifting the burden to others, these developing states may be able to gain some benefit from a better environment while avoiding an obstacle to economic growth and possible cuts to military expenditures. A realist strategy, however, is not only utilized by developing states. Among developed states, the United States in particular, has been motivated by this approach. In regard to climate change, the United States has consistently made it very clear over the past couple of decades that it will accept only a climate change regime based on voluntary reductions. Although the United States did take a leadership role in addressing the ozone layer in the 1980s, it was not entirely motivated by altruistic reasons. Their position was also influenced by the availability of CFC substitutes and the potential to gain a global market share in the production of these substitutes of CFCs and other ozone-depleting substances (Sprinz and Vaahtoranta 1994). In explaining the lack of international action on air pollution, realists would suggest that states have viewed it primarily as a local issue and have not found enough utility in international regulations to address the problem to accept such constraints on their sovereignty and economic development.

Despite realists' traditional lack of attention to the environment in international affairs, if the environment becomes more connected to state security, it should become a more significant aspect of the realist foreign policy agenda. One possibility has to do with the harmful effect that climate change and air pollution could have on their populations. A rise in natural disasters, or an increase in health damage from air pollution, could convince states to place an even greater priority on these issues in international affairs. Another possibility would be the establishment of a link between climate change and conflict. Research at this point, however, has not indicated much support for the view that climate change influences armed conflict. Gleditsch (2012: 7) notes, however, that "framing climate change as a security issue may influence the perceptions of the actors in local and regional conflict and lead to militarized responses and thus perhaps contribute to a self-fulfilling prophecy." Because the environment has an indirect influence on state security, it may not be a strong possibility that realists will elevate the environment as an international relations issue, but the idea has some promise.

Neoliberal Institutionalism

Neoliberal institutionalists place an emphasis on the need for institutions to solve collective action problems such as the environment. An institution can centralize coordination among the national governments. It can also enhance the credibility of states making commitments to address the environment by specifying rules that they are expected to follow. The Vienna Convention for the Protection of the Ozone Layer, the Montreal Protocol, and its subsequent amendments demonstrate a successful case of how an international institution can be created that can help solve a global problem. These agreements were a framework to structure international interactions in addressing the ozone layer. They also called for specific obligations by member states to reduce and later, phase out the chemicals that were depleting the ozone layer. In comparison, air pollution is becoming a growing problem for global health because it lacks such an international institution to assist states in their coordination and commitments to solve the issue. Outside of the states that are members of LRTAP, or that have made commitments in bilateral arrangements, there is little international regulation. The implication is that a focal point for interaction on air pollution and specific commitments by states is generally lacking in this area. This weak institutionalization for air pollution can help explain why the non-binding air quality guidelines of the WHO have been considerably ineffective at addressing air pollution in the urban areas of developing countries.

The issue of climate change creates an interesting puzzle for neoliberal institutionalists. According to von Stein (2008), the Kyoto Protocol is relatively hard law for developed countries compared to the UNFCCC. They have a legally binding commitment to fix greenhouse gas emissions with a quantified target, and the COP can monitor their implementation and compliance of these commitments. As noted, however, the Kyoto Protocol has not been a particularly effective instrument in addressing climate change. One solution could be to amend the Kyoto Protocol or create a new instrument that would carry over these hard law commitments to developing countries. This solution, however, could be politically problematic even from an institutionalist perspective. Keohane and Victor (2011) have suggested that climate change is governed by a regime complex. This concept means that governance is not hierarchical but is rather organized into several different weakly connected forums. In the area of climate change, the UNFCCC and the Kyoto Protocol are but one forum for governance. They also describe other climate change forums such as international "clubs" (i.e., the G20); bilateral partnerships (such as the U.S.-China climate accord in 2014); expert assessments by the IPCC, the World Bank, the EU, subnational actors (i.e., the state of California's emission limits); and industrial standards. They argue that this form of governance is unlikely to change due to the diversity of interests, the lack of a hierarchical authority in this area, and uncertainty about the effect of climate change, as well as the level of commitment and burden-sharing. As a consequence, it may not be feasible to create a strong international institution to govern climate change. Rather, Keohane and Victor (2011: 20) find that "at the present juncture, however, both political reality and the need for flexibility and diversity suggest that it is preferable to work for a loosely linked but effective regime complex for climate change."

Constructivism

Constructivists emphasize that the framing of the environment as a political problem by political and scientific elites will be a driving factor in how global governance responds to health hazards posed by the environment. The ozone layer case represents an example where a very strong norm emerged that compelled states to commit to taking steps to resolve the problem. As mentioned earlier, Haas (1992) gave the epistemic community much credit in using scientific findings as persuasive evidence to convince policy-makers to accept CFC emission reductions. In another constructivist approach, Hoffmann (2005b) utilized an analysis based on a norm life cycle approach to explain how universal participation became the accepted remedy to ozone layer depletion. In 1986, less than thirty states began negotiating the Montreal Protocol. By 1989, however, almost 100 states participated in the first session to amend it. Hoffmann attributes an evolving norm of universal participation to explaining this development. The ozone layer issue has initially been framed as a global problem that required a solution devised by developed states. UNEP, however, led by Mostafa Tolba, used its influence as an agenda-setter for negotiations, as well as a series of informal meetings, to convince developing states to participate in negotiations and for these states to be accepted as relevant stakeholders by developed countries. As the norm of universal participation became stronger during ozone layer negotiations, it became the accepted practice for the outset of climate change negotiations in the early 1990s.

While developing a norm for a comprehensive global response to ozone layer depletion has been much stronger than climate change and air pollution, norms in these other environmental areas are beginning to emerge as well. Over the past two decades, the Kyoto Protocol has demonstrated the acceptance of some states to accept quantifiable reductions on their greenhouse gas emissions. While most states, have not accepted this restriction, the Copenhagen, Cancun, and Paris agreements illustrate a universal acknowledgment of the need to limit global warming and make efforts to reduce greenhouse gas emissions. In comparison, while the construction of air pollution is largely based on it as a local issue rather than a global issue, the WHO resolution indicates an early step to recognize it as more of an international problem due to more scientific evidence indicating that it is a significant hazard to human health. Progress in scientific knowledge on the deleterious effects of climate change and air pollution, in addition to support by civil society and influential policy-makers, will have a major impact on whether the norms in these areas will continue to develop over time and lead to more viable global responses to these problems.

Marxism

Marxist and neo-Marxist perspectives view the greatest challenge for resolving global environment problems and their corresponding impacts on health to be the capitalist structure of the global economy and its resulting economic inequalities. The pursuit of economic profit facilitated the process of global warming and continues to motivate opposition to climate change policies and complicate an acceptable allocation of burden-sharing. Although climate change has adverse costs for all, developing countries will receive a far more negative impact. These countries have much weaker capabilities to respond to the adverse environmental and health consequences of climate change in comparison to states with developed economies. Developing countries also have greater incentives to permit significant emissions in greenhouse gases and air pollution as a trade-off to improve their economic development in a capitalist global economy.

The capitalist structure of the state and the global economy give fossil fuel companies, especially coal and oil, a privileged position in politics according to Newell and Patterson (1998). As capitalism has become increasingly the norm for most societies, policy-makers have been very sensitive to the interests of the fossil fuel industry because of its key role in economic growth. Without an alternative economic interest to rival this industry in lobbying policy-makers, or a societal change to promote greater acceptance of social welfare interests over the interests of the market, national governments will be constrained in their capability to address climate change and air pollution.

From this perspective, the power of the coal and oil industry will make it difficult for robust international agreements to be concluded to address these environmental hazards to health.

CONCLUSION

A significant amount of the global burden of disease and ill health can be linked to the environment. Nevertheless, global health governance has not paid a great deal of attention to environmental issues. A couple of reasons can account for this situation. First, global health governance has tended to address environmental issues in a reactionary manner. In this respect, it relied on preexisting treatment and health security mechanisms to address these problems. Second, the response of global governance to the environment has been outside the sphere of the health arena. Its hub has been with the institutional support of UNEP and the key international environmental agreements, the Montreal Protocol, the UNFCCC, and the Kyoto Protocol, none of which direct much of their attention to a health objective. The WHO has played a secondary role in global environmental politics, but it does appear to be more active within the past decade with stronger advocacy regarding the link between health and the environment, as well as passing two significant resolutions on climate change and air pollution.

Climate change has emerged to become the dominant issue for global governance and the environment. Other atmospheric threats to human health such as the depletion of the ozone layer and air pollution have received international attention as well. Theories of international relations can provide different perspectives as to how effective global governance can manage these environmental challenges. From a realist perspective, until these environmental issues exhibit a threat to national security, the environment will not be a high-priority interest for national governments. Commitments to international environmental regulations constrain state sovereignty, and as long as the environment is not accepted as a security threat, states will be reluctant to make significant concessions to addressing these issues. Neoliberal institutionalists suggest that a robust international regime for the environment could help to resolve this issue at the global level. While such a response was developed to address the depletion of the ozone layer, climate change has proven to be much more problematic. Diverging interests of national governments in terms of responsibility and burden-sharing and a fragmented governance system have made a strong institutional response to climate change very challenging. A constructivist approach would emphasize the development of international norms to compel states to develop a strong institutional response. Such a norm was effectively cultivated in the case of ozone layer depletion. Norms for climate change and air pollution are not as nearly as established at the present time, but political activity over the past decade has at least indicated a growing international consensus on these issues. Marxist perspectives emphasize that these environmental problems are created and connected to the structure of capitalist power. To effectively address these issues, the market and private sector interests must be curtailed on favor of greater state regulation.

A common aspect of all these approaches is the development of scientific knowledge and the recognition of the increasing costs of environmental degradation by policy-makers, which provides an opportunity to advance global environmental cooperation forward. Greater certainty regarding the harmful economic, ecological, and health effects of climate change and air pollution and a stronger political consensus accepting this connection could motivate policy-makers to overcome the obstacles suggested by these different perspectives and develop a more effective response to these environmental issues and associated health problems at the global level.

DISCUSSION QUESTIONS

1. Why was relatively little notice paid to environmental issues in global governance, with the exception of conservation, until the 1960s?
2. What is sustainable development? How has this concept evolved as a principle in global environmental politics after the Rio Conference (or Earth Summit) in 1992?
3. What is the connection between the environment and public health? How might global governance be more effective in providing good health by managing transnational environmental issues?
4. What are some negative effects on health associated with the issues of climate change, ozone layer depletion, and air pollution? Has global governance effectively addressed these issues? Why or Why not?
5. Based on one or more theories of international relations, can global health be improved through the current system of global environmental governance?

SUGGESTED READINGS

Bodansky, Daniel. 2010a. *The Art and Craft of International Environmental Law*. Cambridge, MA: Harvard University Press.
This book provides a detailed account of international environmental law in global governance.
Sprinz, Detlef, and Tapani Vaahtoranta. 1994. "The interest-based explanation of international environmental policy." *International Organization* 48(1): 77–105.

Analysis of the success and failure of international environmental regulations using an interest-based approach.
Watts, Nick, W. et al. 2015. "Health and climate change policy: Policy responses to protect public health." *Lancet* 386: 1861–1894.
A comprehensive report by health experts describing the impact of climate change on health and providing policy suggestions.
Wiley, Lindsay F. 2010. "Moving global health law upstream: A critical appraisal of global health law as a tool for health adaptation to climate change." *Georgetown International Environmental Law Review* 22: 439–489.
A good examination of utilizing global health law to address the future health problems associated with climate change.

Bibliography

Aaronson, Susan A. and Jamie M. Zimmerman. 2006. "Fair Trade?: How Oxfam Presented a Systemic Approach to Poverty, Development, Human Rights, and Trade." *Human Rights Quarterly* 28 (4): 998–1030.

Abbasi, Kamran. 1999. "The World Bank and World Health: Changing Sides." *British Medical Journal* 318 (7187): 865–869.

Abbott, Frederick M. 2002. "The TRIPS Agreement, Access to Medicines, and the WTO Doha Ministerial Conference." *Journal of World Intellectual Property* 5: 15–52.

Abbott, Frederick M. 2005. "The WTO Medicines Decision: World Pharmaceutical Trade and the Protection of Public Health." *American Journal of International Law* 99: 317–358.

Abbott, Kenneth W. and Duncan Snidal. 1998. "Why States Act thorough Formal International Organizations." *Journal of Conflict Resolution* 42 (1): 3–32.

Abbott, Kenneth W. and Duncan Snidal. 2000. "Hard and Soft Law in International Governance." *International Organization* 54 (3): 421–456.

Adler, Emanuel and Michael Barnett. 1998. *Security Communities*. Cambridge, UK: Cambridge University Press.

Ahmad, Khabir. 2004. "MSF Tuberculosis Report Criticises DOTS Strategy." *Lancet Infectious Diseases* 4 (12): 719.

Akin, John, Nancy Birdsall, and Davide de Ferranti. 1987. *Financing Health Services in Developing Countries: An Agenda for Reform*. Washington, DC: World Bank.

Aldis, William. 2008. " Health Security as a Public Health Concept: A Critical Analysis." *Health Policy and Planning* 23 (6): 369–375.

Ali, Sofia, Olivia Gugliemini, Serena Harber, Alexandra Harrison, Lauren Houle, Javarcia Ivory, and Sierra Kersten, et al. 2017. "Environmental and Social Change Drive the Explosive Emergence of Zika Virus in the Americas." *PLOS Neglected Tropical Diseases* 11 (2): e0005135.

Alston, Philip and Gerard Quinn. 1987. "The Nature and Scope of States Parties' Obligations under the International Covenant of Economic, Social and Cultural Rights." *Human Rights Quarterly* 9 (2): 156–229.

Anderson, Peter. 2004. "The Beverage Alcohol Industry's Social Aspects Organizations: A Public Health Warning." *Addiction* 20 (99): 1376–1377.

Anheier, Helmut K. and Siobhan Daly. 2005. *The Politics of Foundations: Comparative Perspectives from Europe and Beyond*. London: Routledge.

The Antiretroviral Therapy Cohort Collaboration. 2017. "Survival of HIV-Positive Patients Starting Antiretroviral Therapy between 1996 and 2013: A Collaborative Analysis of Cohort Studies." *Lancet HIV* 4: e349–356.

Archibugi, Daniele and Kim Bizzarri. 2005. "The Global Governance of Communicable Diseases: The Case for Vaccine R&D." *Law and Policy* 27 (1): 33–51.

Asher, Robert E. and Edward S. Mason. 1973. *The World Bank since Bretton Woods*. Washington, DC: Brookings Institution.

Associated Press. 1999. "Charity Created by Gates Is Now Largest in U.S." *New York Times*. August 23, 1999. http://www.nytimes.com/1999/08/23/us/charity-created-by-gates-is-now-largest-in-us.html (accessed August 2, 2014).

Associated Press. 2015. "CDC: Uninsured Drop by 11M since Passage of Obama's Law." *U.S. News*. March 24, 2015. https://www.usnews.com/news/politics/articles/2015/03/24/cdc-uninsured-drop-by-11m-since-passage-of-obamas-law (accessed March 15, 2017).

Attaran, Amir, Karen I. Barnes, Christopher Curtis, Umberto d'Alessandro, Caterina I. Fanello, Mary R. Galinski, and Gilbert Kokwaro, et al. 2004. "WHO, the Global Fund, and Medical Malpractice in Malaria Treatment." *The Lancet* 363 (9404): 237–240.

Baer, Britta, Andrew Ball, Helena Nygren-Krug, Aafje Rietveld, and Diana Weil. 2013. "Human Rights-Based Approaches to HIV, Tuberculosis, and Malaria." In *Advancing the Human Right to Health*, edited by Jose M. Zuniga, Stephen P. Marks, and Lawrence O. Gostin, 245–259. New York: Oxford University Press.

Baggot, Rob. 2013. *Partnerships for Public Health and Well-Being*. New York: Palgrave Macmillan.

Baldwin, David A. 1997. "The Concept of Security." *Review of International Studies* 23 (1): 5–26.

Barnard, David. 2002. "In the High Court of South Africa, Case No. 4138/98: The Global Politics of Access to Low-Cost AIDS Drugs in Poor Countries." *Kennedy Institute of Ethics Journal* 12 (2): 159–174.

Barnett, Michael and Raymond Duvall. 2005. "Power in Global Governance." In *Power in Global Governance*, edited by Michael Barnett and Raymond Duvall, 1–32. Cambridge, UK: Cambridge University Press.

Barnett, Michael and Martha Finnemore. 2004. *Rules for the World: International Organizations in Global Politics*. Ithaca, NY: Cornell University Press.

Barnett, Tony and Alan Whiteside. 2006. *AIDS in the Twenty-First Century: Disease and Globalization*. Second Edition. New York: Palgrave Macmillan.

Barraclough, Simon. 2009. "Chronic Diseases and Global Health Governance: The Contrasting Cases of Food and Tobacco." In *Global Health Governance: Crisis, Institutions, and Political Economy*, edited by Adrian Kay and Owain Williams, 102–128. New York: Palgrave Macmillan.

Bartsch, Sonja. 2007. "The Global Fund to Fight AIDS, Tuberculosis, and Malaria." In Global *Health Governance and the Fight against HIV/AIDS*, edited by Wolfgang

Hein, Sonja Bartsch, and Lars Kohlmorgen, 146–171. New York: Palgrave Macmillan.

Bartsch, Sonja and Lars Kohlmorgen. 2007. "The Role of Civil Society Organizations in Global Health Governance." In *Global Health Governance and the Fight against HIV/AIDS*, edited by Wolfgang Hein, Sonja Bartsch, and Lars Kohlmorgen, 92–118. New York: Palgrave Macmillan.

Basilico, Matthew, Jonathan Weigal, Anjali Motgi, Jacob Bor, and Salmaan Keshavjee. 2013. "Health for All? Competing Theories and Geopolitics." In *Reimagining Global Health: An Introduction*, edited by Paul Farmer, Jim Young Kim, Arthur Kleinman, and Matthew Basilico, 74–110. Berkeley: University of California Press.

Baumberg, Ben and Peter Anderson. 2008. "Trade and Health: How World Trade Organization (WTO) Law Affects Alcohol and Public Health." *Addiction* 103: 1952–1958.

Beall, Reed and Randall Kuhn. 2012. "Trends in Compulsory Licensing of Pharmaceuticals since the Doha Declaration: A Database Analysis." *PLoS Med* 9 (1): e1001154. doi:10.1371/journal.pmed.1001154.

Belsky, Leah, Reidar Lie, Aaditya Mattoo, Ezekiel J. Emanuel, and Gopal Sreenivasan. 2004. "The General Agreement on Trade in Services: Implications for Health Policymakers." *Health Affairs* 23 (3): 137–145.

Benedick, Richard E. 1998. *Ozone Diplomacy: New Directions in Safeguarding the Planet*. Enlarged edition. Cambridge, MA: Harvard University Press.

Bernstein, Steven. 2013. "Rio+20: Sustainable Development in a Time of Multilateral Decline." *Global Environmental Politics* 13 (4): 12–21.

Bill and Melinda Gates Foundation. 2018. "2016 Annual Report." https://www.gatesfoundation.org/Who-We-Are/Resources-and-Media/Annual-Reports/Annual-Report-2016 (accessed January 20, 2018).

Birn, Anne-Emmanuelle and Elizabeth Free. 2013. "The Rockefeller Foundation and the International Health Agenda." *The Lancet* 381 (9878): 1618–1619.

Black, Maggie. 1992. *A Cause for Our Times: Oxfam—The First 50 Years*. Oxford: Oxford University Press.

Bodansky, Daniel. 2010a. *The Art and Craft of International Environmental Law*. Cambridge, MA: Harvard University Press.

Bodansky, Daniel. 2010b. "The Copenhagen Climate Change Conference: A Postmortem." *American Journal of International Law* 104 (2): 230–240.

Boseley, Sarah. 2015. "Hon Lik Invented the E-Cigarette to Quit Smoking—But Now He's a Dual User." *The Guardian*. June 9, 2015. https://www.theguardian.com/society/2015/jun/09/hon-lik-e-cigarette-inventor-quit-smoking-dual-user (accessed on January 29, 2018).

Boyle, Alan, "Human Rights and the Environment: Where Next?" *The European Journal of International Law* 23 (3): 613–642.

Breidenich, Clare, Daniel Magraw, Anne Rowley, and James W. Rubin. 1998. "The Kyoto Protocol to the United Nations Framework on Climate Change." *American Journal of International Law* 92 (2): 315–331.

Brenton, Tony. 1994. *The Greening of Machiavelli: The Evolution of International Environmental Politics*. London: Royal Institute of International Affairs.

Brown, Garrett Wallace. 2009. "Multisectoralism, Participation, and Stakeholder Effectiveness: Increasing the Role of Nonstate Actors in the Global Fund to Fight AIDS, Tuberculosis, and Malaria." *Global Governance* 15 (2):169–177.

Brown, Garrett Wallace. 2010. "Safeguarding Deliberative Global Governance: The Case of The Global Fund to Fight AIDS, Tuberculosis and Malaria." *Review of International Studies* 36 (2): 511–530.

Brown, Theodore, Marcus Cueto, and Elizabeth Free. 2006. "The World Health Organization and the Transition from 'International' to 'Global' Public Health." *American Journal of Public Health* 96 (1): 62–72.

Brownell, Kelly D. and Kenneth E. Warner. 2009. "The Perils of Ignoring History: Big Tobacco Played Dirty and Millions Died. How Similar Is Big Food?" *Milbank Quarterly* 87 (1): 259–94.

Brundtland, Gro Harlem. 2003. "Global Health and International Security." *Global Governance* 9 (4): 417–423.

Buse, Kent and Catherine Gwin. 1998. "World Health: The World Bank and Global Cooperation in Health : The Case of Bangladesh." *The Lancet* 351 (9103): 665–669.

Buse, Kent and Andrew M. Harmer. 2007. "Seven Habits of Highly Effective Global Public-Private Health Partnerships: Practice and Potential." *Social Science and Medicine* 64 (2): 259–271.

Buse, Kent and Gill Walt. 2000. "Global Public-Private Partnerships: Part I—A New Development in Health?" *Bulletin of the World Health Organization* 78 (4): 549–561.

Buzan, Barry, Ole Wæver, and Jaap de Wilde. 1998. *Security: A New Framework for Analysis*. Boulder, CO: Lynne Rienner.

Cabrera, Oscar A. and Lawrence O. Gostin. 2013. "Global Tobacco Control: A Vital Component of the Right to Health." In *Advancing the Human Right to Health*, edited by Jose M. Zuniga, Stephen P. Marks, and Lawrence O. Gostin, 261–274. New York: Oxford University Press.

Cameron, Alexandra, Margaret Ewen, Dennis Ross-Degnan, Douglas Ball, and Richard Laing. 2009. "Medicine Prices, Availability, and Affordability in 36 Developing and Middle-Income Countries: A Secondary Analysis." *The Lancet* 373 (9659): 240–249.

Cannon, Geoffrey. 2004. "Why the Bush Administration and the Global Sugar Industry Are Determined to Demolish the 2004 WHO Global Strategy on Diet, Physical Activity and Health." *Public Health Nutrition* 7 (3): 369–380.

Cardoso, Fernando H. and Enzo Faletto. 1979. *Dependency and Development in Latin America*. Berkeley: University of California Press.

Carroll, Aaron E. 2015. "Drink to Your Health (in Moderation), the Science Says." *New York Times*. December 21, 2015. https://www.nytimes.com/2015/12/22/upshot/alcohols-effect-on-health-what-the-science-says.html (accessed January 29, 2018).

Carter, Stacy M. 2002. "Mongoven, Biscoe & Duchin: Destroying Tobacco Control Activism from the Inside." *Tobacco Control* 11 (2): 112–118.

Carus, W. Seth. 2015. "The History of Biological Weapons Use: What We Know and What We Don't." *Health Security* 13 (4): 219–255.

Casswell, Sally and Thaksaphon Thamarangsi. 2009. "Reducing Harm from Alcohol: Call to Action." *The Lancet* 373 (9682): 2247–2257.

Centers for Disease Control and Prevention. 2010. "The 2009 H1N1 Pandemic Summary Highlights, April 2009-April 2010." http://www.cdc.gov/h1n1flu/cdcresponse.htm (accessed September 9, 2013).

Centers for Disease Control and Prevention. 2016. "Global Health Security Agenda: Action Packages." http://www.cdc.gov/globalhealth/healthprotection/ghs/pdf/ghsa-action-packages_24-september-2014.pdf (accessed July 15, 2016).

Centers for Disease Control and Prevention. 2017. "Electronic Cigarettes." https://www.cdc.gov/tobacco/basic_information/e-cigarettes/index.htm (accessed January 29, 2018).

Chapman, Audrey R. 1996. "A 'Violations Approach' for Monitoring the International Covenant of Economic, Social and Cultural Rights." *Human Rights Quarterly* 18 (1): 23–66.

Charnovitz, Steve. 2006. "Nongovernmental Organizations and International Law." *American Journal of International Law* 100 (2): 348–372.

Chayes, Abram and Antonia H. Chayes. 1995. *The New Sovereignty: Compliance with International Regulatory Agreements*. Cambridge, MA: Harvard University Press.

Checkel, Jeffrey. 1998. "The Constructivist Turn in International Relations Theory." *World Politics* 50 (2): 324–348.

Chorev, Nitsan. 2012. *The World Health Organization between North and South*. Ithaca, NY: Cornell University Press.

Clemencon, Raymond. 2016. "The Two Sides of the Paris Climate Agreement: Dismal Failure or Historic Breakthrough." *Journal of Environment and Development* 25 (1): 3–24.

Clinton, Chelsea and Devi Sridhar. 2017. *Governing Global Health: Who Runs the World and Why?* New York: Oxford University Press.

Cockerham, Geoffrey B. and William C. Cockerham. 2010. *Health and Globalization*. Cambridge, UK: Polity.

Cohn, Theodore. 2016. *Global Political Economy*. Seventh Edition. New York: Routledge.

Collin, Jeff. 2004. "Tobacco Politics." *Development* 47 (2): 91–96.

Collin, Jeff. 2010. "Global Health, Equity and the WHO Framework Convention on Tobacco Control." *Global Health Promotion* 17 (1 Suppl): 73–75.

Commission on Global Governance. 1995. *Our Global Neighborhood: The Report of the Commission of Global Governance*. Oxford: Oxford University Press.

Committee on Economic, Social, and Cultural Rights. 2000. "General Comment 14: The Right to the Highest Attainable Standard of Health," UN Doc. E/C.12/2000/4, August 11, 2000.

Committee on Economic, Social and Cultural Rights. 2008. " Concluding Observations of the Committee on Economic, Social and Cultural Rights: India," UN Doc. E/C.12/IND/CO/5, August 8, 2008.

Constitution of the World Health Organization. Opened for signature July 22, 1946. *United Nations Treaty Series* 14:185. https://treaties.un.org/doc/Treaties/1948/04/19480407%2010-51%20PM/Ch_IX_01p.pdf

Cooper, Alice H. and Paulette Kurzer. 2003. "Rauch ohne Feuer: Why Germany Lags in Tobacco Control." *German Politics and Society* 21 (68): 24–47.

Coovadia, Hoosen, Rachel Jewkes, Peter Barron, David Sanders, and Diane McIntyre. 2009. "The Health and Health System of South Africa: Historical Roots of Current Public Health Challenges." *The Lancet* 374: 817–834.

Correa, Carlos María. 2006. "Implications of Bilateral Free Trade Agreements on Access to Medicines." *Bulletin of the World Health Organization* 84 (5): 399–404.

Cortell, Andrew P. and Susan Peterson. 2006. "Dutiful Agents, Rogue Actors or Both? Staffing, Voting Rules, and Slack in the WHO and WTO." In *Delegation and Agency in International Organizations*, edited by Darren G. Hawkins, David A. Lake, Daniel L. Nielson, and Michael J. Tierney, 229–254. Cambridge, UK: Cambridge University Press.

Costello, Anthony, Mark Maslin, Hugh Montgomery, Anne M. Johnson, and Paul Ekins. 2011. "Global Health and Climate Change: Moving from Denial and Catastrophic Fatalism to Positive Action." *Philosophical Transactions: Mathematical, Physical and Engineering Sciences* 369: 1866–1882.

Cox, Robert W. 1987. *Production, Power, and World Order*. New York: Columbia University Press.

Craven, Matthew. 1995. *The International Covenant of Economic, Social and Cultural Rights: A Perspective on Its Development*. New York: Oxford University Press.

Crow, Melissa E. 2005. "The Human Rights Responsibilities of Multinational Tobacco Companies." *Tobacco Control* 14 (Suppl ii): ii14–ii18.

Csete, Joanne. 2007. "Rhetoric and Reality: HIV/AIDS as a Human Rights Issue." In *The Global Politics of AIDS*, edited by Paul G. Harris and Patricia D. Siplon, 247–261. Boulder, CO: Lynne Rienner.

Cueto, Marcos. 2004. "The Origins of Primary Health Care and Selective Primary Health Care." *American Journal of Public Health* 94 (11): 1864–1874.

Cumming-Bruce, Nick. 2014. "W.H.O. Chief Calls Ebola Outbreak a 'Crisis for International Peace'." *New York Times*. October 13, 2014. https://www.nytimes.com/2014/10/14/world/africa/ebola-virus-outbreak.html (accessed January 30, 2018).

Daniel, Thomas M. 2006. "The History of Tuberculosis." *Respiratory Medicine* 100 (11): 1862–1870.

Das, Pam and Udani Samarasekera. 2008. "What's Next for UNAIDS?" *The Lancet* 372 (9656): 2099–2102.

Davey, Eleanor. 2011. "Famine, Aid, and Ideology: The Political Activism of Médecins sans Frontières in the 1980s." *French Historical Studies* 34 (3): 529–558.

Davies, Sara E. 2010. *Global Politics of Health*. Cambridge, UK: Polity.

Davis, Peter. 2013. *Corporations, Global Governance and Post-Conflict Reconstruction*. New York: Routledge.

Dawood, Fatimah S. A. Danielle Iuliano, Carrie Reed, Martin I. Meltzer, David K. Shay, Po-Yung Cheng, and Don Bandaranayake, et al. 2012. "Estimated Global Mortality Associated with the First 12 Months of 2009 Pandemic Influenza A H1N1 Virus Circulation: A Modelling Study." *The Lancet Infectious Diseases* 12 (9): 687–695.

Declaration of the United Nations Conference on the Human Environment. 1972. http://www.un-documents.net/unchedec.htm (accessed July 10, 2018).

Demmers, Jolle, Alex E. Fernandez Jilberto, and Barbara Hogenboom. 2004. "Good Governance and Democracy in a World of Neoliberal Regimes." In *Good*

Governance in the Era of Neoliberalism: Conflict and Depolitisation in Latin America, Eastern Europe, Asia, and Africa, edited by Jolle Demmers, Alex E. Fernandez Jilberto, and Barbara Hogenboom, 1–32. London: Routledge.

Den Elzen, Michel G. J., Andries F. Hof, and Mark Roelfsema. 2013. "Analysing the Greenhouse Gas Emission Reductions of the Mitigation Action Plans by Non-Annex I Countries by 2020." *Energy Policy* 56: 633–643.

Detomasi, David Antony. 2007. "The Multinational Corporation and Global Governance." *Journal of Business Ethics* 71 (3): 321–334.

Di Cesare, Mariachiara, Young-Ho Khang, Perviz Asaria, Tony Blakely, Melanie J. Cowan, Farshad Farzadfar, and Ramiro Guerrero, et al. 2013. "Inequalities in Non-Communicable Diseases and Effective Responses." *The Lancet* 381 (9866): 585–597.

Doremus, Paul N., William W. Keller, Louis W. Pauly, and Simon Reich. 1998. *The Myth of the Global Corporation*. Princeton, NJ: Princeton University Press.

Doshi, Peter. 2013. "The 2009 Influenza Pandemic." *The Lancet Infectious Diseases* 13 (3): 193.

Dresler, Carolyn, Harry Lando, Nick Schneider, and Hitakshi Sehgal. 2013. "Human Rights-Based Approach to Tobacco Control." In *Health and Human Rights in a Changing World*, edited by Michael A. Grodin et al., 472–482. New York: Routledge.

Drewnowski, Adam and Barry M. Popkin. 1997. "The Nutrition Transition: New Trends in the Global Diet." *Nutrition Reviews* 55: 31–43.

Drezner, Daniel. 2007. *All Politics Are Global: Explaining International Regulatory Regimes*. Princeton, NJ: Princeton University Press.

Duggal, Ravi. 2013. "Health and Development in India: Moving towards the Right to Health." In *Advancing the Human Right to Health*, edited by Jose M. Zuniga, Stephen P. Marks, and Lawrence O. Gostin, 113–126. New York: Oxford University Press.

Dye, Christopher and Martien Borgdorff. 2008. "Global Epidemiology and Control of Tuberculosis." In *Handbook of Tuberculosis: Clinics, Diagnostics, Therapy and Epidemiology*, edited by Stefan H. E. Kaufmann and Paul van Helden, 1–21. London: Wiley-VCH.

Dye, Christopher and Katherine Floyd. 2006. "Tuberculosis." In *Disease Control Priorities in Developing Countries*. Second Edition, edited by Dean T. Jamison et al. Washington, DC: World Bank.

Dyer, Owen. 2004. "United States Wins More Time to Lobby against WHO Diet Plan." *British Medical Journal* 328: 45.

Eckl, Julian. 2014. "The Power of Private Foundations: Rockefeller and Gates in the Struggle against Malaria." *Global Social Policy* 14 (1): 91–116.

Ehlermann, Claus-Dieter and Lothar Ehring. 2005. "Decision-Making in the World Trade Organization: Is the Consensus Practice of the World Trade Organization Adequate for Making, Revising and Implementing Rules on International Trade?" *Journal of International Economic Law* 8 (1): 51–75.

Eichengreen, Barry and Peter B. Kenen. 1994. "Managing the World Economy under the Bretton Woods System: An Overview." In *Managing the World Economy: Fifty Years after Bretton Woods*, edited by Peter B. Kenan. Washington, DC: Institute for International Economics.

Elbe, Stefan. 2010. *Security and Global Health*. Cambridge, UK: Polity.

Elzinga, Gijs, Mario C. Raviglione, and Dermot Maher. 2004. "Scale Up: Meeting Targets in Global Tuberculosis Control." *The Lancet* 363 (9411): 814–819.

Emslie, John J. 2005. "Labeling Programs as a Reasonably Available Least Restrictive Trade Measure under Article XX's Nexus Requirement." *Brooklyn Journal of International Law* 30: 485–545.

European Commission. 2018. "Fertility Statistics." http://ec.europa.eu/eurostat/statistics-explained/index.php/Fertility_statistics (accessed January 29, 2018).

Evans, Tony. 2002. "A Human Right to Health?" *Third World Quarterly* 23 (2): 197–215.

Farrar, Jeremy J. and Peter Piot. 2014. "The Ebola Emergency—Immediate Action, Ongoing Strategy." *New England Journal of Medicine* 371 (16): 1545–1546.

Fauci, Anthony S. 2017. "The Ebola Epidemic of 2014–2015: A Perfect Storm." In *Global Management of Infectious Disease after Ebola*, edited by Sam F. Halabi, Lawrence O. Gostin, and Jeffrey S. Crowley, 21–32. New York: Oxford University Press.

Fee, Elizabeth and Manon Parry. 2008. "Jonathan Mann, HIV/AIDS, and Human Rights." *Journal of Public Health Policy* 29 (1): 54–71.

Feldmann, Heinz and Thomas W. Geisbert. 2011. "Ebola Haemorrhagic Fever." *The Lancet* 377 (9678): 849–862.

Fidler, David P. 1999. *International Law and Infectious Disease*. Oxford: Clarendon Press.

Fidler, David P. 2001. "The Globalization of Public Health: The First 100 Years of International Health Diplomacy." *Bulletin of the World Health Organization* 79 (9): 842–849.

Fidler, David P. 2004. *SARS, Governance and the Globalization of Disease*. New York: Palgrave Macmillan.

Fidler, David P. 2005. "From International Sanitary Conventions to Global Health Security: The New International Health Regulations." *Chinese Journal of International Law* 4 (2): 325–392.

Fidler, David P. 2007. "A Pathology of Public Health Securitism." In *Governing Global Health: Challenges, Response, Innovation*, edited by Andrew F. Cooper, John Kirton, and Ted Schrecker, 41–64. Aldershot, UK: Ashgate Publishing.

Fidler, David P. 2009. "H1N1 after Action Review: Learning from the Unexpected, the Success and the Fear." *Future Microbiology* 4 (7): 767–769.

Fidler, David P. 2010. *The Challenges of Global Health Governance*. Council of Foreign Relations Working Paper. New York: Council on Foreign Relations.

Fidler, David P. 2017. "Global Health Diplomacy and the Ebola Outbreak." In *Global Management of Infectious Disease after Ebola*, edited by Sam F. Halabi, Lawrence O. Gostin, and Jeffrey S. Crowley, 133–147. New York: Oxford University Press.

Fidler, David P. and Lawrence O. Gostin. 2006. "The New International Health Regulations: An Historic Development for International Law and Public Health." *Journal of Law, Medicine, and Ethics* 34 (1): 85–94.

Fidler, David P. and Lawrence O. Gostin. 2008. *Biosecurity in the Global Age: Biological Weapons, Public Health and the Rule of Law*. Palo Alto, CA: Stanford University Press.

Filho, Armando De Negri. 2013. "Brazil: A Long Journey towards a Universal Healthcare System." In *Advancing the Human Right to Health*, edited by Jose M. Zuniga, Stephen P. Marks, and Lawrence O. Gostin, 173–179. New York: Oxford University Press.

Finnemore, Martha. 1993. "International Organizations as Teachers of Norms: The United Nations Educational, Scientific, and Cultural Organization." *International Organization* 47 (4): 565–597.

Finnemore, Martha. 1996. *National Interests in International Society*. Ithaca, NY: Cornell University Press.

Finnemore, Martha and Kathryn Sikkink. 1998. "International Norm Dynamics and Political Change." *International Organization* 52 (4): 887–917.

Flanagin, Jack. 2014. "Australia's Little Guantánamos." *New York Times*. November 7, 2014.

Fleck, Fiona. 2003. "How SARS Changed the World in Less than Six Months." *Bulletin of the World Health Organization* 81 (8): 625–626.

Flint, Adrian. 2011. *HIV/AIDS in Sub-Saharan Africa: Politics, Aid, and Globalization*. New York: Palgrave Macmillan.

Ford, Nicole D., Shivani A. Patel, and K. M. Venkat Narayan. 2017. "Obesity in Low and Middle-Income Countries: Burden, Drivers, and Emerging Challenges." *Annual Reviews of Public Health* 38: 145–164.

Forero, Juan. 2000. "$5 Billion Puts Gates Fund in First Place." *New York Times*, January 25, 2000. http://www.nytimes.com/2000/01/25/us/5-billion-puts-gates-fund-in-first-place.html (accessed August 2, 2014).

Forsythe, David P. 2005. *The Humanitarians: The International Committee of the Red Cross*. Cambridge, UK: Cambridge University Press.

Fountain, Henry, Jugal K. Patel, and Nadja Popovich. 2018. "2017 Was One of the Hottest Years on Record. And That Was without El Niño." *New York Times*. January 18, 2018. https://www.nytimes.com/interactive/2018/01/18/climate/hottest-year-2017.html (accessed on January 29, 2018).

Fox, Renee. 2014. *Doctors Without Borders: Humanitarian Quests, Impossible Dreams of Médecins Sans Frontières*. Baltimore, MD: Johns Hopkins University Press.

Franco-Giraldo, Alvaro, Marco Palma, and Carlos Alvarez-Dardet. 2006. "The Effect of Structural Adjustment on Health Conditions in Latin America and the Caribbean, 1980–2000. *Pan American Journal of Health* 19 (5): 291–299.

Freeman, Jody and Andre Guzman. 2009. "Climate Change and U.S. Interests." *Columbia Law Review* 109 (6): 1531–1601.

Freeman, Michael. 2011. *Human Rights: An Interdisciplinary Approach*. Second Edition. Cambridge, UK: Polity.

Frieden, Thomas R., Jordan W. Tappero, Scott F. Dowell, Nguyen T. Hien, Florence D. Guillaume, and Jane R. Aceng. 2014. "Safer Countries through Global Health Security." *The Lancet* 383: 764–766.

Friedman, Eric A. and Lawrence O. Gostin. 2012. "Pillars for Progress on the Right to Health: Harnessing the Potential of Human Rights through a Framework Convention on Global Health." *Health and Human Rights* 14 (1): 1–16.

Fuchs, Doris. 2007. *Business Power in Global Governance*. Boulder, CO: Lynne Rienner.

Galizzi, Paolo. 2005. "From Stockholm to New York, via Rio and Johannesburg: Has the Environment Lost Its Way on the Global Agenda?" *Fordham International Law Journal* 29 (5): 952–1008.

Garrett, Laurie. 2005. "The Lessons of HIV/AIDS." *Foreign Affairs* 84 (4): 51–64.

GAVI Alliance. 2018a. "History of GAVI." http://www.gavialliance.org/about/mission/history/ (accessed January 20, 2018).

GAVI Alliance. 2018b. "GAVI's Strategy." http://www.gavialliance.org/about/strategy/ (accessed January 20, 2018).

GAVI Alliance. 2018c. *2016 Progress Report*. http://www.gavialliance.org/library/publications/gavi-progress-reports/gavi-alliance-progress-report-2013 (accessed August 9, 2014).

Gilmore, Anna B. and Martin McKee. 2004. "Moving East: How the Transnational Tobacco Industry Gained Entry to the Emerging Markets of the former Soviet Union. Part I: Establishing Cigarette Imports. *Tobacco Control* 13: 143–150.

Gilpin, Robert. 1987. *The Political Economy of International Relations*. Princeton, NJ: Princeton University Press.

Gilpin, Robert. 2001. *Global Political Economy: Understanding the International Economic Order*. Princeton, NJ: Princeton University Press.

Gilpin, Robert. 2002. "A Realist Perspective on International Governance." In *Governing Globalization*, edited by David Held and Andrew McGrew, 237–248. Cambridge, UK: Polity.

Glantz, Stanton A., Deborah E. Barnes, Lisa Bero, Peter Hanauer, and John Slade. 1995. "Looking through a Keyhole at the Tobacco Industry: The Brown and Williamson Documents." *Journal of the American Medical Association* 274 (3): 219–224.

Gleditsch, Nils Petter. 2012. "Whither the Weather? Climate Change and Conflict: Introduction." *Journal of Peace Research* 49 (1): 3–9.

Global Environment Facility. 2018. "About Us." https://www.thegef.org/gef/whatisgef (accessed March 10, 2018).

Global Fund for AIDS, Tuberculosis, and Malaria. 2017. *Results Report 2017*. Geneva: Global Fund for AIDS, Tuberculosis and Malaria. https://www.theglobalfund.org/media/6773/corporate_2017resultsreport_report_en.pdf?u=636486806780000000 (accessed January 20, 2018).

Global Health Security Agenda. 2016. "About Global Health Security Agenda." https://ghsagenda.org/about (accessed July 15, 2016).

Godlee, Fiona. 1998. "Change at Last at WHO: But Will the Regions Play Ball?" *BMJ* 317 (7154): 296.

Goertz, Gary. 2003. *International Norms and Decision Making*. Oxford: Rowman & Littlefield Publishers.

Goodchild, Mark, Nigar Nargis, and Edouard Tursan d'Espaignet 2017. "Global Economic Cost of Smoking-Attributable Diseases." *Tobacco Control* 27 (1): 58–64.

Gostin, Lawrence O. 2007. "Meeting the Survival Needs of the World's Least Healthy People: A Proposed Model for Global Health Governance." *Journal of the American Medical Association* 298 (2): 225–228.

Gostin, Lawrence O. 2014. *Global Health Law*. Cambridge, MA: Harvard University Press.

Gostin, Lawrence O. and Eric A. Friedman. 2014. "Ebola: A Crisis in Global Health Leadership." *The Lancet* 384 (9951): 1323–1325.

Gostin, Lawrence O. and Rebecca Katz. 2017. "The International Health Regulations: The Governing Framework for Global Health Security." In *Global Management of Infectious Disease after Ebola*, edited by Sam F. Halabi, Lawrence O. Gostin, and Jeffrey S. Crowley, 101–132. New York: Oxford University Press.

Gostin, Lawrence O. and Zita Lazzarini. 1997. *Human Rights and Public Health in the AIDS Pandemic*. New York: Oxford University Press.

Grana, Rachel, Neal Benowitz, and Stanton A. Glantz. 2014. "E-Cigarettes: A Scientific Review." *Circulation* 129 (19): 1972–1986.

Grange, John M. 1999. 'The Global Burden of Tuberculosis." In *Tuberculosis: An Interdisciplinary Perspective*, edited by John D. H. Porter and John M. Grange, 3–31. London: Imperial College Press.

Gravely, Shannon, Gary A. Giovino, Lorraine Craig, Alison Commar, Edouard Tursan D'Espaignet, Kerstin Schotte, Geoffrey T. Fong. 2017. "Implementation of Key Demand-Reduction Measures of the WHO Framework Convention on Tobacco Control and Change in Smoking Prevalence in 126 Countries: An Association Study." *The Lancet Public Health* 2: 166–174.

Greene, Jeremy, Marguerite Thorp Basilico, Heidi Kim, and Paul Farmer. 2013. "Colonial Medicine and Its Legacies." In *Reimagining Global Health: An Introduction*, edited by Paul Farmer, Jim Young Kim, Arthur Kleinman, and Matthew Basilico, 33–73. Berkeley: University of California Press.

Grieco, Joseph. 1988. "Anarchy and the Limits of Cooperation: A Realist Critique of the Newest Liberal Institutionalism." *International Organization* 42 (3): 485–507.

Griswold, Eliza. 2012. "How 'Silent Spring' Ignited the Environmental Movement." *New York Times*. September 21, 2012. http://www.nytimes.com/2012/09/23/magazine/;how-silent-spring-ignited-the-environmental-movement.html?_r=0 (accessed July 27, 2015).

Grüning, Thilo, Heide Weishaar, Jeff Collin, and Anna B. Gilmore. 2011. "Tobacco Industry Attempts to Influence and Use the German Government to Undermine the WHO Framework Convention on Tobacco Control." *Tobacco Control* 21 (1): 30–38.

Gruskin, Sofia, Edward J. Mills, and Daniel Tarantola. 2007. "History, Principles and Practice of Health and Human Right." *The Lancet* 370: 449–455.

Guillemin, Jeanne. 2005. *Biological Weapons: From the Invention of State-Sponsored Programs to Contemporary Bioterrorism*. New York: Columbia University Press.

Gunter, Valerie J. and Craig K. Harris. 1998. "Noisy Winter: The DDT Controversy in the Years before *Silent Spring*." *Rural Sociology* 63 (2): 179–198.

Haas, Ernst. 1958. *The Uniting of Europe*. Stanford: Stanford University Press.

Haas, Peter. 1992. "Banning Chlorofluorocarbons: Epistemic Community Efforts to Protect Stratospheric Ozone." *International Organization* 46 (1): 187–224.

Hafner-Burton, Emilie M. and Kiyoteru Tsutsui. 2007. "Justice Lost! The Failure of International Human Rights Law to Matter Where Needed Most." *Journal of Peace Research* 44 (4): 407–425.

Hammond, Ross. 1998. "Consolidation in the Tobacco Control Industry," *Tobacco Control* 7: 426–428.

Harman, Sophie. 2009. "The World Bank and Health." In *Global Health Governance: Crisis, Institutions, and Political Economy*, edited by Adrian Kay and Owain Williams, 227–243. New York: Palgrave Macmillan.

Harman, Sophie. 2010. *The World Bank and HIV/AIDS*. London: Routledge.

Harman, Sophie. 2012. *Global Health Governance*. New York: Routledge.

Harrison, Graham. 2004. *The World Bank and Africa: The Construction of Governance States*. London: Routledge.

Hawkes, Corinna. 2005. "The Role of Foreign Direct Investment in the Nutrition Transition." *Public Health Nutrition* 8 (4): 357–365.

Hawkes, Corinna. 2006. "Uneven Dietary Development: Linking the Policies and Processes of Globalization with the Nutrition Transition, Obesity and Diet-related Chronic Diseases." *Globalization and Health* 2: 4.

Hawkes, Corinna and Barry M. Popkin. 2015. "Can the Sustainable Development Goals Reduce the Burden of Nutrition-related Non-Communicable Diseases without Truly Addressing Major Food System Reforms?" *BMC Medicine* 13: 143.

Hawkins, Darren G., David A. Lake, Daniel L. Nielson, and Michael J. Tierney. 2006. "Delegation under Anarchy: States, International Organizations, and Principal-Agent Theory." In *Delegation and Agency in International Organizations*, edited by Darren G. Hawkins, David A. Lake, Daniel L. Nielson, and Michael J. Tierney, 3–38. Cambridge, UK: Cambridge University Press.

He, Peisen, Takeaki Takeuchi, and Eiji Yano. 2012. "An Overview of the China National Tobacco Corporation and State Tobacco Monopoly Administration." *Environmental Health and Preventive Medicine* 18 (1): 85–90.

Heins, Volker. 2008. *Nongovernmental Organizations in International Society: Struggle over Recognition*. New York: Palgrave Macmillan.

Held, David and Andrew McGrew. 2002. "Introduction." In *Governing Globalization*, edited by David Held and Andrew McGrew, 1–24. Cambridge, UK: Polity.

Henkin, Louis. 1990. *The Age of Rights*. New York: Columbia University Press.

Heymann, David L., John S. Mackenzie, and Malik Peiris. 2013. "SARS Legacy: Outbreak Reporting Is Expected and Respected." *The Lancet* 381 (9869): 779–781.

Heywood, Mark. 2002. "Drug Access, Patents and Global Health: 'Chaffed and Waxed Sufficient'." *Third World Quarterly* 23 (2): 217–231.

Hoekman, Bernard M. and Michel M. Kostecki. 2001. *The Political Economy of the World Trading System: From GATT to WTO*. Second Edition. New York: Oxford University Press.

Hoffman, Steven J. 2010. "The Evolution, Etiology and Eventualities of the Global Health Security Regime." *Health Policy and Planning* 25 (6): 510–522.

Hoffman, Steven J. and John-Arne Røttingen. 2013. "Dark Sides of the Proposed Framework Convention on Global Health's Many Virtues: A Systematic Review and Critical Analysis." *Health and Human Rights* 15 (1): 117–134.

Hoffmann, Matthew J. 2005a. "Constructing Global Governance." In *Contending Perspectives on Global Governance: Coherence, Contestation, and World Order*, edited by Alice D. Ba and Matthew J. Hoffmann, 110–128. London: Routledge.

Hoffmann, Matthew J. 2005b. *Ozone Depletion and Climate Change: Constructing a Global Response*. Albany: State University of New York Press.

Hogerzeil, Hans V., Melanie Samson, Jaume Vidal Casanovas, and Ladan Rahmani-Ocora. 2006. "Is Access to Essential Medicines as Part of the Fulfilment of the Right to Health Enforceable through the Courts?" *The Lancet* 368 (9532): 305–311.

Homedes, Núria and Antonio Ugalde. 2005. "Why Neoliberal Health Reforms Have Failed in Latin America." *Health Policy* 71: 83–96.

Hopf, Ted. 1998. "The Promise of Constructivism in International Relations." *International Security* 23 (1): 171–200.

Horiomoto, Taisuke and Yoshihiro Kawaoka. 2001. "Pandemic Threat Posed by Avian Influenza A Viruses." *Clinical Microbiology Review* 14 (1): 129–149.

Horton, Richard. 2005. "The Neglected Epidemic of Chronic Diseases." *The Lancet* 366: 1514.

Horton, Richard and Udani Samarasekera. 2016. "WHO's Director-General Candidates: Visions and Priorities." *The Lancet* 388 (10056): 2072–2095.

Hotez, Peter J., Alan Fenwick, Lorenzo Savioli, and David H. Molyneux. 2009. "Rescuing the Bottom Billion through Control of Neglected Tropical Diseases." *The Lancet* 373: 1570–1575.

Howard-Jones, Norman. 1975. *The Scientific Background to the International Sanitary Conferences 1851–1938*. Geneva: World Health Organization.

Howard-Jones, Norman. 1978. *International Public Health between the Two World Wars: The Organizational Problems*. Geneva: World Health Organization.

Htenas, Aira Maria, Yurie Tanimichi-Hoberg, and Lynn Brown. 2017. *An Overview of Links between Obesity and Food Systems : Implications for the Agriculture GP Agenda*. Washington, DC: World Bank Group. http://documents.worldbank.org/curated/en/222101499437276873/An-overview-of-links-between-obesity-and-food-systems-implications-for-the-agriculture-GP-agenda (accessed March 10, 2018).

Hulme, Mike. 2009. *Why We Disagree about Climate Change: Understanding Controversy, Inaction, and Opportunity*. Cambridge, UK: Cambridge University Press.

Human Rights Committee. 1982. *General Comment No. 6, The Right to Life (Art.6)*. UN Doc. HR1/GEN/Rev.1, April 30, 1982.

Ingram, Alan. 2009. "The International Political Economy of Global Responses to HIV/AIDS." In *Global Health Governance: Crisis, Institutions, and Political Economy*, edited by Adrian Kay and Owain Williams, 81–101. New York: Palgrave Macmillan.

Intergovernmental on Climate Change. 2013. "Summary for Policymakers." In *Climate Change 2013: The Physical Science Basis. Contribution of Working Group I to the Fifth Assessment Report of the Intergovernmental Panel on Climate Change*, edited by Thomas F. Stocker, Dahe Qin, Gian-Kasper Plattner, Melinda Tignor, Simon K. Allen, Judith Boschung, Alexander Nauels, Yu Xia, Vincent Bex, and Pauline M. Midgley. Cambridge: Cambridge University Press.

Intergovernmental Panel on Climate Change. 2014. "Summary for Policymakers." In *Climate Change 2014: Mitigation of Climate Change. Contribution of Working Group III to the Fifth Assessment Report of the Intergovernmental Panel on Climate Change*, edited by Ottmar Edenhofer, Ramon Pichs-Madruga, Youba

Sokona, Ellie Farahani, Susanne Kadner, Kristin Seyboth, and Anna Adler, et al. Cambridge, UK: Cambridge University Press.

International Covenant on Economic, Social, and Cultural Rights. Opened for signature December 16, 1966. *United Nations Treaty Series* 999: 3. https://treaties.un.org/doc/Treaties/1976/01/19760103%2009-57%20PM/Ch_IV_03.pdf

International Monetary Fund. 2015. *The Managing Director's Statement on the Role of the Fund in Addressing Climate Change*. November 25, 2015. http://www.imf.org/external/np/pp/eng/2015/112515.pdf (accessed May 21, 2016).

International Monetary Fund. 2018. "IMF Response to the Ebola Crisis." http://www.imf.org/external/np/fad/ebola/ (accessed January 15, 2018).

Irwin, Douglas A. 1995. "GATT in Historical Perspective." *American Economic Review* 323–328.

Ivanova, Maria. 2010. "Moving Forward by Looking Back: Learning from UNEP's History." In *Green Planet Blues: Four Decades of Global Environmental Politics*, edited by Ken Conca and Geoffrey D. Dabelko, 143–160. Boulder, CO: Westview Press.

Ivanova, Maria. 2013. "The Contested Legacy of Rio+20." *Global Environmental Politics* 13 (4): 1–11.

James, W. Phillip T. 2008. "WHO Recognition of the Global Obesity Epidemic." *International Journal of Obesity* 32: S120–S126.

James, Phillip T., Neville Rigby, and Rachael Leach. 2004. "The Obesity Epidemic, Metabolic Syndrome and Future Prevention Strategies." *European Journal of Cardiovascular Prevention and Rehabilitation* 11 (1): 3–8.

Jansen, Hugo-Jan, Florence J. Breeveld, Cornelis Stijnis, and Martin P. Grobusch. 2014. "Biological Warfare, Bioterrorism, and Biocrime." *Clinical Microbiology and Infection* 20: 488–496.

Jargon, Julie. 2011. "Subway Runs Past McDonald's Chain." *Wall Street Journal*. March 8.

Jernigan, David H. 2009. "The Global Alcohol Industry: An Overview." *Addiction* 104 (Suppl 1): 6–12.

Jha, Prabhat. 2009. "Avoidable Cancer Deaths and Total Deaths from Smoking." *Nature Reviews Cancer* 9: 655–664.

Jha, Prabhat and Frank Chaloupka. 2000. *Tobacco Control in Developing Countries*. Oxford: Oxford University Press.

Joy, Robert J. T. 1999. "Malaria in American Troops in the South and Southwest Pacific in World War II." *Medical History* 43 (2): 192–207.

Kaasa, Stine Madland. 2007. "The UN Commission on Sustainable Development: Which Mechanisms Explain Its Accomplishments?" *Global Environmental Politics* 7 (3): 107–129.

Kaldor, Mary. 2003. *Global Civil Society: An Answer to War*. Cambridge, UK: Polity.

Kamradt-Scott, Adam. 2016. "WHO's to Blame? The World Health Organization and the 2014 Ebola Outbreak in West Africa." *Third World Quarterly* 37 (3): 401–418.

Kamradt-Scott, Adam, and McInnes, Colin. 2012. "The Securitisation of Pandemic Influenza: Framing, Security and Public Policy." *Global Public Health* 7(S2), S95–S110.

Kapur, Devesh, John Prior Lewis, and Richard Charles Webb. 1997. *The World Bank. Its First Half Century. Volume I: History*. Washington, DC: Brookings Institution.

Karns, Margaret P. and Karen A. Mingst. 2015. *International Organizations: The Politics and Processes of Global Governance*. Third Edition. Boulder, CO: Lynne Rienner.

Katz, James E. 2005. "Individual Rights Advocacy in Tobacco Control Policies: An Assessment and Recommendation." *Tobacco Control* 14 (Suppl ii): ii31–ii37.

Katz, Rebecca and Julie Fischer. 2010. "The Revised International Health Regulations: A Framework for Global Pandemic Response." *Global Health Governance* 3 (2): 1–18.

Katz, Rebecca, Erin M. Sorrell, Sarah A. Kornblet, and Julie E. Fischer. 2014. "Global Health Security Agenda and the International Health Regulations: Moving Forward." *Biosecurity and Bioterrorism* 12 (5): 231–238.

Keck, Margaret E. and Kathryn Sikkink. 1998. *Activists beyond Borders: Advocacy Networks in International Politics*. Ithaca, NY: Cornell University Press.

Keith, Linda Camp. 1999. "The United Nations International Covenant on Civil and Political Rights: Does It Make a Difference in Human Rights Behavior?" *Journal of Peace Research* 36 (1): 95–118.

Kellman, Barry. 2001. "Biological Terrorism: Legal Measures for Preventing Catastrophe." *Harvard Journal of Law and Public Policy* 24: 417–488.

Ken, Ivy. 2014. "A Healthy Bottom Line: Obese Children, a Pacified Public, and Corporate Legitimacy." *Social Currents* 1 (2): 130–148.

Keohane, Robert O. 1984. *After Hegemony: Cooperation and Discord in the World Political Economy*. Princeton, NJ: Princeton University Press.

Keohane, Robert O. 1989. *International Institutions and State Power: Essays in International Relations Theory*. Boulder, CO: Westview Press.

Keohane, Robert O. 2001. "Governance in a Partially Globalized World." *American Political Science Review* 95 (1): 1–13.

Keohane, Robert O. and Joseph S. Nye. 1977. *Power and Interdependence: World Politics in Transition*. Boston: Little Brown.

Keohane, Robert O. and David G. Victor. 2011. "The Regime Complex for Climate Change." *Perspectives on Politics* 9 (1): 7–23.

Kim, Jim Yong, Aaron Shakow, Arachu Castro, Chris Vanderwanker, and Paul Farmer. 2003. "Tuberculosis Control." In *Global Public Goods for Health*, edited by Richard D. Smith, Robert Beaglehole, David Woodward, and Nick Drager, 54–72. Oxford: Oxford University Press.

Kindhauser, Mary Kay, Tomas Allen, Veronika Frank, Ravi Shankar Santhana, and Christopher Dye. 2016. "Zika: The Origin and Spread of a Mosquito-borne Virus." *Bulletin of the World Health Organization* 94: 675–686C.

Kirkup, Alex and Tony Evans. 2009. "The Myth of Western Opposition to Economic, Social, and Cultural Rights? A Reply to Whelan and Donnelly." *Human Rights Quarterly* 31 (1): 221–238.

Kiss, Alexandre and Dinah L. Shelton 2007. *Guide to International Environmental Law*. The Hague: Martinus Nijhoff Publishers.

Kiszewski, Anthony, Benjamin Johns, Allan Schapira, Charles Delacollette, Valerie Crowell, Tessa Tan-Torres, Birkinesh Ameneshewa, Awash Teklehaimanot, and Fatoumata Nafo-Traoré. 2007. "Estimated Global Resources Needed To Attain International Malaria Control Goals." *Bulletin of the World Health Organization* 85: 623–630.

Klotz, Audie. 1995. *Norms in International Relations: The Struggle Against Apartheid.* Ithaca, NY: Cornell University Press.

Knell, A. J. 1991. *Malaria.* Oxford: Oxford University Press.

Koblentz, Gregory D. 2012. "From Biodefence to Biosecurity: The Obama Administration's Strategy for Countering Biological Threats." *International Affairs* 88 (1): 131–148.

Kohlmorgen, Lars. 2007. "International Governmental Organization and Global Health Governance: the Role of the World Health Organization, World Bank, and UNAIDS." In *Global Health Governance and the Fight against HIV/AIDS*, edited by Wolfgang Hein, Sonja Bartsch, and Lars Kohlmorgen, 119–145. New York: Palgrave Macmillan.

Kohr, Martin. 2010. "The Real Tragedy of Copenhagen." *Economic and Political Weekly* 45 (1): 10–13.

Krasner, Stephen D. 1976. "State Power and the Structure of International Trade." *World Politics* 28 (3): 317–347.

Krasner, Stephen D. 1982. "Structural Causes and Regime Consequences: Regimes as Intervening Variables." *International Organization* 36 (2): 185–205.

Krasner, Stephen D. 2004. "Sharing Sovereignty: New Institutions for Collapsed and Failing States." *International Security* 29 (2): 85–120.

Labonté, Ronald. 2008. "Global Health in Public Policy? Finding the Right Frame?" *Critical Public Health* 18 (4): 467–482.

Lancet. 2005. "Reversing the Failures of Roll Back Malaria." *Lancet* 365 (9469): 1439.

Lancet. 2014. "Ebola: What Lessons for the International Health Regulations?" *Lancet* 384: 1321.

Lanoszka, Anna. 2003. "The Global Politics of Intellectual Property Rights and Pharmaceutical Drug Policies in Developing Countries." *International Political Science Review* 24 (2): 181–197.

Lauren, Paul Gordon. 1996. *Power and Prejudice: The Politics and Diplomacy of Racial Discrimination.* Second edition. Boulder, CO: Westview.

Lauren, Paul Gordon. 2007. "To Preserve and Build on Its Achievements and to Redress Its Shortcomings: The Journey from the Commission on Human Rights to the Human Rights Council." *Human Rights Quarterly* 29 (2): 307–345.

Lee, Kelley. 2006. "Global Health Promotion: How Can We Strengthen Government and Build Effective Strategies?" *Health Promotion International* 21 (Suppl 1): 42–50.

Lee, Kelley. 2009. *The World Health Organization (WHO).* New York: Routledge.

Lee, Kelley and Meri Koivusalo. 2005. "Trade and Health: Is the Health Community Ready for Action?" *PLoS Medicine* 2 (1): e8.

Leeder, Stephen, Susan Raymond, Henry Greenburg, Hui Liu, and Kathy Esson. 2004. *A Race against Time: The Challenge of Cardiovascular Disease in Developing Economies.* New York: Columbia University.

Lencucha, Raphael, Anita Kothari, and Ronald Labonté. 2011. "The Role of Non-Governmental Organizations in Global Health Diplomacy: Negotiating the Framework Convention on Tobacco Control." *Health Policy and Planning* 26 (5): 405–412.

Levy, David L. and Aseem Prakash. 2003. "Bargains Old and New: Multinational Corporations in Global Governance." *Business and Politics* 5 (2): 131–150.

Lob-Levyt, Julian. 2011. "Contribution of the GAVI Alliance to Improving Health and Reducing Poverty." *Philosophical Transactions of the Royal Society B: Biological Sciences* 366 (1579): 2743–2747.

Luke, Douglass A. and Melissa Krauss. 2004. "Where There's Smoke There's Money: Tobacco Industry Campaign Contributions and U.S. Congressional Voting." *American Journal of Preventive Medicine* 27 (5): 363–372.

Ma, Zhenkun, Christian Lienhardt, Helen McIlleron, Andrew J. Nunn, and Xiexiu Wang. 2010. "Global Tuberculosis Drug Development Pipeline: The Need and the Reality." *The Lancet* 375 (9731): 2100–2109.

Mamudu, Hadii M. 2014. "The Interlocking World of Global Health Governance: The Tobacco Industry, Bilateral Investment Treaties, and Health Policy." In *Law and Global Health: Current Legal Issues Volume 16*, edited by Michael Freeman, Sarah Hawkes, and Belinda Bennett, 532–558. Oxford, UK: Oxford University Press.

Mamudu, Hadii M., Ross Hammond, and Stanton A. Glantz. 2008. "Project Cerberus: Tobacco Industry Strategy to Create an Alternative to the Framework Convention on Tobacco Control." *American Journal of Public Health* 98 (9): 1630–1642.

Mamudu, Hadii M., Ross Hammond, and Stanton A. Glantz. 2011. "International Trade versus Public Health during the FCTC Negotiations, 1999–2003." *Tobacco Control* 20 (1): e3.

Mann, Jonathan M. 1999. "Human Rights and AIDS: The Future of the Pandemic." In *Health and Human Rights: A Reader*, edited by Jonathan M. Mann, Sofia Gruskin, Michael A. Grodin, and George J. Annas, 216–226. New York: Routledge.

Mann, Jonathan M., Lawrence O. Gostin, Sofia Gruskin, Troyen Brennan, Zita Lazzarini, and Harvey V. Fineberg. 1994. "Health and Human Rights." *Health and Human Rights* 1 (1): 7–23.

Mann, Jonathan and Kathleen Kay. 1991. "Confronting the Pandemic: The World Health Organization: The World Health Organization's Global Programme on AIDS, 1986–1989." *AIDS 5* (Suppl 2): S221–S229.

Marquez, Patricio V. and Blanca Moreno-Dodson. 2017. *Tobacco Tax Reform at the Crossroads of Health and Development: A Multisectoral Perspective*. Washington DC: World Bank.

Mathers, Colin D. and Dejan Loncar. 2006. "Projections of Global Mortality and Burden of Disease from 2002 to 2030." *PLoS Medicine* 3 (11): e442.

Mathews, Jessica T. 1997. "Power Shift." *Foreign Affairs* 76 (1): 50–66.

McCormick, John. 1991. *Reclaiming Paradise: The Global Environmental Movement*. Bloomington: Indiana University Press.

McCoy, David, Sudeep Chand, and Devi Sridhar. 2009a. "Global Health Funding: How Much, Where It Comes From and Where It Goes." *Health Policy and Planning* 24 (6): 407–417.

McCoy, David, Gayatri Kembhavi, Jinesh Patel, Akish Luintel. 2009b. "The Bill & Melinda Gates Foundation's Grant-making Programme for Global Health." *The Lancet* 373: 1645–1653.

McInnes, Colin. 2006. "HIV/AIDS and Security." *International Affairs* 82 (2): 315–326.

McInnes, Colin. 2015. "WHO's Next? Changing Authority in Global Health Governance after Ebola." *International Affairs* 91 (6): 1299–1316.

McInnes, Colin, Adam Kamradt-Scott, Kelley Lee, Anne Roemer-Mahler, Simon Rushton, and Owain David Williams. 2014. *The Transformation of Global Health Governance*. New York: Palgrave Macmillan.

McInnes, Colin and Kelley Lee. 2006. "Health, Security, and Foreign Policy." *Review of International Studies* 32 (1): 5–23.

McInnes, Colin and Kelley Lee. 2012. *Global Health and International Relations*. Cambridge, UK: Polity.

McInnes, Colin and Simon Rushton. 2010. "HIV, AIDS and Security: Where Are We Now?" *International Affairs* 86 (1): 225–245.

McInnes, Colin and Simon Rushton. 2013. "HIV/AIDS and Securitization Theory." *European Journal of International Relations* 19 (1): 115–138.

McKinsey Global Institute. 2014. "Overcoming Obesity: An Initial Economic Analysis." https://www.mckinsey.com/~/media/McKinsey/Business%20Functions/Economic%20Studies%20TEMP/Our%20Insights/How%20the%20world%20could%20better%20fight%20obesity/MGI_Overcoming_obesity_Full_report.ashx (accessed January 30, 2018).

McMichael, Anthony J., Robyn Lucas, Anne-Louise Ponsonby, and Sally J. Edwards. 2003. "Stratospheric Ozone Depletion, Ultraviolet Radiation, and Health." In *Climate Change and Human Health: Risks and Responses*, edited by Anthony McMichael, Diarmid Campbell-Lendrum, Carlos F. Corvalan, Kristie L. Ebi, Andrew K. Githeko, Joel D. Scheraga, and Alistair Woodward, 159–180. Geneva: World Health Organization.

McMichael, Anthony J., Maria Neira, Roberto Bertollini, Diarmid Campbell-Lendrum, and Simon Hales. 2009. "Climate Change: A Time of Need and Opportunity for the Health Sector." *Lancet* 374: 2123–2125.

McNeil, Donald G. 2002. "New Drug for Malaria Pits U.S. against Africa." *New York Times*. May 28, 2002. http://www.nytimes.com/2002/05/28/health/new-drug-for-malaria-pits-us-against-africa.html (accessed January 20, 2018).

McNeil, Donald G. 2008. "Gates Foundation's Influence Criticized." *New York Times*, February 16, 2008. http://www.nytimes.com/2008/02/16/science/16malaria.html (accessed August 3, 2014).

McNeil, Donald G. 2014. "Ebola, Killing Scores in Guinea, Threatens Nearby Nations." *New York Times*. March 24, 2014. https://www.nytimes.com/2014/03/25/health/ebola-killing-scores-in-guinea-threatens-nearby-nations.html (accessed March 20, 2018).

McNeil, Donald G. 2016. "Zika Is No Longer a Global Emergency, W.H.O. Says." *New York Times*. November 18, 2016. https://www.nytimes.com/2016/11/19/health/who-ends-zika-global-health-emergency.html (accessed January 30, 2018).

McNeil, Donald G. and Rick Lyman. 2006. "Buffett's Billions Will Aid Fight against Disease." *New York Times*, June 27, 2006. http://www.nytimes.com/2006/06/27/us/27gates.html (accessed August 2, 2014).

Mearsheimer, John. 1994/1995. "The False Promise of International Institutions." *International Security* 19 (3): 5–49.

Mearsheimer, John J. 2001. *The Tragedy of Great Power Politics*. New York: W. W. Norton.

Médecins Sans Frontières. 1996. "Chantilly Principles." http://association.msf.org/sites/default/files/rst_library_item/Principles%20Chantilly%20EN.pdf (accessed August 6, 2014).

Médecins Sans Frontières. 2014. "MSF Charter and Principles." http://www.msf.org/msf-charter-and-principles (accessed July 25, 2014).

Meier, Benjamin Mason. 2010. "Global Health Governance and the Contentious Politics of Human Rights: Mainstreaming the Right to Health for Public Health Advancement." *Stanford Journal of International Law* 46: 1–50.

Mendis, Kamini, Aafje Rietveld, Marian Warsame, Andrea Bosman, Brian Greenwood, and Walther H. Wernsdorfer. 2009. "From Malaria Control to Eradication: The WHO Perspective." *Tropical Medicine and International Health* 14 (7): 1–7.

Merson, Michael H. Jeffrey O'Malley, David Serwadda, Chantawipa Apisuk. 2008. "The History and Challenge of HIV Prevention." *Lancet* 372 (9637): 475–488.

Mitchell, Ronald B. 1994. "Regime Design Matters: Intentional Oil Pollution and Treaty Compliance." *International Organization* 48 (3): 425–458.

Mitchell, Ronald B. 1998. "Sources of Transparency: Information Systems in International Regimes." *International Studies Quarterly* 42: 109–130.

Mitrany, David A. 1966. *A Working Peace System*. Chicago: Quadrangle Books.

Monteiro, Carlos A., Jean-Claude Moubarac, Geoffrey Cannon, Shu Wen Ng, and Barry M. Popkin. 2013. "Ultra-Processed Products Are Becoming Dominant in the Global Food System." *Obesity Reviews* 14 (Suppl. 2): 21–28.

Moodie, Rob, David Stuckler, Carlos Monteiro, Nick Sheron, Bruce Neal, Thaksaphon Thamarangsi, Paul Lincoln, Sally Casswell, and Lancet NCD Action Group. 2013. "Profits and Pandemics: Prevention of Harmful Effects of Tobacco, Alcohol, and Ultra-Processed Food and Drink Industries." *Lancet* 381 (9867): 670–679.

Moran, Michael and Michael Stevenson. 2013. "Illumination and Innovation: What Philanthropic Foundations Bring to Global Health Governance." *Global Society* 27 (2): 117–137.

Moravscik, Andrew. 1995. "Explaining International Human Rights Regimes: Liberal Theory and Western Europe." *European Journal of International Relations* 1 (2): 157–189.

Morgenthau, Hans. 1967. *Politics among Nations: The Struggle for Power and Peace*. Fourth Edition. New York: Knopf.

Morsink, Johannes. 1999. *The Universal Declaration of Human Rights: Origins, Drafting, and Intent*. Philadelphia: University of Pennsylvania Press.

Mukherjee, Joia S. 2013. "Financing Governments: Towards Achieving the Right to Health." In *Advancing the Human Right to Health*, edited by Jose M. Zuniga, Stephen P. Marks, and Lawrence O. Gostin 411–422. New York: Oxford University Press.

Murphy, Craig. N. 1994. *International Organizations and Industrial Change*. New York: Oxford University Press.
Murphy, Craig. N. 2000. "Global Governance: Poorly Done and Poorly Understood." *International Affairs* 76 (4): 789–804.
Murray, Christopher, Lisa C. Rosenfeld, Stephen S. Lim, Kathryn G. Andrews, Kyle J. Foreman, Diana Haring, Nancy Fullman, Mohsen Naghavi, Rafael Lozano, and Alan D. Lopez. 2012. "Global Malaria Mortality between 1980 and 2010: A Systematic Analysis." *Lancet* 379 (9814): 4–10.
Nabarro, David N. and Elizabeth M. Taylor. 1998. "The Roll Back Malaria Campaign." *Science* 280 (5372): 2062–2068.
Nájera, Jose A., Matiana González-Silva, and Pedro L. Alonso. 2011. "Some Lessons for the Future from the Global Malaria Eradication Programme (1955–1969)." *PLoS Medicine* 8 (1): e1000412. 1371/journal.pmed.1000412.
Nanda, Ved P. and George (Rock) Pring. 2013. *International Environmental Law and Policy for the 21st Century*. Second Edition. Leiden, The Netherlands: Martinus Nijhoff.
National Center for Health Statistics. 2015. *Prevalence of Obesity among Adults and Youth: United States, 2011–2014*, NCHS Data Brief No. 219. Washington, DC: National Center for Health Statistics.
Navarro, Vicente. 1976. *Medicine under Capitalism*. New York: Prodist.
Navarro, Vicente. 2002. "The World Health Report 2000: Can Health Care Systems Be Compared Using a Single Measure of Performance?" *American Journal of Public Health* 92 (1): 31–34.
Navarro, Vicente and Leiyu Shi. 2001. "The Political Context of Social Inequalities and Health." *Social Science and Medicine* 52 (3): 481–491.
Newell, Peter and Matthew Paterson. 1998. "A Climate for Business: Global Warming, the State, and Capital." *Review of International Political Economy* 5 (4): 679–703.
NGO Branch, Office for ECOSOC Support and Coordination, and UN Department of Economic and Social Affairs. 2018. "NGO Branch." http://csonet.org/ (accessed January 19, 2018).
Ngwena, Charles, Rebecca Cook, and Ebenezer Durojaye. 2013. "The Right to Health in Post-Apartheid Era South Africa." In *Advancing the Human Right to Health*, edited by Jose M. Zuniga, Stephen P. Marks, and Lawrence O. Gostin 129–141. New York: Oxford University Press.
Norum, Kaare R. 2005. "World Health Organization's Global Strategy on Diet, Physical Activity and Health: The Process behind the Scenes." *Scandinavian Journal of Nutrition* 49: 83–88.
Nowotny, Thomas. 2011. *Diplomacy and Global Governance: The Diplomatic Service in an Age of Worldwide Interdependence*. New Brunswick, Canada: Transaction Publishers.
Oaks, Stanley C., Violaine S. Mitchell, Greg W. Pearson, and Charles C. J. Carpenter. 1991. *Malaria: Obstacles and Opportunities*. Washington, DC: National Academy Press.
Office of the United Nations High Commissioner for Human Rights and the Joint United Nations Programme on HIV/AIDS. 2006. *International Guidelines on HIV/*

AIDS and Human Rights: 2006 Consolidated Version. Geneva, Switzerland: Office of the United Nations High Commissioner for Human Rights and the Joint United Nations Programme on HIV/AIDS. http://www.ohchr.org/Documents/Publications/HIVAIDSGuidelinesen.pdf (accessed June 13, 2015).

Ogden, Jessica, Gill Walt, and Louisiana Lush. 2003. "The Politics of 'Branding' in Policy Transfer: The Case of DOTS for Tuberculosis Control." *Social Science and Medicine* 57 (1): 179–188.

Okowa, Phoebe. 2009. "The Legal Framework for the Protection of the Environment against Transboundary Air Pollution: A Reflection of Customary and Treaty Law." In *The Protection of Ambient Air in International and European Law*, edited by Harry Post, 53–72. AJ Utrecht, The Netherlands: Eleven International Publishing.

Olivier, Jos, Greet Janssens-Maenhout, Marilena Muntean, and Jeroen A. H. W. Peters. 2015. "Trends in Global CO_2 Emissions: 2015 Report." *PBL Netherlands Environmental Assessment Agency*. http://edgar.jrc.ec.europa.eu/news_docs/jrc-2015-trends-in-global-co2-emissions-2015-report-98184.pdf (accessed May 9, 2016).

Olson, Mancur. 1968. *The Logic of Collective Action*. New York: Schocken.

O'Manique, Colleen. 2004. *Neoliberalism and the AIDS Crisis in Sub-Saharan Africa*. New York: Palgrave Macmillan.

Orgad, Liav. 2010. "The Preamble in Constitutional Interpretation." *International Journal of Constitutional Law* 8 (4): 714–738.

Organization for Economic Cooperation and Development. 2017. *Health at a Glance 2017: OECD Indicators*. http://www.oecd.org/els/health-systems/Health-at-a-Glance-2017-Chartset.pdf (accessed January 30, 2018).

Ostrom, Elinor. 1990. *Governing the Commons: The Evolution of Institutions for Collective Action*. Cambridge, UK: Cambridge University Press.

Oxfam International. 2014a. "Why Do We Care about Trade?" http://www.oxfam.org/en/campaigns/trade/about (accessed July 29, 2014).

Oxfam International. 2014b. "Put Public First, and Provide HealthCare for All." http://www.oxfam.org/en/campaigns/health-education/primary-healthcare-services (accessed July 29, 2014).

Packard, Randall M. 1997. "Malaria Dreams: Postwar Visions of Health and Development in the Third World." *Medical Anthropology* 17 (3): 279–296.

Packard, Randall M. 2007. *The Making of a Tropical Disease: A Short History of Malaria*. Baltimore, MD: Johns Hopkins University Press.

Pagano, Heather and Marc Poncin. 2017. "Treating, Containing, Mobilizing: The Role of Médecins Sans Frontières in the West African Ebola Epidemic Response." In *Global Management of Infectious Disease after Ebola*, edited by Sam F. Halabi, Larence O. Gostin, and Jeffrey S. Crowley, 33–53. New York: Oxford University Press.

Paim, Jairnilson, Claudia Travassos, Celia Almeida, Ligia Bahia, and James Macinko. 2011. "The Brazilian Health System: History, Advances, and Challenges." *Lancet* 377: 1778–1797.

Parker, Elizabeth Rindskopf and Bryan Pate. 2005. "Implementing UN Security Council Resolution 1540 to Combat the Proliferation of Biological Weapons." *Biosecurity and Bioterrorism* 3 (2):166–173.

Patterson, Amy S. 2007. "The UN and the Fight against HIV/AIDS." In *The Global Politics of AIDS*, edited by Paul G. Harris and Patricia D. Siplon, 203–224. Boulder, CO: Lynne Rienner.

Peterson, Susan. 2002/2003. "Epidemic Disease and National Security." *Security Studies* 12 (2): 43–81.

Pinson, Lauren, Mila Johns, and Gary Ackerman. 2013. "Ricin Letters Mailed to President and Senator." https://www.start.umd.edu/sites/default/files/files/publications/br/STARTBackgroundReport_RicinMailings_April2013.pdf (accessed September 20, 2016).

Poku, Nana K. 2002. "Global Pandemics: HIV/AIDS." In *Governing Globalization*, edited by David Held and Anthony McGrew, 111–126. Cambridge, UK: Polity.

Popkin, Barry M. 1998. "The Nutrition Transition and Its Health Implications in Low-Income Countries." *Public Health Nutrition* 1 (1): 5–21.

Popkin, Barry M. 2006. "Global Nutrition Dynamics: The World Is Shifting Rapidly toward a Diet Linked with Noncommunicable Diseases." *American Journal of Clinical Nutrition* 84 (2): 289–298.

Popkin, Barry M. 2011. "Does Global Obesity Represent a Public Health Challenge?" *American Journal of Clinical Nutrition* 93 (2): 232–233.

Porter, John, Kelley Lee, and Jessica Ogden. 2002. "The Globalisation of DOTS: Tuberculosis in a Global Emergency." In *Health Policy in a Globalising World*, edited by Kelley Lee, Kent Buse, and Suzanne Fustukian, 181–194. Cambridge: Cambridge University Press.

Powell, Robert. 1991. "Absolute and Relative Gains in International Relations Theory." *American Political Science Review* 85 (4): 1303–1320.

President's Emergency Plan for AIDS Relief. 2017. "PEPFAR Funding." https://www.pepfar.gov/documents/organization/252516.pdf (accessed January 29, 2018).

Price-Smith, Andrew T. 2009. *Contagion and Chaos: Disease, Ecology, and National Security in the Era of Globalization*. Cambridge, MA: MIT Press.

Pring, George (Rock). 2002. "The 2002 Johannesburg World Summit on Sustainable Development: International Environmental Law Collides with Reality, Turning Jo'Burg into 'Joke'Burg'." *Denver Journal of International Law and Policy* 30 (3): 410–419.

Quarmby, Katherine. 2005. "Why Oxfam Is Failing Africa." *New Statesmen*. http://www.newstatesman.com/world-affairs/world-affairs/2014/04/why-oxfam-failing-africa (accessed August 13, 2014).

Rajamani, Lavanya. 2009. "Addressing the 'Post-Kyoto' Stress Disorder: Reflections on the Emerging Legal Architecture of the Climate Change Regime." *The International and Comparative Law Quarterly* 58 (4): 803–834.

Ramlogan, Rajendra. 2011. *Sustainable Development: Towards a Judicial Interpretation*. The Hague, The Netherlands: Martinus Nijhoff Publishers.

Rassy, Dunia and Richard D. Smith. 2013. "The Economic Impact of H1N1 on Mexico's Tourist and Pork Sectors." *Health Economics* 22 (7): 824–834.

Raviglione, Mario, Ben Marais, Katherine Floyd, Knut Lönnroth, Haileyesus Getahun, Giovanni B. Migliori, and Anthony D. Harries, et al. 2012. "Scaling Up Interventions to Achieve Global Tuberculosis Control: Progress and New Developments." *Lancet* 379 (9829): 1902–1913.

Raviglione, Mario C. and Antonio Pio. 2002. "Evolution of WHO policies for Tuberculosis Control, 1948–2001." Lancet 359: 775–780.

Rayner, Geof, Corinna Hawkes, Tim Lang, and Walden Bello. 2006. "Trade Liberalization and the Diet Transition: A Public Health Response." *Health Promotion International* 21 (Suppl 1): 67–74.

Rehm, Jürgen, Colin Mathers, Svetlana Popova, Montarat Thavorncharoensap, Yot Teerawattananon, and Jayadeep Patra. 2009. "Global Burden of Disease and Injury and Economic Cost Attributable to Alcohol Use and Alcohol-use Disorders." *Lancet* 373 (9682): 2223–2233.

Reimann, Kim D. 2006. "A View From the Top: International Politics, Norms, and the Worldwide Growth of NGOs." *International Studies Quarterly* 50 (1): 45–67.

Reuters. 2014. "Ebola Still Spreading, W.H.O. Reports." *New York Times*. December 31, 2014. https://www.nytimes.com/2015/01/01/world/africa/ebola-still-spreading-who-reports.html (accessed January 30, 2018).

Risse, Thomas and Kathryn Sikkink. 1999. "The Socialization of International Human Rights Norms and Domestic Change: Introduction." In *The Power of Human Rights: International Norms and Domestic Change*, edited by Thomas Risse, Stephen C. Ropp, and Kathryn Sikkink, 1–38. Cambridge, UK: Cambridge University Press.

Roach, Brian. 2005. "A Primer on Multinational Corporations." In *Leviathans: Multinational Corporations and the New Global History*, edited by Alfred D. Chandler and Bruce Mazlish, 19–44. Cambridge, UK: Cambridge University Press.

Roemer, Ruth, Allyn L. Taylor, and Jean Lariviere. 2005. "Origins of the WHO Framework Convention on Tobacco Control." *American Journal of Public Health* 95: 936–938.

Rogelj, Joeri, Gunnar Luderer, Robert C. Pietzcker, Elmar Kriegler, Michiel Schaeffer, Volker Krey, and Keywan Riahi. 2015. "Energy System Transformations for Limiting End-of-Century Warming to below 1.5°C." *Nature Climate Change* 5: 519–527.

Romero, Sergio and John M. Broder. 2012. "Progress on Sidelines as Rio Conference Ends." *New York Times*. June 23, 2012. http://www.nytimes.com/2012/06/24/world/americas/rio20-conference-ends-with-some-progress-on-the-sidelines.html (accessed August 11, 2015).

Room, Robin. 1984. "The World Health Organization and Alcohol Control." *British Journal of Addiction* 79: 85–92.

Room, Robin. 2005. "Negotiating the Place of Alcohol in Public Health: The Arguments at the Interface." *Addiction* 100: 1396–1397.

Rosen, Amanda. 2015. "The Wrong Solution at the Right Time: The Failure of the Kyoto Protocol on Climate Change." *Politics and Policy* 43 (1): 30–58.

Rosenau, James N. 1990. *Turbulence in World Politics*. Princeton, NJ: Princeton University Press.

Rosenau, James N. 2005. "Global Governance as Disaggregated Complexity." In *Contending Perspectives on Global Governance: Coherence, Contestation, and World Order*, edited by Alice D. Ba and Matthew J. Hoffmann, 131–153. London: Routledge.

Rosenau, William. 2001. "Aum Shinrikyo's Biological Weapons Program: Why Did It Fail?" *Studies in Conflict and Terrorism* 24: 289–301.

Roser. Max. 2017. "Fertility Rate." *Our World in Data*. https://ourworldindata.org/fertility-rate (accessed March 10, 2018).

Rothschild, Emma. 1995. "What Is Security?" *Daedalus* 124 (3): 53–98.

Rowlands, Ian H. 1995. *The Politics of Global Atmospheric Change*. New York: Manchester University Press.

Ruger, Jennifer Prah. 2005. "The Changing Role of the World Bank in Global Health." *American Journal of Public Health* 95: 50–70.

Rushton, Simon. 2010. "AIDS and International Security in the United Nations System." *Health Policy and Planning* 25: 495–504.

Sabot, Oliver, Justin M. Cohen, Michelle S. Hsiang, James G. Kahn, Suprotik Basu, Linhua Tang, and Bin Zheng, et al. 2010. "Costs and Financial Feasibility of Malaria Elimination." *Lancet* 376 (9752): 6–12.

Sack, Kevin, Sheri Fink, Pam Belluck, and Adam Nossiter. 2014. "How Ebola Roared Back." *New York Times*. December 29, 2014. https://www.nytimes.com/2014/12/30/health/how-ebola-roared-back.html (accessed January 20, 2018).

Salerno, Reynolds M., Jennifer Gaudioso, Rebecca L. Frerichs, and Daniel Estes. 2004. "A BW Risk Assessment: Historical and Technical Perspectives." *The Nonproliferation Review* (Fall/Winter): 25–55.

Sands, Philippe and Jacqueline Peel. 2012. *Principles of International Environmental Law*. Third Edition. Cambridge, UK: Cambridge University Press.

Saspin, Jason W., Theresa M. Thompson, Lesley Stone, and Katherine E. De Land. 2003. "International Trade, Law, and Public Health Advocacy." *Journal of Law, Medicine, and Ethics* 31: 546–556.

Schelling, Thomas C. 2002. "What Makes Greenhouse Sense? Time to Rethink the Kyoto Protocol." *Foreign Affairs* 81 (3): 2–9.

Selgelid, Michael J. 2008. "Ethics, Tuberculosis and Globalization." *Public Health Ethics* 1 (1): 10–20.

Sell, Susan K. 2007. "TRIPS-Plus Trade Agreements and Access to Medicines." *Liverpool Law Review* 28: 41–75.

Sending, Ole Jacob and Iver B. Neumann. 2006. "Governance to Governability: Analyzing NGOs, States, and Power." *International Studies Quarterly* 50 (3): 651–672.

Sengupta, Somini. 2015. "Effort on Ebola Hurt W.H.O. Chief." *New York Times*. January 6, 2015. https://www.nytimes.com/2015/01/07/world/leader-of-world-health-organization-defends-ebola-response.html (accessed January 18, 2018).

Shear, Michael D. 2017. "Trump Will Withdraw U.S. from Paris Climate Agreement." *New York Times*. June 1, 2017. https://www.nytimes.com/2017/06/01/climate/trump-paris-climate-agreement.html (accessed January 29, 2018).

Shepard, Benjamin Heim. 2007 "Shifting Priorities in US AIDS Policy." In *The Global Politics of AIDS*, edited by Paul G. Harris and Patricia D. Siplon, 171–199. Boulder, CO: Lynne Rienner.

Shimkin, Michael B. 1946. "The World Health Organization." *Science* 104 (2700): 281–283.

Simon, Roger. 1982. *Gramsci's Political Thought*. London: Lawrence Wilson.

Sims, Nicholas A. 2011. "A Simple Treaty, a Complex Fulfillment: A Short History of the Biological Weapons Fulfillment Conferences." *Bulletin of the Atomic Scientists* 67 (3): 8–15.

Smith, Randall. 2014. "As His Foundation Has Grown, Gates Has Slowed His Donations." *New York Times*, May 26, 2014. http://dealbook.nytimes.com/2014/05/26/as-his-foundation-has-grown-gates-has-slowed-his-donations/ (accessed August 3, 2014).

Soltau, Friedrich. 2009. *Fairness in Climate Change Law and Policy*. Cambridge, UK: Cambridge University Press.

Son, Kyung-Bok and Tae-Jin Lee. 2017. "Compulsory Licensing of Pharmaceuticals Reconsidered: Current Situation and Implications for Access to Medicines." *Global Public Health* 1–11.

Sprinz, Detlef and Tapani Vaahtoranta. 1994. "The Interest-Based Explanation of International Environmental Policy." *International Organization* 48 (1): 77–105.

Sterling-Folker, Jennifer. 2005. "Realist Global Governance: Revisiting Cave! Hic Dragones and Beyond." In *Contending Perspectives on Global Governance: Coherence, Contestation, and World Order*, edited by Alice D. Ba and Matthew J. Hoffmann, 17–38. London: Routledge

Stolberg, Sheryl Gay. 2008. "In Global Battle on AIDS, Bush Creates Legacy." *New York Times*. January 5, 2008.

Strickman, Daniel, Stephen P. Frances, and Mustapha Debboun. 2009. *Prevention of Bug Bites, Stings, and Disease*. New York: Oxford University Press.

Stroup, Sarah S. 2012. *Borders among Activists: International NGOs in the United States, Britain, and France*. Ithaca, NY: Cornell University Press.

Stubbs, Thomas, Alexander Kentikelenis, David Stuckler, Martin McKee, and Lawrence King. 2017. "The Impact of IMF Conditionality on Government Health Expenditure: A Cross-National Analysis of 16 West African Nations." *Social Science and Medicine* 174: 220–227.

Stuckler, David, Corinna Hawkes, and Derek Yach. 2009. "Governance of Chronic Diseases." In *Making Sense of Global Health Governance*, edited by Kent Buse, Wolfgang Hein, and Nick Drager, 268–293. New York: Palgrave Macmillan.

Stuckler, David, Sanjay Basu, and Martin McKee. 2011. "International Monetary Fund and Aid Displacement." *International Journal of Health Services* 41 (1): 67–76.

Studlar, Donley T. 2008. "U.S. Tobacco Control: Public Health, Political Economy, or Morality Policy?" *Review of Policy Research* 25 (5): 393–410.

Tannenwald, Nina. 1999. "The Nuclear Taboo: The United States and the Normative Basis of Nuclear Non-Use." *International Organization* 53 (3): 433–468.

Taylor, Allyn L., Frank J. Chaloupka, Emmanuel Guindon, and Michaelyn Corbett. 2000. "Trade Policy and Tobacco Control." In *Tobacco Control in Developing Countries*, edited by Prabhat Jha and Frank Chaloupka, 343–364. Oxford: Oxford University Press.

Taylor, Allyn L. and Ibadat Dhillon. 2013. "An International Legal Strategy for Alcohol Control: Not a Framework Convention—At Least Not Yet." *Addiction* 108: 450–455.

Teschke, Benno. 2008. "Marxism." In *The Oxford Handbook of International Relations*, edited by Christian Reus-Smit and Duncan Snidal, 163–187. New York: Oxford University Press.

Thomas, Caroline and Martin Weber. 2004. "The Politics of Global Governance: Whatever Happened to 'Health for All by the Year 2000." *Global Governance* 10: 187–205.

Thucydides. 1972. *History of the Peloponnesian War*, translated by Rex Warner. Harmondsworth, UK: Penguin.

Tobin, John. 2012. *The Right to Health in International Law*. New York: Oxford University Press.

Tomasevski, Katarina, Sofia Gruskin, Zita Lazzarini, and Aart Hendriks. 1992. "AIDS and Human Rights." In *AIDS in the World*, edited by Jonathan Mann, Daniel J. M. Tarantola, and Thomas W. Netter, 537–573. Cambridge, MA: Harvard University Press.

UNAIDS. 2016. *Global AIDS Update 2016*. Geneva: UNAIDS. http://www.who.int/hiv/pub/arv/global-AIDS-update-2016_en.pdf?ua=1 (accessed January 29, 2018).

UNAIDS. 2017. *UNAIDS Data 2017*. Geneva: UNAIDS. http://www.unaids.org/sites/default/files/media_asset/20170720_Data_book_2017_en.pdf (accessed January 29, 2018).

United Nations. 1972. *Report of the United Nations Conference on the Human Environment*. UN Doc. A/CONF.48/14/Rev.1.

United Nations. 1989. *Convention on the Rights of the Child*. New York: United Nations.

United Nations. 2013. "About the UN Global Compact." http://www.unglobalcompact.org/AboutTheGC/index.html (accessed June 13, 2014).

United Nations. 2015a. "Millennium Development Goals: 2015 Progress Chart." http://www.un.org/millenniumgoals/2015_MDG_Report/pdf/MDG%202015%20PC%20final.pdf. (accessed June 22, 2016).

United Nations. 2015b. *The Millennium Goals Report 2015*. New York: United Nations. http://www.un.org/millenniumgoals/2015_MDG_Report/pdf/MDG%202015%20rev%20(July%201).pdf (accessed June 22, 2016).

United Nations Environmental Programme. 2014. "Ozone Layer on Track to Recovery: Success Story Should Encourage Action on Climate." https://www.unenvironment.org/news-and-stories/press-release/ozone-layer-track-recovery-success-story-should-encourage-action (accessed May 28, 2016).

United Nations Environmental Programme. 2015. "About UNEP." http://www.unep.org/about/ (accessed July 29, 2015).

United Nations General Assembly. 1972. *Institutional and Financial Commitments for International Environmental Cooperation*, A/RES/27/2997 (December 15). http://www.un-documents.net/a27r2997.htm

United Nations General Assembly. 1979. *Health as an Integral Part of Development*, A/RES/34/58 (November 29) http://www.un.org/documents/ga/res/34/a34res58.pdf

United Nations General Assembly. 2001. *Declaration of Commitment on HIV/AIDS*, A/RES/S-26/2 (June 27) http://www.un.org/ga/aids/docs/aress262.pdf

United Nations General Assembly. 2006a. *Human Rights Council*, A/RES/60/251 (March 15) http://www.un.org/en/ga/search/view_doc.asp?symbol=A/RES/60/251

United Nations General Assembly. 2006b. *Political Declaration on HIV/AIDS*, A/RES/60/262 (June 2) http://www.un.org/en/ga/search/view_doc.asp?symbol=A/RES/60/262&Lang=E

United Nations General Assembly. 2010. *Prevention and Control of Non-Communicable Diseases*, A/RES/64/265 (May 20) http://www.who.int/nmh/events/2011/UN_resolution_prevention_control_ncds.pdf

United Nations General Assembly. 2011. *Political Declaration on HIV and AIDS: Intensifying Our Efforts to Eliminate HIV and AIDS*, A/RES/70/266 (June 8) http://www.un.org/en/ga/search/view_doc.asp?symbol=A/RES/70/266

United Nations General Assembly. 2014. *Measures to Contain and Combat the Recent Ebola Outbreak in West Africa*, A/RES/69/1 (September 19) http://www.un.org/en/ga/search/view_doc.asp?symbol=A/RES/69/1

United Nations Security Council. 2011. *Resolution 1983*, S/RES/1983 (June 7) http://www.un.org/en/ga/search/view_doc.asp?symbol=S/RES/1983(2011)

United Nations Security Council. 2014. *Resolution 2177*, S/RES/2177 (September 18) http://www.un.org/en/ga/search/view_doc.asp?symbol=S/RES/2177%20(2014)

United Nations Treaty Collection. 2018. "Chapter IV: Human Rights." https://treaties.un.org/pages/Treaties.aspx?id=4&subid=A&lang=en (accessed January 29, 2018).

Vienna Convention for the Protection of the Ozone Layer. Opened for signature March 22, 1985. *United Nations Treaty Series* 1513: 293. https://treaties.un.org/doc/Treaties/1988/09/19880922%2003-14%20AM/Ch_XXVII_02p.pdf (accessed May 26, 2016).

Volberding, Paul A. and Steven G. Deeks. 2010. "Antiretroviral Therapy and Management of HIV Infection." *Lancet* 376 (9734): 49–62.

Volger, John. 2003. "Taking Institutions Seriously: How Regime Analysis Can Be Relevant to Multilevel Environmental Governance." *Global Environmental Politics* 3 (2): 25–39.

von Stein, Jana. 2008. "The International Law and Politics of Climate Change: Ratification of the United Nations Framework Convention and the Kyoto Protocol." *The Journal of Conflict Resolution* 52 (2): 243–268.

Voon, Tania. 2013. "Flexibilities in WTO Law to Support Tobacco Control Regulation." *American Journal of Law and Medicine* 39: 199–217.

Wagner, Theodore L., Michael Siegel, and Belinda Borrelli. 2012. "Electronic Cigarettes: Achieving a Balanced Perspective." *Addiction* 107: 1545–1548.

Waldman, Amy. 2002. "Gates Offers India $100 Million to Fight AIDS." *New York Times*, November 12, 2002. http://www.nytimes.com/2002/11/12/world/gates-offers-india-100-million-to-fight-aids.html (accessed August 2, 2014).

Wallerstein, Immanuel. 1974. "The Rise and Future Demise of the World Capitalist System: Concepts for Comparative Analysis." *Comparative Studies in Society and History* 16 (4): 387–415.

Walsh, Julia A. and Kenneth Walsh. 1979. "Selective Primary Health Care—An Interim Strategy for Disease Control in Developing Countries." *New England Journal of Medicine* 301: 967–974.

Walt, Gill. 1999. "The Politics of Tuberculosis: The Role of Process and Power." In *Tuberculosis: An Interdisciplinary Perspective*, edited by John D. H. Porter and John M. Grange, 67–98. London: Imperial College Press.

Waltz, Kenneth. 1979. *Theory of International Politics*. Reading, MA: Addison-Wesley.

Waltz, Susan. 2001. "Universalizing Human Rights: The Role of Small States in the Construction of the Universal Declaration of Human Rights." *Human Rights Quarterly* 23 (1): 44–72.

Warner, Kenneth E. 2005. "The Role of Research in International Tobacco Control." *American Journal of Public Health* 95 (6): 976–984.

Warrick, Joby. 2010. "FBI Investigation of 2001 Anthrax Attacks Concluded; U.S. Releases Details." *Washington Post*, February 20, 2010. Available at http://www.washingtonpost.com/wp-dyn/content/article/2010/02/19/AR2010021902369.html (accessed September 25, 2016).

Watson, James L. 2006. *Golden Arches East: McDonald's in East Asia*. Second Edition. Stanford, CA: Stanford University Press.

Watts, Nick, W. Neil Adger, Paolo Agnolucci, Jason Blackstock, Peter Byass, Wenjia Cai, and Sarah Chaytor, et al. 2015. "Health and Climate Change Policy: Policy Responses to protect Public Health." *Lancet* 386: 1861–1894.

Weir, Lorna. 2015. "Inventing Global Health Security, 1994–2005." In *The Routledge Handbook of Global Health Security*, edited by Simon Rushton and Jeremy Youde, 18–31. London: Routledge.

Weishaar, Heide, Jeff Collin, Katherine Smith, Thilo Grüning, Sema Mandal, and Anna Gilmore. 2012. "Global Health Governance and the Commercial Sector: A Documentary Analysis of Tobacco Company Strategies to Influence the WHO Framework Convention on Tobacco Control." *PLoS Medicine* 9(6): e1001249.

Weiss, Thomas G. 2000. "Governance, Good Governance and Global Governance: Conceptual and Actual Challenges." *Third World Quarterly* 21 (5): 795–814.

Wendt, Alexander. 1992. "Anarchy Is What States Make of It: The Social Construction of Power Politics." *International Organization* 46 (2): 391–425.

West, Keith P., Benjamin Caballero, and Robert E. Black. 2006. "Nutrition." In *International Public Health: Diseases, Programs, Systems, and Policies*. Second Edition, edited by Michael H. Merson, Robert E. Black, and Anne J. Mills, 187–272. Sudbury, MA: Jones and Bartlett Publishers.

Whelan, Daniel J. and Jack Donnelly. 2007. "The West, Economic and Social Rights and the Global Human Rights Regime: Setting the Record Straight." *Human Rights Quarterly* 29 (4): 908–949.

The White House. 2016. "Fact Sheet: The Global Health Security Agenda." https://www.whitehouse.gov/the-press-office/2015/07/28/fact-sheet-global-health-security-agenda (accessed July 15, 2016).

WHO Ebola Response Team. 2016. "After Ebola in West Africa—Unpredictable Risks, Preventable Epidemics." *New England Journal of Medicine* 375: 587–596.

Wiley, Lindsay F. 2010. "Moving Global Health Law Upstream: A Critical Appraisal of Global Health Law as a Tool for Health Adaptation to Climate Change." *Georgetown International Environmental Law Review* 22: 439–489.

Willetts, Peter. 2011. *Non-Governmental Organizations in World Politics*. New York: Routledge.

Wipfli, Heather and Grace Huang. 2011. "Power of the Process: Evaluating the Impact of the Framework Convention on Tobacco Control Negotiations." *Health Policy* 100: 107–115.

Wise, Jacqui. 2006. "Access to AIDS Medicines Stumbles on Trade Rules." *Bulletin of the World Health Organization* 84 (5): 342–344.

Wohlforth, William. 2008. "Realism." In *The Oxford Handbook of International Relations*, edited by Christian Reus-Smit and Duncan Snidal, 131–149. New York: Oxford University Press.

Wolfers, Arnold. 1952. "'National Security' as an Ambiguous Symbol." *Political Science Quarterly* 67 (4): 481–502.

Wolff, Jonathan. 2012. *The Human Right to Health*. New York: W.W. Norton.

Woods, Ngaire. 2002. "Global Governance and the Role of Institutions." In *Governing Globalization*, edited by David Held and Andrew McGrew, 25–45. Cambridge, UK: Polity.

Woodward, David. 2005. "The GATS and Trade in Health Services: Implications for Health Care in Developing Countries." *Review of International Political Economy* 12 (3): 511–534.

World Bank. 1993. *World Development Report 1993: Investing in Health*. Washington, DC: World Bank.

World Bank. 1999. *Curbing the Epidemic: Governments and the Economics of Tobacco Control*. Washington, DC: World Bank.

World Bank. 2007. *Healthy Development: The World Bank Strategy for Health, Nutrition, and Population Results*. Washington, DC: World Bank.

World Bank. 2012. *Human Rights and Economics: Tensions and Positive* Relationships. Washington, DC: World Bank. http://siteresources.worldbank.org/PROJECTS/Resources/40940133106826855 8/Report_Development_Fragility_Human_Rights.pdf (accessed January 29, 2018).

World Bank. 2015. "Funding Boost for Climate Action." http://www.worldbank.org/en/news/feature/2015/10/10/funding-boost-for-climate-action (accessed May 21, 2016).

World Bank. 2016a. "2014–2015 West Africa Ebola Crisis: Impact Update." http://www.worldbank.org/en/topic/macroeconomics/publication/2014-2015-west-africa-ebola-crisis-impact-update (accessed January 30, 2018).

World Bank. 2016b. "Overview." http://www.worldbank.org/en/topic/climatefinance/overview (accessed May 21, 2016).

World Bank. 2016c. "World Development Indicators: CO2 Emissions (kt)." http://data.worldbank.org/indicator/EN.ATM.CO2E.KT/countries (accessed May 5, 2016).

World Bank. 2017. "Universal Health Coverage." http://www.worldbank.org/en/topic/universalhealthcoverage (accessed January 13, 2018).

World Commission on Environment and Development. 1987. *Our Common Future*. Oxford: Oxford University Press.

World Health Assembly. 1977. *Technical Cooperation*, WHA30.43 (May 19) http://apps.who.int/iris/handle/10665/93206

World Health Assembly. 1979. *Development of the WHO Programme on Alcohol-related Problems*, WHA32.40 (May 25) http://www.who.int/substance_abuse/en/WHA32.40.pdf

World Health Assembly. 2005. *Public-Health Problems Caused by Harmful Use of Alcohol*, WHA58.26 (May 25), http://www.who.int/substance_abuse/wha58_26_en.pdf

World Health Assembly. 2008. *Strategies to Reduce the Harmful Use of Alcohol*, WHA61.4 (May 24), http://apps.who.int/gb/ebwha/pdf_files/WHA61-REC1/A61_Rec1-part2-en.pdf

World Health Organization. 1978. *Declaration of Alma-Ata*. Geneva: World Health Organization.

World Health Organization. 1993. *A Global Strategy for Malaria Control*. Geneva: World Health Organization.

World Health Organization. 1998a. *Global Tuberculosis Control: WHO Report 1998*. Geneva: World Health Organization.

World Health Organization. 1998b. "Environmental Matters: Climate Change and Human Health—WHO Participation in the Interagency Climate Agenda." WHO Doc. A51/21. *Report by the Director-General*. March 5, 1998.

World Health Organization. 2003a. "Severe Acute Respiratory Syndrome (SARS)—Multi-Country Outbreak—Update, 15 March 2003." http://www.who.int/csr/don/2003_03_16/en/index.html (accessed September 5, 2013).

World Health Organization. 2003b. "Severe Acute Respiratory Syndrome (SARS)—Multi-Country Outbreak—Update, 1 April 2003." http://www.who.int/csr/don/2003_03_16/en/index.html (accessed September 5, 2013).

World Health Organization. 2003c. "Update 92-Chronology of Travel Recommendations, Areas with Local Transmission, 1 July 2003." http://www.who.int/csr/don/2003_07_01/en/index.html (accessed September 5, 2013).

World Health Organization 2003d. *WHO Framework Convention on Tobacco Control*. World Health Organization: Geneva.

World Health Organization. 2005. "Access to HIV Treatment Continues to Accelerate in Developing Countries, But Bottlenecks Persist, Says WHO/UNAIDS Report." http://www.who.int/3by5/progressreportJune2005/en/ (accessed November 5, 2017).

World Health Organization. 2007. *The World Health Report 2007: A Safer Future: Global Public Health Security in the 21st Century*. Geneva: World Health Organization.

World Health Organization. 2008a. *The Global Burden of Disease: 2004 Update*. Geneva: World Health Organization.

World Health Organization. 2008b. *WHO Report on the Global Tobacco Epidemic 2008: The MPOWER Package*. Geneva: World Health Organization. Available at http://www.who.int/tobacco/mpower/gtcr_download/en/ (accessed January 27, 2018).

World Health Organization. 2008c. *World Health Report: Primary Health Care-Now More than Ever*. Geneva: World Health Organization.

World Health Organization. 2009. *Global Health Risks: Mortality and Burden of Disease Attributable to Selected Major Risks*. Geneva: World Health Organization. Available at http://www.who.int/healthinfo/global_burden_disease/GlobalHealthRisks_report_full.pdf (accessed January 27, 2018).

World Health Organization. 2010. *Global Strategy to Reduce the Harmful Use of Alcohol*. Geneva: World Health Organization.

World Health Organization. 2011. *WHO Public Health and Environment Global Strategy Overview 2011*. http://www.who.int/phe/publications/PHE_2011_global_strategy_overview_2011.pdf (accessed July 22, 2015).

World Health Organization. 2012a. *Accelerating Work to Overcome the Global Impact of Neglected Tropical Diseases*. Geneva: World Health Organization. Available at http://www.who.int/neglected_diseases/resources/WHO_HTM_NTD_2012.1/en/ (accessed January 29, 2018).

World Health Organization. 2012b. "Ebola Haemorrhagic Fever." http://www.who.int/mediacentre/factsheets/fs103/en/ (accessed September 9, 2013).

World Health Organization. 2014a. "WHO Statement on the Meeting of the International Health Regulations Emergency Committee regarding the 2014 Ebola Outbreak in West Africa." August 8, 2014. http://who.int/mediacentre/news/statements/2014/ebola-20140808/en/ (accessed January 19, 2015).

World Health Organization. 2014b. *Global Status Report on Noncommunicable Diseases 2014*. Geneva. World Health Organization.

World Health Organization. 2014c. *Global Status Report on Alcohol and Health 2014*. Geneva: World Health Organization.

World Health Organization. 2014d. *Quantitative Risk Assessment of the Effects of Climate Change on Selected Causes of Death, 2030s and 2050s*. Geneva: World Health Organization.

World Health Organization. 2014e. *Burden of Disease from Ambient Air Pollution*. http://www.who.int/phe/health_topics/outdoorair/databases/AAP_BoD_results_March2014.pdf?ua=1 (accessed May 30, 2016).

World Health Organization. 2014f. "7 Million Premature Deaths Annually Linked to Air Pollution." http://www.who.int/mediacentre/news/releases/2014/air-pollution/en/ (accessed May 30, 2016).

World Health Organization. 2015a. *World Tuberculosis Report 2015*. Geneva: World Health Organization.

World Health Organization. 2015b. *WHO Report on the Global Tobacco Epidemic, 2015*. Geneva: World Health Organization. http://www.who.int/tobacco/global_report/2015/en/ (accessed January 30, 2018).

World Health Organization 2015c. "World Health Assembly Closes, Passing Resolutions on Air Pollution and Epilepsy." http://www.who.int/mediacentre/news/releases/2015/wha-26-may-2015/en/ (accessed May 31, 2016).

World Health Organization. 2016a. *International Health Regulations (2005)*. Third Edition. Geneva: World Health Organization. http://www.who.int/ihr/publications/9789241580496/en/ (accessed January 30, 2018).

World Health Organization. 2016b. *Zika Strategic Response Plan Quarterly Update, October 2016*. Geneva: World Health Organization. http://apps.who.int/iris/bitstream/10665/250626/1/WHO-ZIKV-SRF-16.4-eng.pdf?ua=1 (accessed January 29, 2018).

World Health Organization. 2016c. *Global Report on Diabetes*. Geneva: World Health Organization. http://www.who.int/diabetes/global-report/en/ (accessed January 30, 2018).

World Health Organization. 2016d. *Preventing Disease through Healthy Environments: A Global Assessment of the Burden of Disease from Environmental Risks*. Geneva: World Health Organization.

World Health Organization. 2016e. "WHO Global Urban Ambient Air Pollution Database." http://www.who.int/phe/health_topics/outdoorair/databases/cities/en/ (accessed May 30, 2016).

World Health Organization. 2017a. *Programme Budget 2018–2019*. Geneva: World Health Organization. http://www.who.int/about/finances-accountability/budget/en/ (accessed January 30, 2018).

World Health Organization. 2017b. "The Top 10 Causes of Death." http://www.who.int/mediacentre/factsheets/fs310/en/ (accessed January 29, 2018).

World Health Organization. 2017c. *World Malaria Report 2017*. Geneva: World Health Organization.

World Health Organization. 2017d. *World Tuberculosis Report 2017*. Geneva: World Health Organization.

World Health Organization. 2017e. "Zika Response Funding July 2016 to December 2017." http://www.who.int/emergencies/zika-virus/response/contribution/en/ (accessed January 30, 2018).

World Health Organization. 2017f. *WHO Report on the Global Tobacco Epidemic, 2017*. Geneva: World Health Organization. http://www.who.int/tobacco/global_report/2017/en/ (accessed January 26, 2018).

World Health Organization. 2017g. *Noncommunicable Diseases Progress Monitor 2017*. Geneva: World Health Organization. http://apps.who.int/iris/bitstream/10665/258940/1/9789241513029-eng.pdf?ua=1 (accessed January 27, 2018).

World Health Organization. 2018a. "Cumulative Number of Confirmed Human Cases for Avian Influenza A(H5N1) Reported to WHO, 2003–2018." http://www.who.int/influenza/human_animal_interface/2018_01_25_tableH5N1.pdf?ua=1 (accessed January 30, 2018).

World Health Organization. 2018b. "Obesity and Overweight Fact Sheet." http://www.who.int/mediacentre/factsheets/fs311/en/ (accessed March 10, 2018).

World Health Organization. 2018c. "Ambient (outdoor) air quality and health." http://www.who.int/en/news-room/fact-sheets/detail/ambient-(outdoor)-air-quality-and-health (accessed July 10, 2018).

World Health Organization and Food and Agriculture Organization. 2003. *Diet, Nutrition and the Prevention of Chronic Diseases*. Geneva: World Health Organization.

World Health Organization and World Trade Organization. 2002. *WTO Agreements and Public Health: A Joint Study by the WHO and WTO Secretariat*. Geneva: World Trade Organization.

Yach, Derek. 2014. "The Origins, Development, Effects, and Future of the WHO Framework Convention on Tobacco Control: A Personal Perspective." *Lancet* 383: 1771–1789.

Yach, Derek, Corinna Hawkes, Joanne Eping-Jordan, and Sarah Galbraith. 2003. "The World Health Organization's Framework Convention on Tobacco Control: Implications for the Global Epidemics of Food-Related Deaths and Disease." *Journal of Public Health Policy* 24 (2–3): 274–290.

Yach, Derek, Heather Wipfli, Ross Hammond, and Stanton Glantz. 2007. "Globalization and Tobacco." In *Globalization and Health*, edited by Ichiro Kawachi and Sarah Wamala, 39–67. New York: Oxford University Press.

Yamey, Gavin. 2002. "The World's Most Neglected Diseases." *BMJ* 325 (7360): 176–177.

Yamey, Gavin and Peter J. Hotez. 207. "Neglected Tropical Diseases." *BMJ* 335 (7614): 269–270.

Yamin, Alicia Ely and Jean Connolly Carmalt. 2013. "The United States: Right to Health Obligations in the Context of Disparity and Reform." In *Advancing the Human Right to Health*, edited by Jose M. Zuniga, Stephen P. Marks, and Lawrence O. Gostin 231–241. New York: Oxford University Press.

Youde, Jeremy. 2013. "The Rockefeller and Gates Foundations in Global Health Governance." *Global Society* 27 (2): 139–158.

Youde, Jeremy. 2016. "High Politics, Low Politics, and Global Health." *Journal of Global Security Studies* 1 (2): 157–170.

Young, Oran. 1999. *Governance in World Affairs*. Ithaca, NY: Cornell University Press.

Young, Oran. 2001. "The Behavioral Effects of Environmental Regimes: Collective-Action vs. Social Practice Models." *International Environmental Agreements: Politics, Law, and Economics* 1 (1): 9–29.

Zarcostas, John. 2004. "WHO Waters Down Draft Strategy on Diet and Health." *Lancet* 363: 1373.

Zeigler, Donald. 2013. "On delaying a Framework Convention on Alcohol Control: Regrettably Agreeing but Calling for Strategic Action to Accelerate the Process." *Addiction* 108 (3): 457–459.

Zeltner, Thomas, Kessler, David A., Anke Martiny, and Fazel Randera. 2000. *Tobacco Industry Strategies to Undermine Tobacco Control Activities at the World Health Organization*. Geneva: World Health Organization.

Zhang, Yong-Xiang, Qing-Chen Chao, Qiu-Hong Zheng, and Lei Huang. 2017. "The Withdrawal of the U.S. from the Paris Agreement and Its Impact on Global Climate Change Governance." *Advances in Climate Change Research* 8 (4): 213–219.

Zhong, Fei and Eiji Yano. 2007. "British American Tobacco's Tactics during China's Accession to the World Trade Organization." *Tobacco Control* 16 (2): 133–137.

Index

About the Author

Geoffrey B. Cockerham is Associate Professor of Political Science at Utah Valley University in Orem, Utah. Dr. Cockerham received his Ph.D. in Political Science from the University of Arizona with a specialization in international relations. He also received a J.D. degree from Louisiana State University. His research and teaching interests include global health, international cooperation, international institutions, international law and global governance.

www.ingramcontent.com/pod-product-compliance
Ingram Content Group UK Ltd.
Pitfield, Milton Keynes, MK11 3LW, UK
UKHW012035150926
475560UK00001B/30

9 781786 608482